Bio-Functional Natural Products in Edible Resources for Human Health and Beauty

Bio-Functional Natural Products in Edible Resources for Human Health and Beauty

Editor

Toshio Morikawa

MDPI • Basel • Beijing • Wuhan • Barcelona • Belgrade • Manchester • Tokyo • Cluj • Tianjin

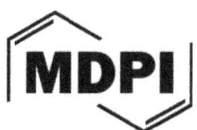

Editor
Toshio Morikawa
Pharmaceutical Research and
Technology Institute
Kindai University
Osaka
Japan

Editorial Office
MDPI
St. Alban-Anlage 66
4052 Basel, Switzerland

This is a reprint of articles from the Special Issue published online in the open access journal *Molecules* (ISSN 1420-3049) (available at: www.mdpi.com/journal/molecules/special_issues/Bio-functional_Natural_Products).

For citation purposes, cite each article independently as indicated on the article page online and as indicated below:

LastName, A.A.; LastName, B.B.; LastName, C.C. Article Title. *Journal Name* **Year**, *Volume Number*, Page Range.

ISBN 978-3-0365-5072-5 (Hbk)
ISBN 978-3-0365-5071-8 (PDF)

© 2022 by the authors. Articles in this book are Open Access and distributed under the Creative Commons Attribution (CC BY) license, which allows users to download, copy and build upon published articles, as long as the author and publisher are properly credited, which ensures maximum dissemination and a wider impact of our publications.

The book as a whole is distributed by MDPI under the terms and conditions of the Creative Commons license CC BY-NC-ND.

Contents

About the Editor vii

Toshio Morikawa
Bio-Functional Natural Products in Edible Resources for Human Health and Beauty
Reprinted from: *Molecules* 2022, 27, 5060, doi:10.3390/molecules27165060 1

GuoLiang Li, Zhaomiao Lin, Hong Zhang, Zhonghua Liu, Yongqing Xu and Guochun Xu et al.
Anthocyanin Accumulation in the Leaves of the Purple Sweet Potato (*Ipomoea batatas* L.) Cultivars
Reprinted from: *Molecules* 2019, 24, 3743, doi:10.3390/molecules24203743 3

Gabriele Vilkickyte, Raimondas Raudonis, Vida Motiekaityte, Rimanta Vainoriene, Deividas Burdulis and Jonas Viskelis et al.
Composition of Sugars in Wild and Cultivated Lingonberries (*Vaccinium vitis-idaea* L.)
Reprinted from: *Molecules* 2019, 24, 4225, doi:10.3390/molecules24234225 17

Louis P. Sandjo, Marcus V. P. dos Santos Nascimento, Milene de H. Moraes, Luiza Manaut Rodrigues, Eduardo M. Dalmarco and Maique W. Biavatti et al.
NO_x-, IL-1β-, TNF-α-, and IL-6-Inhibiting Effects and Trypanocidal Activity of Banana (*Musa acuminata*) Bracts and Flowers: UPLC-HRESI-MS Detection of Phenylpropanoid Sucrose Esters
Reprinted from: *Molecules* 2019, 24, 4564, doi:10.3390/molecules24244564 33

Mohamed Nadjib Boukhatem, Thangirala Sudha, Noureldien H.E. Darwish, Henni Chader, Asma Belkadi and Mehdi Rajabi et al.
A New Eucalyptol-Rich Lavender (*Lavandula stoechas* L.) Essential Oil: Emerging Potential for Therapy against Inflammation and Cancer
Reprinted from: *Molecules* 2020, 25, 3671, doi:10.3390/molecules25163671 53

Maobi Zhu, Sen Takeda and Tomohiko Iwano
Natural Herbal Estrogen-Mimetics (Phytoestrogens) Promote the Differentiation of Fallopian Tube Epithelium into Multi-Ciliated Cells via Estrogen Receptor Beta
Reprinted from: *Molecules* 2021, 26, 722, doi:10.3390/molecules26030722 71

Lina Raudone, Viktorija Puzeryté, Gabriele Vilkickyte, Aurelija Niekyte, Juozas Lanauskas and Jonas Viskelis et al.
Sea Buckthorn Leaf Powders: The Impact of Cultivar and Drying Mode on Antioxidant, Phytochemical, and Chromatic Profile of Valuable Resource
Reprinted from: *Molecules* 2021, 26, 4765, doi:10.3390/molecules26164765 81

Fah Chueahongthong, Singkome Tima, Sawitree Chiampanichayakul, Cory Berkland and Songyot Anuchapreeda
Co-Treatments of Edible Curcumin from Turmeric Rhizomes and Chemotherapeutic Drugs on Cytotoxicity and FLT3 Protein Expression in Leukemic Stem Cells
Reprinted from: *Molecules* 2021, 26, 5785, doi:10.3390/molecules26195785 99

Shogo Takeda, Kenchi Miyasaka, Sarita Shrestha, Yoshiaki Manse, Toshio Morikawa and Hiroshi Shimoda
Lycoperoside H, a Tomato Seed Saponin, Improves Epidermal Dehydration by Increasing Ceramide in the Stratum Corneum and Steroidal Anti-Inflammatory Effect
Reprinted from: *Molecules* 2021, 26, 5860, doi:10.3390/molecules26195860 115

Peerasak Lerttrakarnnon, Winthana Kusirisin, Pimpisid Koonyosying, Ben Flemming, Niramon Utama-ang and Suthat Fucharoen et al.
Consumption of Sinlek Rice Drink Improved Red Cell Indices in Anemic Elderly Subjects
Reprinted from: *Molecules* **2021**, *26*, 6285, doi:10.3390/molecules26206285 . . . . **133**

Hiroaki Takemoto, Yuki Saito, Kei Misumi, Masaki Nagasaki and Yoshinori Masuo
Stress-Relieving Effects of Sesame Oil Aroma and Identification of the Active Components
Reprinted from: *Molecules* **2022**, *27*, 2661, doi:10.3390/molecules27092661 . . . . **155**

Xiaoyan Xia and Jiao Xiao
Natural Ingredients from Medicine Food Homology as Chemopreventive Reagents against Type 2 Diabetes Mellitus by Modulating Gut Microbiota Homoeostasis
Reprinted from: *Molecules* **2021**, *26*, 6934, doi:10.3390/molecules26226934 . . . . **165**

Olga Babich, Viktoria Larina, Svetlana Ivanova, Andrei Tarasov, Maria Povydysh and Anastasiya Orlova et al.
Phytotherapeutic Approaches to the Prevention of Age-Related Changes and the Extension of Active Longevity
Reprinted from: *Molecules* **2022**, *27*, 2276, doi:10.3390/molecules27072276 . . . . **185**

About the Editor

Toshio Morikawa

Toshio Morikawa is Professor at the Pharmaceutical Research and Technology Institute, Kindai University, Japan. He was born in Kyoto Prefecture, Japan in 1972 and received his Ph.D. under the supervision of Professor Masayuki Yoshikawa at Kyoto Pharmaceutical University in 2002. In 2001, he started his academic career at Kyoto Pharmaceutical University as an Assistant Professor. He became a Lecturer in 2005, an Associate Professor in 2010, and a Professor in 2015 at the Pharmaceutical Research and Technology Institute, Kindai University. He received The Japanese Society of Pharmacognosy (JSP) Award for Young Scientists in 2005, The JSP Award for Scientific Contributions in 2018, and The Pharmaceutical Society of Japan (PSJ) Award for Divisional Scientific Promotion in 2022. His current research program focuses on the search for bioactive constituents from natural resources and the development of new functional foods for the prevention and improvement of lifestyle diseases. He has published over 220 papers in peer reviewed journals and is currently serving on the editorial board members of *Journal of Natural Medicines* (Associate Editor), *Traditional & Kampo Medicine* (Editor-in-Chief, Basic Research), *Japanese Journal of Food Chemistry and Safety*, and *Molecules*.

Editorial

Bio-Functional Natural Products in Edible Resources for Human Health and Beauty

Toshio Morikawa

Pharmaceutical Research and Technology Institute, Kindai University, 3-4-1 Kowakae, Higashiosaka 577-8502, Osaka, Japan; morikawa@kindai.ac.jp

Natural products remain important repositories of promising therapeutic candidates due to their rich chemical and biological diversity. In particular, the development and application of bio-functional natural products from edible resources for the prevention of human diseases, health maintenance, and beauty are attractive for practical research.

The Special Issue "Bio-functional Natural Products in Edible Resources for Human Health and Beauty", published in the journal *Molecules*, includes twelve articles, including ten original and two review articles.

The original papers include 'Anthocyanin accumulation in the leaves of the purple sweet potato (*Ipomoea batatas* L.) cultivars' by Guo Liang Li et al. [1]; 'Composition of sugars in wild and cultivated lingonberries (*Vaccinium vitis-ideaea* L.)' by Gabriele Vilkickyte et al. [2]; 'NO$_x$-, IL-1β-, TNF-α-, and IL-6-inhibiting effects and trypanocidal activity of banana (*Musa acuminata*) bracts and flowers: UPLC-HRESI-MS detection of phenylpropanoid sucrose esters' by Louis P. Sandjo et al. [3]; A new eucalyptol-rich lavender (*Lavandula stoechas* L.) essential oil: emerging potential for therapy against inflammation and cancer' by Mohamed Nadjib Boukhatem et al. [4]; 'Natural herbal estrogen-mimetics (phytoestrogens) promote the differentiation of fallopian tube epithelium into multi-ciliated cells via estrogen receptor beta' by Maobi Zhu et al. [5]; 'Sea buckthorn leaf powders: the impact of cultivar and drying mode on antioxidant, phytochemical, and chromatic profile of valuable resource' by Lina Raudone et al. [6]; 'Co-treatments of edible curcumin from turmeric rhizomes and chemotherapeutic drugs on cytotoxicity and FLT3 protein expression in leukemic stem cells' by Fah Chueahongthong et al. [7]; 'Lycoperoside H, a tomato seed saponin, improves epidermal dehydration by increasing ceramide in the stratum corneum and steroidal anti-inflammatory effects' by Shogo Takeda et al. [8]; 'Consumption of sinlek rice drink improved red cells indices in anemic elderly subjects' by Peerasak Lerttrakarnnon et al. [9]; and 'Stress-relieving effects of sesame oil aroma and identification of the active components' by Hiroaki Takemoto et al. [10].

In addition, two review papers are included, namely 'Natural ingredients from medicine food homology as chemopreventive reagents against type 2 diabetes mellitus by modulating gut microbiota homoeostasis' by Xiaoyan Xia and Jiao Xiao [11] and 'Phytotherapeutic approaches to the prevention of age-related changes and the extension of active longevity', by Olga Babich et al. [12].

As the guest editor of this Special Issue, I hope "Bio-functional Natural Products in Edible Plant for Human Health and Beauty", appearing in the Natural Products Chemistry section of *Molecules*, will be of use to many researchers. I would like to acknowledge all the authors for their valuable contributions and the reviewers for their constructive remarks. Special thanks to the publishing staff of *Molecules* at MDPI for their professional support in all aspects of this Special Issue.

Funding: This research received no external funding.

Conflicts of Interest: The author declares no conflict of interest.

References

1. Li, G.L.; Lin, Z.; Zhang, H.; Liu, Z.; Xu, Y.; Xu, G.; Li, H.; Ji, R.; Luo, W.; Qiu, Y.; et al. Anthocyanin accumulation in the leaves of the purple sweet potato (*Ipomoea batatas* L.) cultivars. *Molecules* **2019**, *24*, 3743. [CrossRef] [PubMed]
2. Vilkickyte, G.; Raudonis, R.; Motiekaityte, V.; Vainoriene, R.; Burdulis, D.; Viskelis, J.; Raudone, L. Composition of sugars in wild and cultivated lingonberries (*Vaccinium vitis-ideaea* L.). *Molecules* **2019**, *24*, 4225. [CrossRef] [PubMed]
3. Sandjo, L.P.; dos Santos Nascimento, M.V.P.; de H. Moraes, M.; Rodrigues, L.M.; Dalmarco, E.M.; Biavatti, M.W.; Steindel, M. NO_x-, IL-1β-, TNF-α-, and IL-6-inhibiting effects and trypanocidal activity of banana (*Musa acuminata*) bracts and flowers: UPLC-HRESI-MS detection of phenylpropanoid sucrose esters. *Molecules* **2019**, *24*, 4564. [CrossRef] [PubMed]
4. Boukhatem, M.N.; Sudha, T.; Darwish, N.H.E.; Chader, H.; Belkadi, A.; Rajabi, M.; Houche, A.; Benkebailli, F.; Oudjida, F.; Mousa, S.A. A new eucalyptol-rich lavender (*Lavandula stoechas* L.) essential oil: Emerging potential for therapy against inflammation and cancer. *Molecules* **2020**, *25*, 3671. [CrossRef] [PubMed]
5. Zhu, M.; Takeda, S.; Iwano, T. Natural herbal estrogen-mimetics (phytoestrogens) promote the differentiation of fallopian tube epithelium into multi-ciliated cells via estrogen receptor beta. *Molecules* **2021**, *26*, 722. [CrossRef] [PubMed]
6. Raudone, L.; Puzeryté, V.; Vilkickyte, G.; Niekyte, A.; Lanauskas, J.; Viskelis, J.; Viskelis, P. Sea buckthorn leaf powders: The impact of cultivar and drying mode on antioxidant, phytochemical, and chromatic profile of valuable resource. *Molecules* **2021**, *26*, 4765. [CrossRef] [PubMed]
7. Chueahongthong, F.; Tima, S.; Chiampanichayakul, S.; Berkland, C.; Anuchapreeda, S. Co-treatments of edible curcumin from turmeric rhizomes and chemotherapeutic drugs on cytotoxicity and FLT3 protein expression in leukemic stem cells. *Molecules* **2021**, *26*, 5785. [CrossRef] [PubMed]
8. Takeda, S.; Miyasaka, K.; Shrestha, S.; Manse, Y.; Morikawa, T.; Shimoda, H. Lycoperoside H, a tomato seed saponin, improves epidermal dehydration by increasing ceramide in the stratum corneum and steroidal anti-inflammatory effects. *Molecules* **2021**, *26*, 5860. [CrossRef] [PubMed]
9. Lerttrakarnnon, P.; Kusirisin, W.; Koonyosying, P.; Flemming, B.; Utama-ang, N.; Fucharoen, S.; Srichairatanakool, S. Consumption of sinlek rice drink improved red cells indices in anemic elderly subjects. *Molecules* **2021**, *26*, 6285. [CrossRef] [PubMed]
10. Takemoto, H.; Saito, Y.; Masumi, K.; Nagasaki, M.; Masuo, Y. Stress-relieving effects of sesame oil aroma and identification of the active components. *Molecules* **2022**, *27*, 2661. [CrossRef] [PubMed]
11. Xia, X.; Xiao, J. Natural ingredients from medicine food homology as chemopreventive reagents against type 2 diabetes mellitus by modulating gut microbiota homoeostasis. *Molecules* **2021**, *26*, 6934. [CrossRef] [PubMed]
12. Babich, O.; Larina, V.; Ivanova, S.; Tarasov, A.; Povydysh, M.; Orlova, A.; Strugar, J.; Sukhikh, S. Phytotherapeutic approaches to the prevention of age-related changes and the extension of active longevity. *Molecules* **2022**, *27*, 2276. [CrossRef] [PubMed]

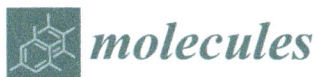

Article

Anthocyanin Accumulation in the Leaves of the Purple Sweet Potato (*Ipomoea batatas* L.) Cultivars

GuoLiang Li, Zhaomiao Lin, Hong Zhang, Zhonghua Liu, Yongqing Xu, Guochun Xu, Huawei Li, Rongchang Ji, Wenbin Luo, Yongxiang Qiu, Sixin Qiu * and Hao Tang

Institute of Crop Sciences, Fujian Academy of Agricultural Sciences, Scientific Observing and Experimental Station of Tuber and Root Crops in South China, Ministry of Agriculture. Fuzhou, Fujian 350013, China; uslgl@126.com (G.L.); linzhaomiao@foxmail.com (Z.L.); teeteeking@163.com (H.Z.); lhl8620@163.com (Z.L.); qingqing0722@126.com (Y.X.); xgc_faas@163.com (G.X.); fjpotato@126.com (H.L.); jrc1976@163.com (R.J.); lwb9630@163.com (W.L.); qyxlm@sohu.com (Y.Q.); tanghao9403@163.com (H.T.)
* Correspondence: qiusixin@faas.cn; Tel.: +86-0591-87572407

Received: 20 September 2019; Accepted: 15 October 2019; Published: 17 October 2019

Abstract: Sweet potato anthocyanins are water-soluble pigments with many physiological functions. Previous research on anthocyanin accumulation in sweet potato has focused on the roots, but the accumulation progress in the leaves is still unclear. Two purple sweet potato cultivars (Fushu No. 23 and Fushu No. 317) with large quantities of anthocyanin in the leaves were investigated. Anthocyanin composition and content were assessed with ultra-performance liquid chromatography diode-array detection (UPLC-DAD) and ultra-performance liquid chromatography/quadrupole time-of-flight mass spectrometry (UPLC-QTOF-MS), and the expressions of genes were detected by qRT-PCR. The two cultivars contained nine cyanidin anthocyanins and nine peonidin anthocyanins with an acylation modification. The acylation modification of anthocyanins in sweet potato leaves primarily included caffeoyl, *p*-coumaryl, feruloyl, and *p*-hydroxy benzoyl. We identified three anthocyanin compounds in sweet potato leaves for the first time: cyanidin 3-*p*-coumarylsophoroside-5-glucoside, peonidin 3-*p*-coumarylsophoroside-5-glucoside, and cyanidin 3-caffeoyl-*p*-coumarylsophoroside-5-glucoside. The anthocyanidin biosynthesis downstream structural genes *DFR4*, *F3H1*, anthocyanin synthase (*ANS*), and UDP-glucose flavonoid 3-O-glucosyltransferase (*UFGT3*), as well as the transcription factor *MYB1*, were found to be vital regulatory genes during the accumulation of anthocyanins in sweet potato leaves. The composition of anthocyanins (nine cyanidin-based anthocyanins and nine peonidin-based anthocyanins) in all sweet potato leaves were the same, but the quantity of anthocyanins in leaves of sweet potato varied by cultivar and differed from anthocyanin levels in the roots of sweet potatoes. The anthocyanidin biosynthesis structural genes and transcription factor together regulated and controlled the anthocyandin biosynthesis in sweet potato leaves.

Keywords: sweet potato; anthocyanin compositions; biosynthesis structural genes; transcription factor

1. Introduction

The sweet potato (*Ipomoea batatas* L.) is an important tropical crop, providing starch, beta-carotene, and anthocyanins for human nutrition and industrial use [1]. Leafy sweet potato is a new type in China that is consumed for its stems and leaves, not the tuberous root. The stems and leaves are nutritious and contain high levels of protein, dietary fiber, calcium, magnesium, iron, zinc, flavonoids, and anthocyanins [2]. In 2003, the first leafy sweet potato cultivar was cultivated in China, called Fushu No. 7-6 [3], but in 2016 there was only one purple leafy sweet potato cultivar being grown in China, Fushu No. 23. Fushu No. 23 has been found to have high levels of anthocyanin in both the stems and leaves (Figure 1).

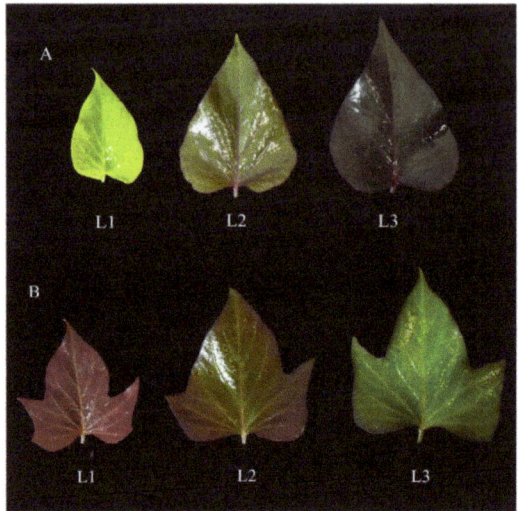

Figure 1. Photographs of sweet potato leaves with differential levels of accumulated anthocyanins. (**A**) Fushu No. 23, (**B**) Fushu No. 317, "L1" indicates the primary leaves (three days old), "L2" indicates the second leaves (five days old), and "L3" indicates the third leaves (seven days old).

Anthocyanins are a group of water-soluble natural pigments that are considered flavonoids with a basic structure of C6–C3–C6. They are responsible for fruit and flower coloration [4]. Previous research on anthocyanins in sweet potato has focused on the roots and found that the basic anthocyanin monomers are cyanidin, peonidin, and pelargonidin. These anthocyanin monomers are often linked to acylated glucoside or sophoroside, and acylation modification comes from caffeic acid, p-coumaric acid, ferulic acid, and p-hydroxybenzoic acid [4–8]. Terahara et al. (1999) identified eight acylated anthocyanins in the roots of the purple Japanese sweet potato cultivar Yamagawamurasaki, and six monomers were identified as diacylated anthocyanins [9]. Tian et al. (2005) identified 26 anthocyanins from the 'Ayamurasaki' line that had been root cultured, and it was first discovered that the purple-fleshed sweet potato contained pelargonidin 3-sophoroside-5-glucoside and pelargonidin 3-feruloylsophoroside-5-glucoside [4]. Lee et al. (2013) separated six pelargonidin-based anthocyanins from Korean purple-fleshed sweet potato cultivar Borami [6], and found that compared with the purple-fleshed root, anthocyanins in sweet potato leaves were relatively less studied. Islam et al. (2002) detected 15 anthocyanin compounds from sweet potato leaves, and eight cyanidin derivatives were identified and measured [10]. Su et al. (2019) identified 14 anthocyanins with a new anthocyanin peonidin 3-caffeoyl-p-coumaryl sophoroside-5-glucoside in the leaves of three sweet potato varieties [11]. Vishnu et al. (2019) found that peonidin derivatives were the major anthocyanins in tubers and the leaves, but that the contents of the cyanidin derivatives were greater in leaves than in tubers [12]. Studies have shown that anthocyanins from sweet potato have good properties regarding scavenging 1,1-diphenyl-2-picrylhydrazyl (DPPH) radicals [13], and protect the liver [14,15], have anti-tumor properties [16], lower blood sugar levels [17], and have other positive physiological functions on the human body [18,19].

In this study, two purple sweet potato cultivars (Fushu No. 23 and Fushu No. 317) with different patterns of anthocyanin accumulation were studied (Figure 1). The content and chemical structures of anthocyanin monomers in the leaves were analyzed and the expression of anthocyanin biosynthetic structural genes and transcription factors were studied.

2. Materials and Methods

2.1. Chemicals

All of the reagents or solvents were of analytical, HPLC, or HPLC-MS grade. Absolute ethanol, acetone, hydrochloric acid (HCl), and sodium hydroxide (NaOH) were obtained from Sinopharm Chemical Reagent Co., Ltd. (Shanghai, China). Methanol and ethanol in LC-MS grade was purchased from Honeywell (Muskegon, MI, USA). Acetonitrile in LC-MS grade was obtained from Merck KgaA (Darmstadt, Germany). Formic acid in LC-MS grade was the product of Fisher Scientific (Waltham, MA, USA). The standard cyanidin 3-O-glucoside was purchased from Sigma-Aldrich (St. Louis, MO, USA). The TransStart Top Green qPCR SuperMix was purchased from Transgen Biotech (Beijing, China).

2.2. Plant Materials

The purple-leaf sweet potato cultivars Fushu No. 23 and Fushu No. 317 were sampled under natural outdoor light and temperature conditions. Two-thirds of samples were stored at −80 °C in a refrigerator (Haier Group Co., Qingdao, China) for later analyses of metabolites. To determine the content of total anthocyanins, the remaining 1/3 of leaves were oven-dried, ground into powder with a diameter less than 0.3 mm, and stored in a vacuum pack (VIP320, Beijing Torch SMT Inc. Co., Beijing, China) at 4 °C.

In order to understand the difference in anthocyanin levels between roots and leaves, some purple-fleshed sweet potatoes were examined, the cultivars Fushu No. 9, Fushu No. 24, Fushu No. 317, Ornamental Purple (OP), Fushu No. 23, and Fushu No. 25 were obtained from the Institute of Crop Sciences, Fujian Academy of Agricultural Sciences, Fuzhou, China, (26°08′ N, 119°28′ E) in August 2018. Yanshu No. 5, Longzishu No. 6, and Longzishu No. 8, were generously provided by the Longyan Institute of Agricultural Sciences, Longyan, China, in August 2018.

2.3. Sample Preparation

Two-thirds of lyophilized samples (50 mg) were grounded by TissueLyser JX-24 (Jingxin, Shanghai, China) with beads at 40 Hz for 4 min, and extracted with 0.5 mL of 70% methanol containing 0.1% formic acid. Samples were then processed for 10 min 100 HZ ultra-sonication in ice water. The mixtures were vortexed for 30 s and left to stand for 2 h at −40 °C. After, samples were centrifuged at 4 °C at 14,000 rpm for 15 min, and 350 μL of supernatant were dried under gentle nitrogen stream and re-dissolved in 90 μL of 70% methanol containing 0.1% formic acid combined with 10 μL of 25 μg/mL lidocaine (internal standard) prior to ultra performance liquid chromatography/quadrupole time-of-flight mass spectrometry (UPLC-QTOF-MS) analysis. Quality control (QC) sample was obtained by isometrically mixing the prepared samples. The injection volume was 1 μL (ESI$^+$).

2.4. Ultra Performance Liquid Chromatography Diode-Array Detection (UPLC-DAD) and UPLC-QTOF-MS Analysis

Chromatographic separation was performed on an ACQUITY UPLC I-Class system (Waters Corporation, Milford, MA, USA) with an ACQUITY UPLC BEH C18 column (100 × 2.1 mm, 1.7 μm, Waters Corporation, Milford, MA, USA) maintained at 45 °C. The injection volume was 3 μL. The mobile phases consisted of water (phase A) and acetonitrile (phase B), both with 0.5% formic acid (v/v). A linear gradient elution was performed using the following program: 0–2 min, 1% B; 3 min, 5% B; 9 min, 20% B; 12 min, 50% B; 15 min, 100% B; 17 min, 100% B; 17.1 min, 1% B, and held for 20 min.

The eluents were analyzed on a Vion IMS QTOF Mass spectrometer (Waters Corporation, Milford, MA, USA) set to ESI$^+$ mode. The capillary voltage was set to 2 kV. The sampling cone voltage and cone gas flow were 40 V and 50 L/h, respectively. The desolvation gas was maintained at a flow rate of 900 L/h and a temperature of 450 °C. The ion source temperature was 115 °C. The TOF-MS scan was operated at a high-resolution with 0.2 s survey scan time and a range of 50–1000 m/z in the continuum mode for both function 1 and 2. To improve the identification of unknown metabolites, MS^E function was also performed to obtain fragment ion information with a ramp collision energy from 20 to 45 eV. The mass accuracy calibration was performed with the 250 ng/mL lock mass leucine-enkephalin at 5 µL/min, with data acquisition frequency set at 30 s. The software for controlling the instrument and collecting data was UNIFI 1.8.1 (Waters Corporation, Milford, MA, USA). Peak picking, alignment, and deconvolution were conducted using Progenesis QI (Nonlinear Dynamics, Newcastle, UK) with default parameters. A suitable quality control sample (QC from pooled samples) from the run was selected as a reference for peak alignment. The structural identification of anthocyanins was performed using UNIFI 1.8.1(Waters Cooperation, Milford, MA, USA). The anthocyanin content was expressed as mg of cyanidin 3-O-glucoside equivalent.

2.5. Quantitative Real-time PCR ANALYSIS of Anthocyanin Biosynthetic Genes in Sweet Potato Leaves

Total RNA was isolated from sweet potato leaves in September using TransZol Plant (Transgen Biotech Inc., Beijing, China) following the manufacturer's instructions. First-strand cDNA were reverse transcribed using a Reverse Transcriptase M-MLV Kit (Promega, Madison, WI, USA). The qRT-PCR assay was performed on an ABI QuantStudio5 Real-time system (ABI, Foster City, CA, USA), and in 10 µL of reaction containing 2× TransStart Top Green qPCR SuperMix (Transgen Biotech Inc., Beijing, China), 10 µM of solution from each primer (Supplementary Table S1), and 100 ng of cDNA. Thermocycling conditions were: initial denaturation at 95 °C for 2 min, followed by 40 cycles for 15 s at 95 °C, and 1 min at 60 °C. The relative expression of anthocyanin biosynthetic genes was assessed by the comparative threshold cycle (Ct) method [20]. The sweet potato actin gene (NCBI accession: EU250003) served as an internal control for signal normalization. Expression levels were evaluated as technical duplicates of biological triplicates from separate plant samples.

3. Results and Discussion

3.1. Total Monomeric Anthocyanin Content in the Leaves of the Cultivars Fushu No. 23 and Fushu No. 317

To further understand the differences between the two purple sweet potato cultivars in the accumulation of anthocyanins, the composition and content of anthocyanins were detected by UPLC-DAD and UPLC-QTOF-MS (Figure 2, Tables 1 and 2). Eighteen anthocyanin monomers were found, which contained a typical anthocyanin spectrum of a maximum absorbance at 520 nm.

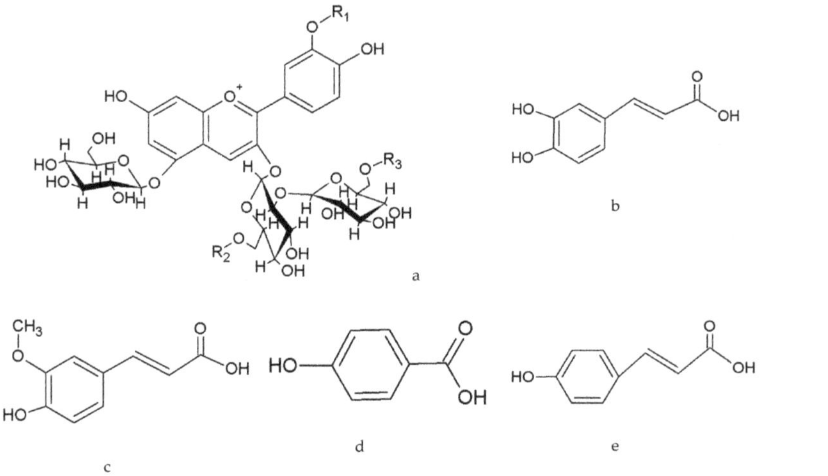

Figure 2. Skeleton structures of anthocyanins in sweet potato leaves. (**a**) Skeleton structures of anthocyanins; (**b**) caffeic acid (*m/z* 180); (**c**) ferulic acid (*m/z* 194); (**d**) *p*-hydro benzoic acid (*m/z* 138); and (**e**) *p*-coumaroyl acid (*m/z* 164).

Table 1. Identification of anthocyanins (1–14) from cultivar Fushu No. 23 and cultivar Fushu No. 317 leaves using ultra performance liquid chromatography/quadrupole time-of-flight mass spectrometry (UPLC-QTOF-MS/MS).

Peak	Rt [a] (min)	Fragment Ions (m/z)			[M]$^+$ (m/z)	Identity [b]
1	4.45	287	449	611	773.2117	Cy 3-soph-5glc
2	4.99	301	463	625	787.2266	Peo 3-soph-5glc
3	5.92	287	449	731	893.2325	Cy 3-p-hydroxybenzoylsoph-5glc
4	6.10	287	449	773	935.2421	Cy 3-caffeylsophsoph-5glc
5	6.63	301	625	745	907.2479	Peo 3-p-hydroxybenzoylsoph-5glc
6	6.77	301	463	787	949.2578	Peo 3-caffeylsophsoph-5glc
7	6.86	287	449	757	919.2477	Cy 3-p-coumarylsoph-5glc
8	6.98	287	449	787	949.2577	Cy 3-feruloylsoph-5glc
9	7.50	301	463	771	933.2634	Peo 3-p-coumarylsoph-5glc
10	7.64	301	463	801	963.2734	Peo 3-feruloylsoph-5glc
11a	7.83	287	449	935	1097.2741	Cy 3-dicaffeylsoph-5glc
11b	7.89	287	449	893	1055.2636	Cy 3-caffeoyl-p-hydroxybenzoylsoph-5glc
12a	8.33	287	449	949	1081.2794	Cy 3-caffeoyl-p-coumarylsoph-5glc
12b	8.35	287	433	919	1111.2898	Cy 3-caffeoyl-feruloylsoph-5glc
13a	8.52	301	463	907	1111.2898	Peo 3-dicaffeoylsoph-5glc
13b	8.62	301	463	949	1069.2791	Peo 3-caffeoyl-p-hydroxybenzoylsoph-5glc
14a	9.05	301	463	933	1095.2942	Peo 3-caffeoyl-p-coumarylsoph-5glc
14b	9.05	301	463	963	1125.3038	Peo 3-caffeoyl-feruloylsoph-5glc

[a] Rt = retention time [b] Cy = cyanidin, Peo = peonidin, soph = sophorside, glc = glucoside.

The m/z ratio of the 18 anthocyanin monomers with daughter fragments was captured within the scanning interval range. Nine cyanidin was detected at m/z 287 and nine peonidin was detected at m/z 301. Cyanidin 3-sophoroside-5-glucoside (Table 1, Figure S1.1, m/z 773) produced three fragments located at m/z 611, 449, and 287. Transition 773 > 611 and 773 > 449 represented the loss of glucose (m/z 162) and sophorose (m/z 324), respectively, while transition 773 > 287 produced cyanidin (m/z 287) aglycone due to the loss of both glucose and sophoroside. Another example for mono- and di-acylated anthocyanin was cyanidin 3-(6″-p-hydroxybenzoylsoph)-5-glucoside (Table 1, Figure S1.3, m/z 893). The transitions from 893 to 731 indicated a loss of glucose [M − 162]$^+$, and from 893 to 449 [M − 162 × 2 − 120]$^+$ indicated a loss of sophoroside and p-hydroxybenzoic acid 120 [p-hydroxybenzoic acid-H2O]$^+$. The remaining anthocyanins were identified in a similar fashion using the LC-MS library and identification results of Tian and Lee et al. [4,6] The m/z ratios of each intact anthocyanin and its daughter fragments are summarized in Table 1. We identified four anthocyanin compounds that were found in the leaves of sweet potato for the first time: cyanidin 3-p-coumarylsophoroside-5-glucoside, peonidin 3-p-coumarylsophoroside-5-glucoside, cyanidin 3-caffeoyl-p-coumarylsophoroside-5-glucoside, and peonidin 3-caffeoyl-p-coumarylsophoroside-5-glucoside.

The composition of anthocyanins in the sweet potato leaves had certain regularity. The first anthocyanin monomers was cyanidin, another anthocyanin monomer peonidin was formed by methylation at the cyanidin R1 position, and other monoacylanthocyanins or diacylanthocyanins were formed by acylation modification at cyanidin or peonidin at the R2 and R3 positions [4–7]. The structure of the acylated anthocyanins was more stable and had stronger physiological activities than nonacylated anthocyanins. The acylation modification of anthocyanin in sweet potato leaves primarily included: caffeoyl, p-coumaroyl, feruloyl, and p-hydroxy benzoyl (Figure 2).

Table 2. Anthocyanin monomer (1–14) content in cultivar Fushu No. 23 and cultivar Fushu No. 317 as determined by ultra performance liquid chromatography (μg/g fresh weight, FW).

Identity [a]	Fushu No. 23			Fushu No. 317		
	Lf1	Lf2	Lf3	Lf1	Lf2	Lf3
Cy 3-soph-5glc	0.93 ± 0.22	1.65 ± 0.10	0.58 ± 0.06	3.47 ± 0.36	1.36 ± 0.17	0.21 ± 0.02
Peo 3-soph-5glc	0.68 ± 0.36	2.31 ± 0.12	1.40 ± 0.21	5.88 ± 0.84	2.76 ± 0.60	0.53 ± 0.05
Cy 3-p-hydroxybenzoylsoph-5glc	2.46 ± 0.50	6.66 ± 0.39	5.71 ± 0.43	10.41 ± 0.10	4.06 ± 1.11	0.63 ± 0.06
Cy 3-caffeylsophsoph-5glc	0.14 ± 0.00	0.40 ± 0.07	0.79 ± 0.11	11.09 ± 1.14	4.55 ± 1.08	0.31 ± 0.02
Peo 3-p-hydroxybenzoylsoph-5glc	0.98 ± 0.49	3.55 ± 0.11	2.85 ± 0.22	5.72 ± 0.05	2.76 ± 1.00	0.45 ± 0.08
Peo 3-caffeylsophsoph-5glc	0.02 ± 0.00	0.11 ± 0.02	0.18 ± 0.01	5.45 ± 1.16	2.00 ± 0.67	0.14 ± 0.01
Cy 3-p-coumarylsoph-5glc	0.06 ± 0.01	0.17 ± 0.04	0.12 ± 0.01	21.23 ± 2.04	7.42 ± 1.91	0.55 ± 0.05
Cy 3-feruloylsoph-5glc	0.21 ± 0.01	0.38 ± 0.03	0.45 ± 0.08	4.65 ± 0.72	1.63 ± 0.19	0.31 ± 0.05
Peo 3-p-coumarylsoph-5glc	0.11 ± 0.01	0.42 ± 0.07	0.31 ± 0.01	15.42 ± 0.79	6.84 ± 2.22	0.35 ± 0.04
Peo 3-feruloylsoph-5glc	0.05 ± 0.03	0.18 ± 0.04	0.20 ± 0.01	4.50 ± 0.85	1.45 ± 0.35	0.33 ± 0.06
Cy 3-dicaffeylsoph-5glc	0.24 ± 0.07	0.71 ± 0.13	3.27 ± 0.66	11.08 ± 0.82	6.34 ± 2.36	0.11 ± 0.01
Cy 3-caffeoyl-p-hydroxybenzoylsoph-5glc	1.43 ± 0.28	4.04 ± 0.61	8.57 ± 1.54	4.52 ± 0.40	2.61 ± 0.95	0.09 ± 0.01
Cy 3-caffeoyl-p-coumarylsoph-5glc	0.02 ± 0.00	0.10 ± 0.03	0.16 ± 0.04	7.24 ± 0.53	4.18±1.27	0.05 ± 0.00
Cy 3-caffeoyl-feruloylsoph-5glc	0.06 ± 0.03	0.21 ± 0.02	0.70 ± 0.22	5.07 ± 0.69	2.14 ± 0.40	0.10 ± 0.00
Peo 3-dicaffeylsoph-5glc	0.02 ± 0.00	0.09 ± 0.01	0.40 ± 0.03	4.81 ± 0.35	2.72 ± 1.11	0.04 ± 0.00
Peo 3-caffeoyl-p-hydroxybenzoylsoph-5glc	0.20 ± 0.09	0.88 ± 0.08	1.56 ± 0.06	2.31 ± 0.14	1.42 ± 0.61	0.04 ± 0.00
Peo 3-caffeoyl-p-coumarylsoph-5glc	-	0.02 ± 0.00	0.02 ± 0.00	2.57 ± 0.28	2.12 ± 0.67	0.01 ± 0.00
Peo 3-caffeoyl-feruloylsoph-5glc	-	0.04 ± 0.01	0.14 ± 0.02	1.92 ± 0.45	0.85 ± 0.24	0.03 ± 0.00
Total anthocyanin	7.62 ± 1.43	21.92 ± 1.25	27.41 ± 2.69	127.33 ± 7.55	57.20 ± 6.75	4.28 ± 0.25
non-acylated anthocyanin	0.98 ± 0.24	1.84 ± 0.14	0.78 ± 0.06	7.97 ± 1.21	2.81 ± 0.51	0.53 ± 0.09
monoacylated anthocyanin	6.01 ± 1.75	17.98 ± 1.48	23.46 ± 3.42	60.99 ± 4.58	29.39 ± 8.78	2.28 ± 0.24
diacylated anthocyanin	0.63 ± 0.13	2.10 ± 0.25	3.17 ± 0.21	58.37 ± 5.93	25.00 ± 7.62	1.48 ± 0.17
cyanidin-based anthocyanin	5.59 ± 1.59	15.66 ± 0.93	12.38 ± 1.11	83.32 ± 7.19	33.37 ± 8.95	3.47 ± 0.38
peonidin-based anthocyanin	2.03 ± 0.52	6.26 ± 0.94	15.03 ± 2.58	44.01 ± 4.52	23.83 ± 7.96	0.81 ± 0.11

[a] Cy = cyanidin, Peo = peonidin, soph = sophorside, glc = glucoside.

3.2. Differential Accumulation of Anthocyanins in the Leaves of the Cultivars Fushu No. 23 and Fushu No. 317

As shown in Figure 1, the anthocyanin accumulation in the leaves of the cultivars Fushu No. 23 and Fushu No. 317 was different. The anthocyanin content in Fushu No. 23 leaves increased with the growth of the first to third leaves (one- to seven-day-old from new leaves), while the anthocyanin content in Fushu No. 317 leaves decreased in that period.

The total anthocyanin content in sweet potato leaves ranged from 4.28 to 127.33 μg/g fresh weight (FW). The accumulation of anthocyanin monomers in the leaves of Fushu No. 23 and Fushu No. 317 was different (Table 2). In Fushu No. 23, the simple structure of anthocyanidin monomers led cyanidin 3-sophoroside-5-glucoside to increase from the first to second leaves, and then decrease from the second to third leaves. Meanwhile, the structurally complex monomers in Fushu No. 317 caused cyanidin 3-(6′,6′′-dicaffeylsophoroside)-5-glucoside to increase from the first to the third leaves.

3.3. Expression of Anthocyanidin Biosynthesis Structural Genes and Transcription Factor

The synthesis precursor of anthocyanin monomers in sweet potato leaves is phenylalanine, and structural genes in the synthesis process include: phenylalanine ammonialyase (PAL), cinnamic acid-4-hydroxylase (C4L), 4-coumarate:CoA ligase (4CL), chalconesynthase (CHS), chalconeisomerase (CHI), flavanone 3-hydroxylase (F3H), flavonoids 3′-hydroxylase (F3′H), dihydrofavonol4-reductase (DFR), and anthocyanin synthase (ANS) [21]. The first anthocyanin monomer was cyanidin, and other acylated anthocyanin monomers formed under the action of the UDP-glucose flavonoid 3-O-glucosyltransferase (UFGT) [22] or anthocyanin 3-O-acyltransferases (3AT) [23,24] genes (Figure 3). DFRs, UFGTs, and 3Ats are mined from two diploid wild relatives of cultivated sweet potato (Ipomoea triloba. L). UFGT1 (3GGT) was found to transfer glucose to glycosylated anthocyanins in purple sweet potato [25], but this is the only UFGT whose function in the sweet potato has been established. The transcription factors in anthocyanin synthesis were MYB, bLHL, and WDR40 [21,26]. IbMYB1 is a key regulatory gene of anthocyanin biosynthesis in the storage roots of purple-fleshed sweet potato [27]. IbMYB60 is homologous to the Arabidopsis R2R3-MYB transcription factor AtMYB60, a transcriptional repressor of anthocyanin biosynthesis in lettuce [28]. *AtMYB75* (*PAP1*) [29,30] and *AtMYB113* (*PAP2*) [31,32] regulate the anthocyanin pathway in *Arabidopsis* seedlings. Two homologous *AtMYB75* genes (*IbMYB75-1* and *IbMYB75-2*) were mined from *Ipomoea triloba* genome, but only one homologous gene *IbMYB113* was found in the *Ipomoea triloba* genome (www.sweetpotato-garden.kazusa.or.jp).

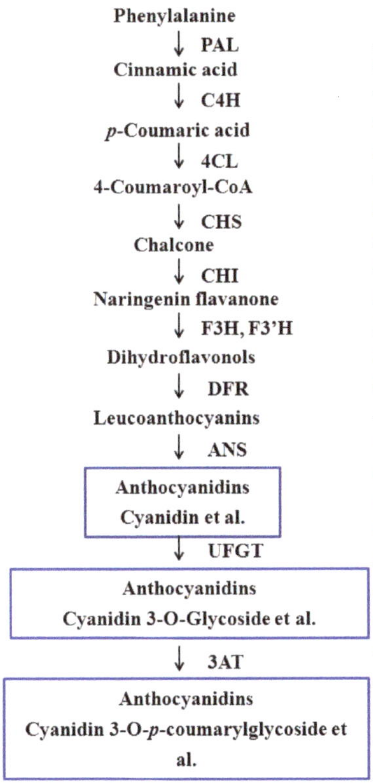

Pathway	Related Genes	Fushu No.23/Fushu No.317 expression ratio					
		Lf1	*p*-value	Lf2	*p*-value	Lf3	*p*-value
Phenylalanine ↓ PAL							
Cinnamic acid ↓ C4H	*PAL*	3.27	0.0060	5.08	0.0236	2.43	0.0060
	4CL	0.77	0.1506	2.80	0.0011	1.11	0.0528
p-Coumaric acid ↓ 4CL	*C4H*	16.07	0.0004	9.16	0.0206	4.87	0.0008
	CHS	12.68	0.0014	2.64	0.0027	78.72	0.0004
4-Coumaroyl-CoA ↓ CHS	*CHI*	2.42	0.0029	1.22	0.0308	6.92	0.0050
	DFR1	5.10	0.0009	5.80	0.0040	2.68	0.0112
Chalcone ↓ CHI	*DFR2*	3.44	0.0001	2.23	0.0193	1.46	0.0082
	DFR3	0.03	0.0001	2.34	0.0012	2.66	0.0013
Naringenin flavanone ↓ F3H, F3'H	*DFR4*	9.44	0.0004	1.25	0.0126	32.72	0.0009
	F3H1	1.40	0.0130	2.46	0.0001	9.70	0.0001
Dihydroflavonols ↓ DFR	*F3H2*	0.17	0.0010	2.73	0.0032	1.23	0.0430
	F3'H	3.19	0.0418	1.00	0.0208	25.88	0.0025
Leucoanthocyanins ↓ ANS	*ANS*	0.08	0.2692	0.88	0.0560	11.21	0.0016
	UFGT1	0.08	0.0002	1.31	0.1776	0.47	0.0001
Anthocyanidins Cyanidin et al. ↓ UFGT	*UFGT2*	0.01	0.0001	2.75	0.0005	0.65	0.0720
	UFGT3	1.85	0.0003	0.87	0.0163	16.21	0.0004
	UFGT4	0.05	0.0003	1.16	0.2244	0.35	0.0001
Anthocyanidins Cyanidin 3-O-Glycoside et al. ↓ 3AT	*3AT1-1*	0.04	0.0005	2.37	0.0008	1.73	0.0001
	3AT1-2	0.01	0.0001	1.92	0.0219	2.95	0.0038
	3AT1-3	0.12	0.0001	3.22	0.0002	1.68	0.0035
	3AT1-4	0.01	0.0008	0.92	0.0485	0.45	0.0003
Anthocyanidins Cyanidin 3-O-*p*-coumarylglycoside et al.	*3AT1-5*	0.01	0.0008	1.16	0.0485	0.45	0.0003
	3AT1-6	1.85	0.0031	1.48	0.0072	2.10	0.0050
	3AT1-7	0.02	0.0007	5.05	0.0002	1.51	0.0333
	3AT2	0.03	0.0002	2.28	0.0089	0.83	0.1045

(a)

Figure 3. *Cont.*

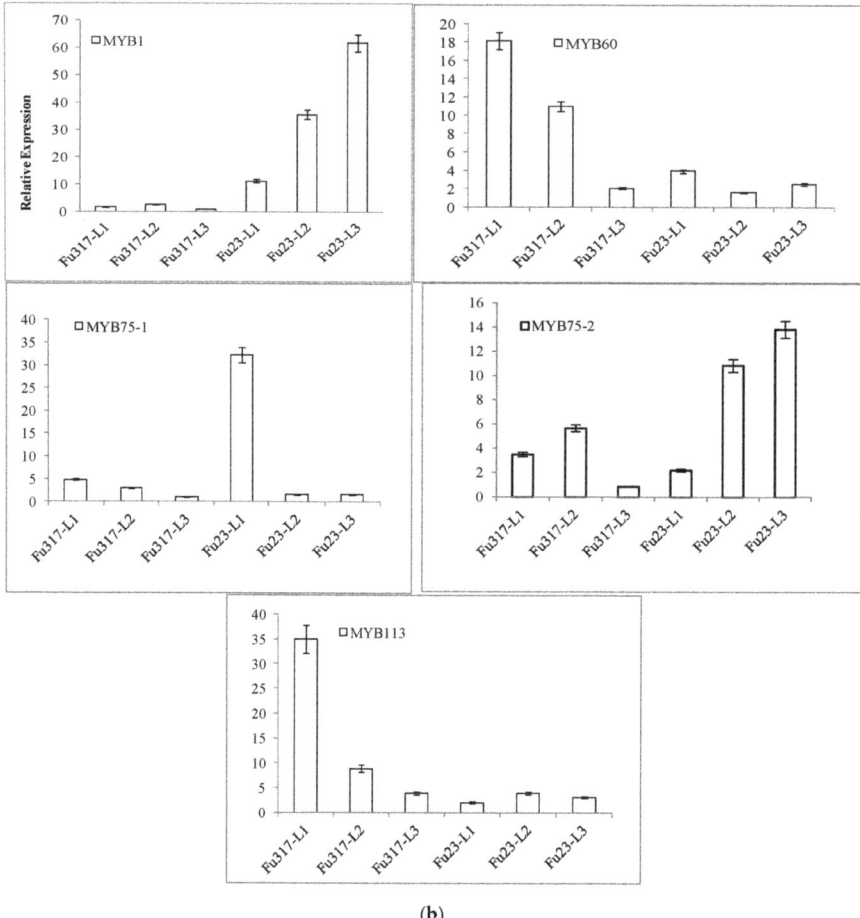

(b)

Figure 3. Expression of anthocyanin structural genes and transcription factors in the purple sweet potato cultivars Fushu No. 23 and Fushu No. 317. (**a**) Simplified model of the anthocyanin biosynthetic pathway and qRT-PCR analysis of the transcript abundance of the anthocyanin biosynthesis-related genes in Fushu No. 23 and Fushu No. 317 leaves. (**b**) Expression of transcription factors *IbMYBs* in sweet potato leaves.

To further clarify the internal connection of anthocyanin content with transcription levels of the genes involved in anthocyanin biosynthesis, 25 anthocyanin structural genes and five transcription factor genes were detected by quantitative real-time PCR. We found there were substantial differences in the expression of anthocyanidin-related genes in Fushu No. 23 and Fushu No. 317, and we found that the two cultivars had an opposite accumulation pattern. From the first to third leaves of Fushu No. 317, *CHS*, *DFRs*, *F3Hs*, *ANS*, *UFGTs*, and *3Ats* had a tendency to first increase and then decrease. Most anthocyanin biosynthesis related-myb transcription factors also had the same pattern. However, *DFRs* were correlated with the increase in anthocyanin content in the first to third leaves of Fushu No. 23.

On comparing the first leaf of Fushu No. 23 to Fushu No. 317, anthocyanin content was greater in Fushu No. 317 than Fushu No. 23, while the expression of *ANS* in the leaf of Fushu No. 23 was lower than in Fushu No. 317. Therefore, we speculate that *ANS* is the key gene for anthocyanin biosynthesis in the first leaf of sweet potato.

The anthocyanin content in the third leaf was also different. Expression of the structural genes: *CHS*, *DFR4*, *F3'H1*, *ANS*, and *UFGT3* were greater in Fushu No. 23 than in Fushu No. 317. Therefore, *CHS*, *DFR4*, *F3'H1*, *ANS*, and *UFGT3* may be vital regulatory genes of anthocyanin biosynthesis in sweet potato leaves.

MYB transcription factors (TFs) have had a long association with anthocyanin biosynthesis. In sweet potato, activation of anthocyanin levels by IbMYB1 was first observed in a functional complementation experiment using a mutant. Mano et al. (2007) reported *IbMYB1* was only expressed in the roots of purple-fleshed sweet potatoes but not in other related-tissues such as stems, leaves, flowers, and the roots of orange-, yellow-, or white-fleshed varieties [24], but we found *IbMYB1* can be highly expressed in the leaves of sweet potato variety Fushu No. 23, and can have very low expression in the leaves of Fushu No. 317. Perhaps the biosynthesis of anthocyanins in the leaves of sweet potato is through more than one metabolic pathway. *MYB60* and *MYB113* decreased from the first to third leaves, while *MYB1* and *MYB75-2* increased from the first to third leaves, possibly due to the fact that MYB has different effects on anthocyanin biosynthesis in different sweet potato leaves.

3.4. Anthocyanins in Roots of Purple-fleshed Sweet Potato Were Different from the Anthocyanins in Sweet Potato Leaves

In order to further determine differences in the composition of anthocyanins between sweet potato leaves and roots, we used the same method to analyze the anthocyanin components of five sweet potato leaves and five sweet potato roots. Fushu No. 317, Fushu No. 25, and OP contained 18 anthocyanin components and Fushu No. 23 and Yanshu No. 5 contained 17 anthocyanin components. However, cyanidin 3-*p*-coumarylsophoroside-5-glucoside and cyanidin 3-caffeoyl-*p*-coumaryl sophoroside-5-glucoside were not found in the any of the roots in this study. Interestingly, Tian et al. (2005) found cyanidin 3-*p*-coumarylsophoroside-5-glucoside and cyanidin 3-caffeoyl-*p*-coumaryl sophoroside-5-glucoside in a PL (purple line) cell line generated from the storage root of the purple-fleshed sweet potato cultivar Ayamurasaki [4], but this has not been identified in any earlier reports on purple-fleshed sweet potato [9,33]. It is possible that these compounds were not found in our study because they existed at such a low level that they could not be detected.

In this study, among five purple-fleshed sweet potatoes in this study, Longzishu No. 6 had the greatest number of anthocyanin monomers in the roots. The total contents of anthocyanins in Longzishu No. 6 roots were 255.75 ± 17.39 µg/g FW (Table 3), not very high. Anthocyanin monomers cyanidin 3-*p*-coumarylsophoroside-5-glucoside, cyanidin 3-caffeoyl-*p*-coumaryl sophoroside-5-glucoside, and cyanidin 3-caffeoyl-feruloylsophoroside-5-glucoside were not found in the roots of Fushu No. 317. The total contents of anthocyanins in Fushu No. 317 leaves (188.81 ± 18.35 µg/g FW) were much lower than that in the roots (1009.29 ± 66.41 µg/g FW). As Su et al. speculated [11], maybe anthocyanin biosynthesis between sweet potato leaves and roots involved different phenotypes. Fushu No. 9 lacked two anthocyanin monomers: peonidin 3-*p*-coumarylsophoroside-5-glucoside and peonidin 3-caffeoyl-*p*-coumarylsophoroside-5-glucoside in roots. Fushu No. 24 and Longzishu No. 4 only contained 13 anthocyanin monomers in the roots. It should be noted that the total anthocyanins in the roots of purple-fleshed sweet potato had greater changes with different varieties, but the total anthocyanins in the leaves of sweet potato showed small changes. A future study to explain the genotype of anthocyanin biosynthesis genes in the leaves and roots of sweet potato may be necessary.

Table 3. Quantity of anthocyanins (1–14) from the leaves and roots of different sweet potato cultivars (μg/g FW).

Identity [a]	Leaves							Roots			
	Fushu No. 23	Fushu No. 317	Fushu No. 25	OP	Yanshu No. 5	Fushu No. 9	Fushu No. 24	Longzishu No. 4	Longzishu No. 6	Fushu No. 317
Cy 3-soph-5glc	3.16 ± 0.27	5.04 ± 0.62	4.27 ± 0.32	7.51 ± 0.46	3.75 ± 0.26	2.82 ± 0.16	3.60 ± 0.25	1.30 ± 0.09	3.21 ± 0.32	42.02 ± 2.54
Peo 3-soph-5glc	4.38 ± 0.46	9.16 ± 0.94	2.62 ± 0.15	5.38 ± 0.32	8.15 ± 0.52	4.82 ± 0.25	4.02 ± 0.35	5.13 ± 0.69	27.41 ± 1.86	57.40 ± 3.68
Cy 3-p-hydroxybenzoylsoph-5glc	14.83 ± 1.98	15.09 ± 2.21	3.58 ± 0.16	2.55 ± 0.15	1.27 ± 0.08	2.87 ± 0.12	3.41 ± 0.27	3.24 ± 0.73	12.62 ± 0.79	112.39 ± 8.52
Cy 3-caffeylsophsoph-5glc	1.33 ± 0.15	15.94 ± 2.66	14.31 ± 0.86	16.64 ± 1.12	14.19 ± 1.03	1.72 ± 0.08	7.51 ± 0.43	16.15 ± 0.89	27.93 ± 1.56	19.97 ± 1.64
Peo 3-p-hydroxybenzoylsoph-5glc	7.39 ± 0.66	8.93 ± 1.04	5.10 ± 0.35	12.33 ± 0.84	6.17 ± 0.46	1.12 ± 0.07	13.84 ± 0.95	1.65 ± 0.06	4.91 ± 0.23	135.07 ± 9.36
Peo 3-caffeylsophsoph-5glc	0.31 ± 0.06	7.58 ± 0.98	3.70 ± 0.21	10.47 ± 0.76	6.75 ± 0.81	0.99 ± 0.11	0.77 ± 0.06	-	3.67 ± 0.28	13.28 ± 1.12
Cy 3-p-coumarylsoph-5glc	0.34 ± 0.07	29.20 ± 1.45	22.26 ± 2.00	40.33 ± 2.38	20.16 ± 1.74	-	-	-	-	-
Cy 3-feruloylsoph-5glc	1.04 ± 0.15	6.59 ± 0.73	8.08 ± 0.19	9.10 ± 0.55	5.87 ± 0.44	11.46 ± 1.34	1.21 ± 0.08	8.53 ± 0.77	19.29 ± 1.64	11.32 ± 0.88
Peo 3-p-coumarylsoph-5glc	0.84 ± 0.11	22.61 ± 1.56	27.73 ± 1.87	31.23 ± 2.53	15.62 ± 1.15	-	4.15 ± 0.41	2.81 ± 0.16	8.47 ± 0.53	51.15 ± 3.63
Peo 3-feruloylsoph-5glc	0.43 ± 0.05	6.27 ± 0.42	7.69 ± 0.23	8.67 ± 0.79	5.58 ± 0.65	19.71 ± 1.74	3.47 ± 0.26	7.84 ± 0.63	61.44 ± 3.86	17.28 ± 1.41
Cy 3-dicaffeylsoph-5glc	4.23 ± 0.51	17.53 ± 2.08	21.49 ± 1.68	24.21 ± 1.82	12.1 ± 1.04	1.04 ± 0.07	3.11 ± 0.22	16.72 ± 0.92	14.07 ± 1.12	41.56 ± 3.76
Cy 3-caffeoyl-p-hydroxybenzoylsoph-5glc	14.04 ± 2.11	7.22 ± 0.55	8.85 ± 0.66	9.97 ± 0.73	6.42 ± 0.47	3.27 ± 0.19	-	3.04 ± 0.23	3.99 ± 0.24	32.23 ± 2.09
Cy 3-caffeoyl-p-coumarylsoph-5glc	0.28 ± 0.05	11.48 ± 0.92	14.07 ± 1.12	15.85 ± 1.75	7.92 ± 0.78	-	-	-	-	-
Cy 3-caffeoyl-feruloylsoph-5glc	0.97 ± 0.10	7.30 ± 0.67	5.06 ± 0.36	10.09 ± 0.95	6.50 ± 0.47	9.15 ± 1.22	0.91 ± 0.04	17.33 ± 0.81	3.77 ± 0.13	82.11 ± 5.49
Peo 3-dicaffeoyl-5glc	0.50 ± 0.07	7.58 ± 0.72	6.37 ± 0.43	10.47 ± 1.07	5.23 ± 0.32	13.07 ± 1.68	10.63 ± 0.78	40.75 ± 2.58	63.36 ± 4.75	37.02 ± 1.83
Peo 3-caffeoyl-p-hydroxybenzoylsoph-5glc	2.64 ± 0.33	3.77 ± 0.21	8.26 ± 0.61	5.21 ± 0.33	3.36 ± 0.23	1.52 ± 0.13	1.00 ± 0.03	18.17 ± 0.94	1.62 ± 0.08	166.51 ± 10.25
Peo 3-caffeoyl-p-coumarylsoph-5glc	0.04 ± 0.01	4.70 ± 0.37	5.76 ± 0.16	6.49 ± 0.49	3.25 ± 0.28	-	-	-	-	181.75 ± 9.58
Peo 3-caffeoyl-feruloylsoph-5glc	0.18 ± 0.02	2.80 ± 0.22	3.43 ± 0.04	3.87 ± 0.22	2.49 ± 0.17	3.75 ± 0.26	-	-	-	8.22 ± 0.63
Total anthocyanin	56.95 ± 7.10	188.81 ± 18.35	172.65 ± 11.41	230.36 ± 17.26	134.8 ± 9.65	77.32 ± 7.42	57.64 ± 4.13	142.66 ± 9.50	255.75 ± 17.39	1009.29 ± 66.41

[a] Cy = cyanidin, Peo = peonidin, soph = sophorside, glc = glucoside.

Supplementary Materials: The following are available online, Figure S1: UPLC-QTOF-MS/MS of anthocyanins in two purple sweetpotato leaves, Table S1: Primer sequences used for detection of genes related to anthocyanin biosynthesis by qRT-PCR.

Author Contributions: Conceptualization, G.L. and S.Q.; methodology, G.L., Z.L. (Zhaomiao Lin) and H.L.; software, G.L.; validation, G.L. and H.Z.; formal analysis, G.L.; investigation, Y.X.; resources, Z.L. (Zhonghua Liu), R.J., W.L. and Y.Q.; data curation, G.L; writing—original draft preparation, G.L.; writing—review and editing, G.L., Z.L. (Zhaomiao Lin), H.Z. and G.X.; visualization, Z.L. (Zhonghua Liu), R.J., W.L. and Y.Q.; supervision, Y.Q. and H.T.; project administration, G.L. and S.Q.; funding acquisition, S.Q. and H.T.

Funding: This work was supported by Natural Science Foundation of Fujian Province of China (2018J01046), Special Fund for the Industrial Technology System Construction of Modern Agriculture of China (CARS-10-B14) and Fujian Academy of Agricultural Sciences Research Project (DC2017-7).

Acknowledgments: We thank LetPub (www.letpub.com) for its linguistic assistance during the preparation of this manuscript.

Conflicts of Interest: The authors declare no conflict of interest.

Abbreviations

PAL	phenylalanine ammonialyase
C4L	cinnamic acid-4-hydroxylase
4CL	4-coumarate:CoA ligase
CHS	chalconesynthase
CHI	chalconeisomerase
F3H	flavanone 3-hydroxylase
F3'H	flavonoids 3'-hydroxylase
DFR	dihydrofavonol 4-reductase
ANS	anthocyanin synthase
UFGT	UDP-glucose flavonoid 3-O-glucosyltransferase
3AT	anthocyanin 3-O-acyltransferases
qRT-PCR	quantitative real time polymerase chain reaction
SD	standard deviation
UPLC-QTOF-MS	ultra-performance liquid chromatography/quadrupole time-of-flight mass spectrometry
UPLC-DAD	ultra-performance liquid chromatography diode-array detection
FW	fresh weight

References

1. Tahara, M. Current developments in breeding, genetics, genomics, and molecular biology applied to sweetpotato improvement. *Breed. Sci.* **2017**, *67*, 1. [CrossRef] [PubMed]
2. Tanaka, M.; Ishiguro, K.; Oki, T.; Okuno, S. Functional components in sweetpotato and their genetic improvement. *Breed. Sci.* **2017**, *67*, 52–61. [CrossRef] [PubMed]
3. Cai, N.T.; Huang, H.K.; Qiu, Y.X.; Zheng, X.; Wu, Q.Y.; Luo, W.B.; Li, G.X. Breeding and cultivate techniques fo new sweetpotato variety Fushu 7-6 used as leaf vegetable. *Fujian J. Agric. Sci.* **2006**, *1*, 12–15.
4. Tian, Q.; Konczak, I.; Schwartz, S.J. Probing anthocyanin profiles in purple sweetpotato cell line (*Ipomoea batatas* L. Cv. Ayamurasaki) by high-performance liquid chromatography and electrospray ionization tandem mass spectrometry. *J. Agric. Food Chem.* **2005**, *53*, 6503–6509. [CrossRef] [PubMed]
5. Truong, V.-D.; Deighton, N.; Thompson, R.T.; McFeeters, R.F.; Dean, L.O.; Pecota, K.V.; Yencho, G.C. Characterization of Anthocyanins and Anthocyanidins in Purple-Fleshed Sweetpotatoes by HPLC-DAD/ESI-MS/MS. *J. Agric. Food Chem.* **2010**, *58*, 404–410. [CrossRef]
6. Lee, M.J.; Park, J.S.; Choi, D.S.; Jung, M.Y. Characterization and quantitation of anthocyanins in purple-fleshed sweetpotatoes cultivated in Korea by HPLC-DAD and HPLC-ESI-QTOF-MS/MS. *J. Agric. Food Chem.* **2013**, *61*, 3148–3158. [CrossRef]
7. Xu, J.; Su, X.; Lim, S.; Griffin, J.; Carey, E.; Katz, B.; Tomich, J.; Smith, J.S.; Wang, W. Characterisation and stability of anthocyanins in purple-fleshed sweetpotato P40. *Food Chem.* **2015**, *186*, 90–96. [CrossRef]

8. He, W.; Zeng, M.; Chen, J.; Jiao, Y.; Niu, F.; Tao, G.; Zhang, S.; Qin, F.; He, Z. Identification and quantitation of anthocyanins in purple-fleshed sweetpotatoes cultivated in china by UPLC-PDA and UPLC-QTOF-MS/MS. *J. Agric. Food Chem.* **2016**, *64*, 171–177. [CrossRef]
9. Terahara, N.; Shimizu, T.; Kato, Y.; Nakamura, M.; Maitani, T.; Yamaguchi, M.-A.; Goda, Y. Six diacylated anthocyanins from the storage roots of purple sweetpotato, (*Ipomoea batatas*). *Biosci. Biotechnol. Biochem.* **1999**, *63*, 1420–1424. [CrossRef]
10. Islam, M.S.; Yoshimoto, M.; Terahara, N.; Yamakawa, O. Anthocyanin compositions in sweetpotato (*Ipomoea batatas* L.) leaves. *Biosci. Biotechnol. Biochem.* **2002**, *66*, 2483–2486. [CrossRef]
11. Su, X.Y.; Griffin, J.; Xu, J.W.; Ouyan, P.; Zhao, Z.H.; Wang, W.Q. Identification and quantification of anthocyanins in purple-fleshed sweet potato leaves. *Heliyon* **2019**, *5*, e01964. [CrossRef] [PubMed]
12. Vishnu, V.R.; Renjith, R.S.; Mukherjee, A.; Anil, S.R.; Sreekumar, J.; Jyothi, A.N. Comparative study on the chemical structure and in vitro antiproliferative activity of anthocyanins in purple root tubers and leaves of sweetpotato (*Ipomoea batatas*). *J. Agric. Food Chem.* **2019**, *67*, 2467–2475. [CrossRef] [PubMed]
13. Sun, H.; Zhang, P.; Zhu, Y.; Lou, Q.; He, S. Antioxidant and prebiotic activity of five peonidin-based anthocyanins extracted from purple sweetpotato (*Ipomoea batatas* (L.) Lam.). *Sci. Rep.* **2018**, *8*, 5018. [CrossRef] [PubMed]
14. Wang, W.; Li, J.; Wang, Z.; Gao, H.; Su, L.; Xie, J.; Chen, X.; Liang, H.; Wang, C.; Han, Y. Oral hepatoprotective ability evaluation of purple sweetpotato anthocyanins on acute and chronic chemical liver injuries. *Cell Biochem. Biophys.* **2014**, *69*, 539–548. [CrossRef]
15. Hwang, Y.P.; Choi, J.H.; Yun, H.J.; Han, E.H.; Kim, H.G.; Kim, J.Y.; Park, B.H.; Khanal, T.; Choi, J.M.; Chung, Y.C.; et al. Anthocyanins from purple sweetpotato attenuate dimethylnitrosamine-induced liver injury in rats by inducing Nrf2-mediated antioxidant enzymes and reducing COX-2 and iNOS expression. *Food Chem. Toxicol.* **2011**, *49*, 93–99. [CrossRef]
16. Zhao, J.G.; Yan, Q.Q.; Lu, L.Z.; Zhang, Y.Q. In vivo antioxidant, hypoglycemic, and anti-tumor activities of anthocyanin extracts from purple sweetpotato. *Nutr. Res. Pract.* **2013**, *7*, 359–365. [CrossRef]
17. Zhu, Y.; Bo, Y.; Wang, X.; Lu, W.; Wang, X.; Han, Z.; Qiu, C. The effect of anthocyanins on blood pressure: A prisma-compliant meta-analysis of randomized clinical trials. *Medince (Baltim.)* **2016**, *95*, e3380. [CrossRef]
18. Zhuang, J.; Lu, J.; Wang, X.; Wang, X.; Hu, W.; Hong, F.; Zhao, X.X.; Zheng, Y.L. Purple sweet potato color protects against high-fat diet-induced cognitive deficits through AMPK-mediated autophagy in mouse hippocampus. *J. Nutr. Biochem.* **2019**, *65*, 35–45. [CrossRef]
19. Zhang, Z.C.; Su, G.H.; Luo, C.L.; Pang, Y.L.; Wang, L.; Li, X.; Wen, J.H.; Zhang, J.L. Effects of anthocyanins from purple sweet potato (*Ipomoea batatas* L. cultivar Eshu No. 8) on the serum uric acid level and xanthine oxidase activity in hyperuricemic mice. *Food Funct.* **2015**, *6*, 3045–3055. [CrossRef]
20. Schmittgen, T.D.; Livak, K.J. Analyzing real-time PCR data by the comparative CT method. *Nat. Protoc.* **2008**, *6*, 1101–1108. [CrossRef]
21. Dixon, R.A.; Liu, C.; Jun, J.H. Metabolic engineering of anthocyanins and condensed tannins in plants. *Curr. Opin. Biotechnol.* **2013**, *24*, 329–335. [CrossRef] [PubMed]
22. Hu, C.; Gong, Y.; Jin, S.; Zhu, Q. Molecular analysis of a UDP-glucose: Flavonoid 3-O-glucosyltransferase (UFGT) gene from purple potato (*Solanum tuberosum*). *Mol. Biol. Rep.* **2011**, *38*, 561–567. [CrossRef]
23. Luo, J.; Nishiyama, Y.; Fuell, C.; Taguchi, G.; Elliott, K.; Hill, L.; Tanaka, Y.; Kitayama, M.; Yamazaki, M.; Bailey, P.; et al. Convergent evolution in the BAHD family of acyl transferases: Identification and characterization of anthocyanin acyl transferases from Arabidopsis thaliana. *Plant J. Cell Mol. Biol.* **2007**, *50*, 678–695. [CrossRef] [PubMed]
24. Unno, H.; Ichimaida, F.; Suzuki, H.; Takahashi, S.; Tanaka, Y.; Saito, A.; Nishino, T.; Kusunoki, M.; Nakayama, T. Structural and mutational studies of anthocyanin malonyltransferases establish the features of BAHD enzyme catalysis. *J. Biol. Chem.* **2007**, *282*, 15812–15822. [CrossRef] [PubMed]
25. Wang, H.; Fan, W.; Wu, Y.; Zhang, P.; Wang, C.; Yang, J.; Appelhagen, I. A novel glycosyltransferase catalyses the transfer of glucose to glucosylated anthocyanins in purple sweetpotato. *J. Exp. Bot.* **2018**, *69*, 5444–5459. [PubMed]
26. Xie, F.; Burklew, C.E.; Yang, Y.; Liu, M.; Xiao, P.; Zhang, B.; Qiu, D. De novo sequencing and a comprehensive analysis of purple sweetpotato (*Ipomoea batatas* L.) transcriptome. *Planta* **2012**, *236*, 101–113. [CrossRef] [PubMed]

27. Mano, H.; Ogasawara, F.; Sato, K.; Higo, H.; Minobe, Y. Isolation of a regulatory gene of anthocyanin biosynthesis in tuberous roots of purple-fleshed sweetpotato. *Plant Physiol.* **2007**, *143*, 1252–1268. [CrossRef]
28. Park, J.S.; Kim, J.B.; Cho, K.J.; Cheon, C.I.; Sung, M.K.; Choung, M.G.; Roh, K.H. *Arabidopsis* R2R3-MYB transcription factor AtMYB60 functions as a transcriptional repressor of anthocyanin biosynthesis in lettuce (*Lactuca sativa*). *Plant Cell Rep.* **2008**, *27*, 985–994. [CrossRef]
29. Teng, S.; Keurentjes, J.; Bentsink, L.; Koornneef, M.; Smeekens, S. Sucrose-specific induction of anthocyanin biosynthesis in *Arabidopsis* requires the MYB75/PAP1 gene. *Plant Physiol.* **2005**, *139*, 1840–1852. [CrossRef]
30. Li, X.; Gao, M.J.; Pan, H.Y.; Cui, D.J.; Gruber, M.Y. Purple canola: *Arabidopsis* PAP1 increases antioxidants and phenolics in Brassica napus leaves. *J. Agric. Food Chem.* **2010**, *58*, 1639–1645. [CrossRef]
31. Gonzalez, A.; Zhao, M.; Leavitt, J.M.; Lloyd, A.M. Regulation of the anthocyanin biosynthetic pathway by the TTG1/bHLH/Myb transcriptional complex in *Arabidopsis* seedlings. *Plant J. Cell Mol. Biol.* **2008**, *53*, 814–827. [CrossRef] [PubMed]
32. Baudry, A.; Caboche, M.; Lepiniec, L. TT8 controls its own expression in a feedback regulation involving TTG1 and homologous MYB and bHLH factors, allowing a strong and cell-specific accumulation of flavonoids in *Arabidopsis thaliana*. *Plant J. Cell Mol. Biol.* **2006**, *46*, 768–779. [CrossRef] [PubMed]
33. Goda, Y.; Shimizu, T.; Kato, Y.; Nakamura, M.; Maitani, T.; Yamada, T.; Terahara, N.; Yamaguchi, M. Two acylated anthocyanins from purple sweet-potato. *Phytochemistry* **1997**, *44*, 183–186. [CrossRef]

Sample Availability: Samples of the compounds are not available from the authors.

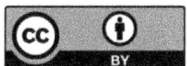

© 2019 by the authors. Licensee MDPI, Basel, Switzerland. This article is an open access article distributed under the terms and conditions of the Creative Commons Attribution (CC BY) license (http://creativecommons.org/licenses/by/4.0/).

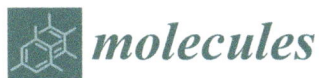

Article

Composition of Sugars in Wild and Cultivated Lingonberries (*Vaccinium vitis-idaea* L.)

Gabriele Vilkickyte [1,*], Raimondas Raudonis [2], Vida Motiekaityte [3], Rimanta Vainoriene [4], Deividas Burdulis [2], Jonas Viskelis [5] and Lina Raudone [1,2]

1. Laboratory of Biopharmaceutical Research, Institute of Pharmaceutical Technologies, Lithuanian University of Health Sciences, Sukileliu av. 13, LT-50162 Kaunas, Lithuania; lina.raudone@lsmuni.lt
2. Department of Pharmacognosy, Lithuanian University of Health Sciences, Sukileliu av. 13, LT-50162 Kaunas, Lithuania; raimondas.raudonis@lsmuni.lt (R.R.); deividas.burdulis@lsmuni.lt (D.B.)
3. Biomedical Sciences Department, Siauliai State College. Ausros av. 40, LT-76241 Siauliai, Lithuania; vmotiek@gmail.com
4. Paitaiciu str, The Botanical Garden of Siauliai University, 4, LT-77175 Siauliai, Lithuania; rimanta.vainoriene@su.lt
5. Laboratory of Biochemistry and Technology, Institute of Horticulture, Lithuanian Research Centre for Agriculture and Forestry, Kauno str. 30, LT-54333 Babtai, Kaunas distr., Lithuania; jonas.viskelis@lammc.lt
* Correspondence: gabriele.vilkickyte@lsmu.lt; Tel.: +370-622-34977

Academic Editor: Toshio Morikawa
Received: 18 October 2019; Accepted: 18 November 2019; Published: 20 November 2019

Abstract: Products of lingonberries are widely used in the human diet; they are also promising beauty and health therapeutic candidates in the cosmetic and pharmaceutical industries. It is important to examine the sugar profile of these berries, due to potential deleterious health effects resulting from high sugar consumption. The aim of this study was to determine the composition of sugars in wild clones and cultivars or lower taxa of lingonberries by HPLC–ELSD method of analysis. Acceptable system suitability, linearity, limits of detection and quantification, precision, and accuracy of this analytical method were achieved. The same sugars with moderate amounts of fructose, glucose, and low amounts of sucrose were found in wild and cultivated lingonberries. Cultivar 'Erntekrone' and wild lingonberries collected from full sun, dry pine tree forests with lower altitude and latitude of the location, distinguished themselves with exclusive high contents of sugars. The changes in the sugar levels during the growing season were apparent in lingonberries and the highest amounts accumulated at the end of the vegetation. According to our findings, lingonberries seem to be an appropriate source of dietary sugars.

Keywords: *Vaccinium vitis-idaea*; lingonberry; sugars; cultivated berries; wild berries; HPLC–ELSD

1. Introduction

As the modern lifestyle and prevalence of chronic diseases have become a relevant issue of concern, functional food ingredients, nutraceuticals, and food supplements have become a significant area of research. Increasing sugar intake is of concern, because it may result in obesity, metabolic disorders, dental caries, and increased risk of noncommunicable diseases—hypertension, dyslipidemia, cardiovascular diseases, type 2 diabetes, cancer and others, which are responsible for more than half of all deaths worldwide [1,2]. Possible harmful cardiometabolic mechanisms of action of dietary sugars include induction of inflammatory processes, oxidative stress, increasing insulin resistance, and impaired β-cell function [3]. Sugars differ from each other in structure, effects, and applications. According to the structure, sugars can be referred to as: (1) Monosaccharides (glucose, fructose, and galactose), which have five or six carbon atoms, sweet taste and can be called reducing sugars; (2) disaccharides (sucrose, lactose, maltose, trehalose), which make up two or more monosaccharide units and may not have reducing properties; and (3) polyols—sugar alcohols (sorbitol, mannitol, lactitol, xylitol, erythritol, isomalt, maltitol). Sugars may naturally present in food or can be added to food additionally by the manufacturer or consumer. The latter is considered to be more dangerous because of the faster absorption and conversion to fats [4–6].

Deleterious health effects may occur if sugars are consumed in large amounts [3]. The same can be said about any macro- or micronutrient. The moderate intake of sugars, which according to WHO should be less than 10% of total energy intake, does not increase the health risk [1]. While excessive amounts of sugars are undoubtedly unhealthy, rational use of sugars can be favorable. Sugars are a prominent constituent of plants, acting as structure matter and molecule signal, regulating growth and enzyme activity [7]. Furthermore, they are the main energy source for the human body and an ubiquitous ingredient of our food, providing a desirable sweet taste [4,8].

It has been suggested that some sugars take part in the anti-adherence activity. Adhesin proteins, fimbriae or pili, expose adhesive lectins on the cell surface, which bind complementary carbohydrates on the tissues of the host, and thus permit *Escherichia coli* bacterial adhesion to the urothelium. Adhesin proteins can be mannose-resistant (p-fimbriae) or mannose-sensitive (type 1 fimbriae). The current hypothesis proposes that proanthocyanidins inhibit the adherence of p-fimbriae, and fructose inhibits adherence of type 1 fimbriae; consequently, uropathogenic bacteria cannot infect mucosal surface and postulate urinary tract infections [9,10]. Hereby, fructose contributes to the disease-preventing properties of the most common bacterial infections, acquired in the community or hospitals [11].

To avoid the harmful impact of sugars and to maintain their positive role, monitoring the concentration of sugars in food is needed, as well as choosing dietary sugars with low energy density that naturally occur in food—vegetables and fruits, including berries. According to this, lingonberries seem to be an appropriate source of dietary sugars [2,4]. Lingonberry (*Vaccinium vitis-idaea* L.) is a native plant to the boreal forest of North Eurasia and North America, nowadays generally accessible in most countries of Europe, especially in Scandinavia. Lingonberries can be consumed fresh, bought at the local markets, or cooked in the form of juices, jams, jellies, compotes, and syrups [12,13]. These berries are widely used in the human diet, especially sweetened products, which are more favorable for most consumers [14]. Fruits of this low-growing, evergreen shrub, belonging to the genus *Vaccinium* L., are popular not only because of their unique taste, but also because of their high level of healthy bioactive compounds. Lingonberries are considered to be a good source of flavonols, anthocyanins, phenolic acids, proanthocyanidins, free amino acids, vitamins, omega-3 fatty acids, and minerals [15,16]. A wide spectrum of biological activities of lingonberries has been determined. Lingonberries exhibit antimicrobial, anti-inflammatory, antioxidant, immunomodulatory, and antiproliferative activities and play a role in bacterial adhesion [12,17]. Products of lingonberries are increasingly marketed as a natural solution for the treatment of various conditions, particularly urinary tract infections [18].

However, the lingonberry's composition and activity have not yet been fully investigated to date. Lingonberry is one of the least studied raw in the *Ericaceae* family; besides that, most studies were conducted in the Nordic countries and focused mainly on phenolic compounds [19]. Considering these berries' popularity in food and health and wellness products, it is necessary to examine their sugar profile, due to potentially adverse effects. Lingonberries have historically been collected from the wild, and this is still mainly the case today. There are some cultivars produced, but there is no large-scale cultivation, and plant breeding of lingonberry is still in its infancy [20]. Cultivation of lingonberry can best meet the increased needs of plant material. To optimize horticulturally important traits, evaluation the phytochemical differences between cultivated and wild lingonberries is needed, as well as emphasis of factors such as optimal collecting time and environmental conditions leading to better yield.

To the best of our knowledge, there have been no comprehensive studies on sugar analysis of many lingonberry coenopopulations, considering phenological growth stages, altitude, and latitude of the berries' collecting locations. The variations of identified sugars have been presented for the first time for the cultivars and lower taxa. This is the first report on sugar composition of *V. vitis-idaea* var. *leucocarpum*, which is a unique white berry-bearing variety that is included in the National Genetic Resources of Lithuania. The obtained results will be really important to breeders for developing new cultivars and, of course, as a part of the ongoing interest in nutritional and nutraceutical properties of food, the content of sugars in lingonberries will be of interest to dietitians and may be used in the pharmaceutical industry in developing new products for consumers with special dietary requirements. Our results can contribute to quality improvement of lingonberry products, leading to increased acceptability of consumers and market size. The findings on the content of fructose in lingonberries may disclose the necessity of further studies on fructose from lingonberries as a natural anti-adhesive agent. The sugar profile and individual sugar ratio can also serve as a fruit authenticity tool to prevent adulterations.

Therefore, our aim was to characterize the sugar composition in wild clones from Lithuania, in seven cultivars ('Erntedank', 'Erntekrone', 'Kostromička', 'Kostromskaja rozovaja', 'Rubin', 'Sanna', 'Sussi') and lower taxa (*V. vitis-idaea* var. *leucocarpum*) of lingonberries, considering genetic and environmental factors.

2. Results

2.1. Method Validation

Linearity for all sugars was evaluated between 0.0625 and 4 mg/mL. Calibration equations with their linearity coefficients of detected sugars in lingonberries presented in Table 1. Limits of detection (LOD) of all tested sugars ranged between 11 and 18 µg/mL, and limits of quantification (LOQ) between 30 and 60 µg/mL. The precision values—repeatability and intermediate precision—were < 2% (relative standard deviation (RSD) of retention times < 1%, and RSD of peak areas < 2%). It could be concluded that our method gave acceptable precision for sugar measurements because the intra- and inter-day variations RSD for sugars were very low. The average recoveries of sugars were 98.08–102.15%, thereby confirming the accuracy of this analytical method. Resolution values were greater than 1.5 and selectivity values were greater than 1, ensuring that the sample components were well separated.

Table 1. The linearity of calibration curves of lingonberry sugars.

Component	Calibration Equation	Coefficient of Determination R^2	Coefficient of Correlation R
Fructose	Y = 1.80 X + 44.9	0.9998	0.9999
Glucose	Y = 2.00 X − 26.3	0.9876	0.9938
Sucrose	Y = 1.77 X + 82.2	0.9999	0.9999

2.2. Qualitative Analysis of Sugars in Wild and Cultivated Lingonberries

Sixteen sugars, including mono- and disaccharides, as well as polyols, were searched in samples of wild and cultivated lingonberries. HPLC–ELSD results showed that only three sugars—fructose, glucose, and sucrose—were detected in all tested samples (Figure 1). Retention times of fructose, glucose, and sucrose were 7.109, 8.132, and 12.251 min, respectively.

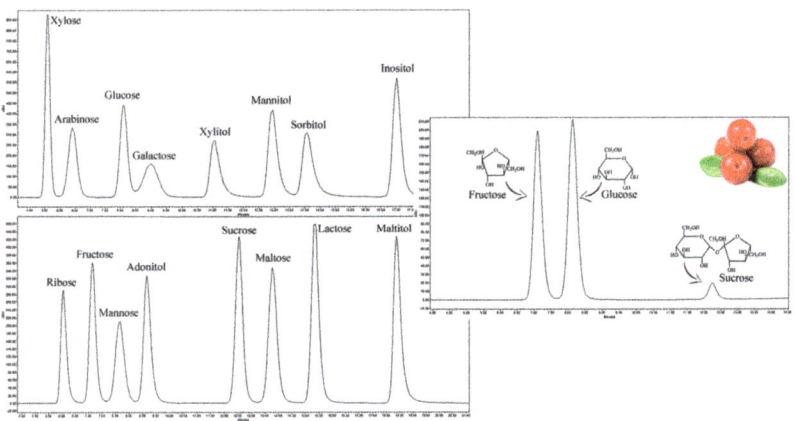

Figure 1. Chromatograms of reference compounds (on the **left**) and analyte (on the **right**).

2.3. Quantitative Analysis of Sugars in Wild Lingonberries

Fructose and glucose were the most abundant sugars in wild lingonberry extracts (Figure 2). These sugars contributed up to 98.01% of total sugars (the sum of identified sugar amounts). Contents of sucrose varied considerably among lingonberries from different collecting locations—the coefficient of variation (CV) was 42.61%—whereas the content of fructose and glucose varied only slightly (CV = 11.78% and 10.58%, respectively). The highest ($p < 0.05$) amounts of fructose were determined in Valkininkai (295.74 ± 13.80 mg/g dry weight (DW)), Gudžiai (286.63 ± 9.40 mg/g DW), and Aukštadvaris (280.58 ± 14.69 mg/g DW) forests, and the lowest ($p < 0.05$) in Juodlė (214.98 ± 6.92 mg/g DW), Jurašiškės (215.97 ± 6.42 mg/g DW), and Gineitiškės (217.10 ± 6.80 mg/g DW) forests. Contents of glucose were quite similar among different collecting locations, with the highest ($p < 0.05$) ones determined in lingonberries from Valkininkai forest (309.83 ± 15.18 mg/g DW), followed by Bingeliai, Aukštadvaris, Rudnia, and Marcinkonys forests. The lowest ($p < 0.05$) amounts of glucose accumulated lingonberries collected from Juodlė, Gineitiškės, and Jurašiškės forests (226.06 ± 7.28, 227.26 ± 7.12, and 236.77 ± 7.04 mg/g DW, respectively). Contents of sucrose ranged between 7.76 ± 0.24 mg/g DW in Gineitiškės forest (contribution 1.72% of total sugars) and 43.01 ± 2.51 mg/g DW in Valkininkai forest (contribution 6.63% of total sugars). Considering the sums of sugars, it was determined that lingonberries from Valkininkai forest accumulated the highest ($p < 0.05$) amount of total sugars (648.59 mg/g DW), meanwhile the lowest ($p < 0.05$) amount was determined in lingonberries from Juodlė, Gineitiškės, and Jurašiškės forests (450.23, 452.13, and 469.29 mg/g DW, respectively). Correlation analysis showed that sugar levels in wild lingonberries negatively correlated ($p < 0.05$) with latitudes and altitudes of their collecting locations.

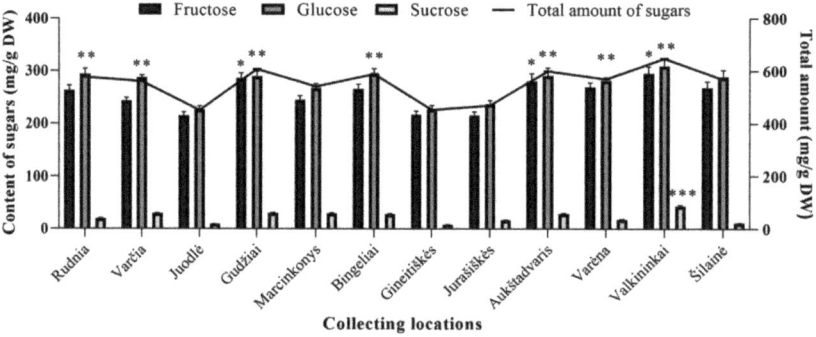

Figure 2. Composition of sugars in wild lingonberries clones. Bars marked with *, **, *** indicate the highest ($p < 0.05$) fructose, glucose, and sucrose amounts in lingonberries, respectively.

The cluster analysis divided lingonberries from different collecting locations into four clusters, which differed statistically significant from each other (Figure 3). The first cluster consisted of the lingonberries from Juodlė, Gineitiškės, and Jurašiškės forests. Lingonberries collected from these forests distinguished themselves by the lowest ($p < 0.05$) amounts of all types of detected sugars. Cluster two was the largest and included lingonberries from Gudžiai, Aukštadvaris, Rudnia, Bingeliai, Varėna, and Šilainė forests. Wild clones from these forests could be characterized by higher than average amounts of fructose and glucose and low amounts of sucrose. Lingonberries from Varčia and Marcinkonys forests were attributed to the third cluster. These lingonberries, on the contrary to the second cluster, accumulated lower than average amounts of fructose and glucose and high amounts of sucrose. Lingonberries from the Valkininkai forest surpassed lingonberries from other collecting locations by the highest ($p < 0.05$) contents of all sugars, and were attributed to the fourth cluster. These results highlight differences between wild clones of lingonberries and their adaptability to growing and environmental conditions in different locations.

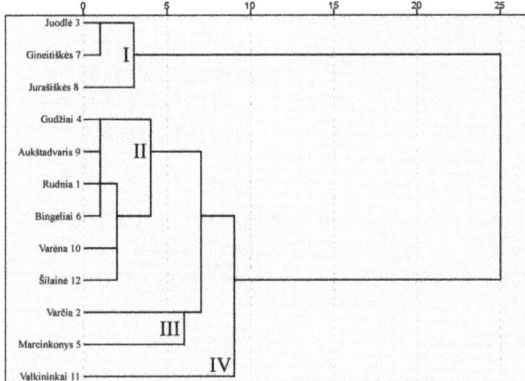

Figure 3. Dendrogram based on the amounts of sugars in wild lingonberry clones from different collecting locations.

2.4. Quantitative Analysis of Sugars in Cultivated Lingonberries

Similarly to wild clones, the predominant sugars in cultivars and lower taxa of lingonberries were fructose and glucose (Figure 4). Fructose contributed 43.51–49.49% and glucose contributed 47.40–50.29% of total sugars in different cultivars and lower taxa of lingonberries. The highest contribution of glucose and fructose was found in *V. vitis-idaea* var. *leucocarpum* (98.16%), and the lowest one in 'Kostromskaja rozovaja' (92.08%). CV of fructose and glucose among tested cultivars and lower taxa were 15.55% and 14.27%, respectively, indicating that the contents of these sugars between cultivated lingonberries did not differ extremely. Significantly the highest contents of fructose were determined in 'Erntedank' (327.64 ± 15.01 mg/g DW), 'Erntekrone' (317.72 ± 16.57 mg/g DW), and 'Sussi' (311.01 ± 11.17 mg/g DW); meanwhile, the lowest ($p < 0.05$) were in 'Sanna' (203.82 ± 7.32 mg/g DW) and 'Rubin' (232.47 ± 8.35 mg/g DW) cultivars of lingonberries. The content of glucose among tested cultivars and lower taxa of lingonberries ranged between 214.78 ± 7.72 mg/g DW (in 'Sanna' cultivar) and 355.24 ± 18.53 mg/g DW (in 'Erntekrone' cultivar). Amounts of sucrose (1.84–7.92% of total sugars in different cultivars and lower taxa of lingonberries) were considerably lower than that of other sugars, but varied within a wide range (CV = 49.85%). Significantly, the highest content of sucrose was found in 'Kostromskaja rozovaja' cultivar (47.29 ± 1.71 mg/g DW), whereas the lowest ($p < 0.05$) in 'Sanna' cultivar (11.46 ± 0.41 mg/g DW) and *V. vitis-idaea* var. *leucocarpum* (10.68 ± 0.54 mg/g DW). It was noticed that 'Erntekrone' cultivar accumulated the highest ($p < 0.05$) amount of total sugars (708.78 mg/g DW), whilst a lower amount of even more than one and a half times was determined in 'Sanna' cultivar.

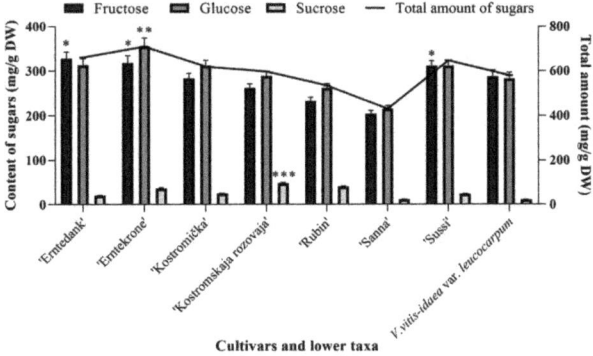

Figure 4. Composition of sugars in cultivated lingonberries. Bars marked with *, **, *** indicate the highest ($p < 0.05$) fructose, glucose, and sucrose amounts in lingonberries, respectively.

After hierarchical cluster analysis, the lingonberry cultivars and lower taxa fruit samples were grouped into four significantly different clusters (Figure 5). The first cluster was distinguished by the highest amounts of total sugars, but the lowest of sucrose. The lingonberry cultivars attributed to this cluster were German cultivar 'Erntedank', Swedish cultivar 'Sussi', and Russian cultivar 'Kostromička'. Lingonberries of Russian ('Rubin') and Swedish origin ('Sanna') accumulated the lowest amounts of fructose and glucose and were attributed to the second cluster, whereas the highest amounts of these two sugars were determined in a cultivar of German origin ('Ertekrone'), which was attributed to the third cluster. The Russian origin 'Kostromskaja rozovaja' was attributed to the fourth cluster, which was characterized by the highest ($p < 0.05$) amount of sucrose and the lowest amount of total sugars. The results of the cluster analysis of cultivated lingonberries indicate genetic variations in the levels of sugars.

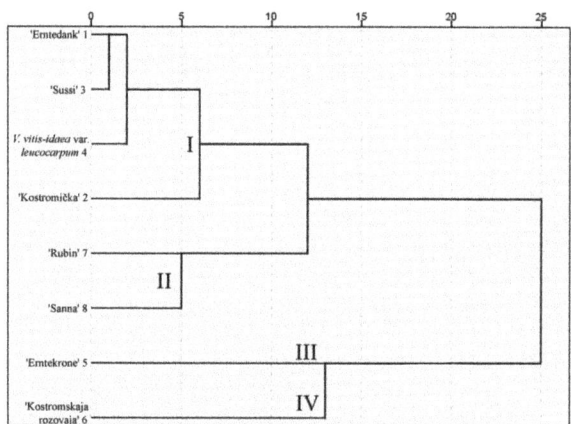

Figure 5. Dendrogram based on the amounts of sugars in cultivated lingonberries.

2.5. Comparison of Sugars Between Wild and Cultivated Lingonberries

The same sugars with dominant fructose and glucose were found either in wild or cultivated lingonberries, collected at the same time—berry formation stage in 2017 (Figure 6). The average amounts of total sugars were 552.58 ± 63.57 mg/g DW in wild and 596.92 ± 85.78 mg/g DW in cultivated lingonberries. Compared with wild lingonberries, cultivated ones accumulated 1.1, 1.1, and 1.2 times higher amounts of glucose, fructose, and sucrose, respectively. Nevertheless, an independent samples t-test showed that there were no statistically significant differences between sugar amounts in the wild and cultivated lingonberries groups. Hence, domestication of lingonberries, genetical changes resulted from human selection, and also presently used constant fertilization, irrigation, and other monitored cultivation conditions had only a slight effect on the accumulation of sugars.

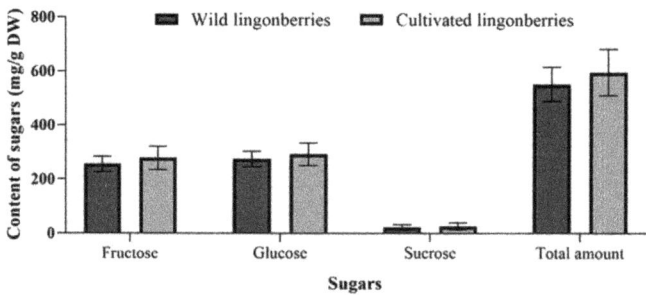

Figure 6. Average amounts of sugars in wild and cultivated lingonberries.

2.6. Sugars of Lingonberries During the Growing Season

The results show that levels of sugars varied unevenly during the growing season (Figure 7). The highest ($p < 0.05$) amount of total sugars was found in lingonberries collected at the end of the vegetation (640.83 mg/g DW). Fructose, glucose, and sucrose levels in berries since the massive blooming stage till the end of the vegetation increased 20.23%, 18.56%, and 26.18%, respectively. Interestingly, the content of sucrose was the highest at the berry formation stage, but this content did not differ statistically significantly from the content accumulated at the end of the vegetation, and had no significant contribution to the total amount of sugars. According to the results, it is apparent that the amounts of sugars are increasing during the growing season, and lingonberries collected at the end of the vegetation are sweeter than those of the beginning of the vegetation.

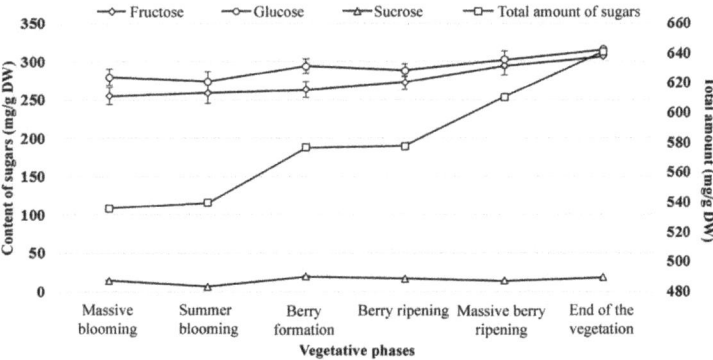

Figure 7. Content of sugars during different vegetative phases of lingonberries.

3. Discussion

Lingonberries are described as very sour and quite tart berries with a little bit of sweetness. The flavor is very similar to cranberries. Organoleptic properties of lingonberries, like other fruits, are mainly determined by volatile compounds, sugars, organic acids, and their ratio [21]. Since sugars in lingonberries affect consumer acceptability, a number of studies have been accomplished.

Mikulic-Petkovsek et al. analyzed various species of berries by the HPLC–RI method of analysis and detected glucose (37.9 ± 1.32 mg/g fresh weight (FW)), fructose (29.2 ± 0.71 mg/g FW), and sucrose (4.10 ± 0.45 mg/g FW) in wild lingonberries. Compared with other tested berries, the sugar level in lingonberries was just moderate. Similar contents of sugars were found in wild blackberries, red gooseberries, black mulberries, goji berries, and wild-grown elderberries [8]. Almost the same amounts of sugars—up to 29, 36, and 2 mg/g FW of glucose, fructose, and sucrose, respectively—were determined earlier in lingonberries, bought from the local retail shop [22]. The sugars were also found in the lingonberry juices, extracted with a hydraulic press. Viljakainen et al., by using the HPLC–RI method of analysis, found that amounts of fructose and glucose in Finnish lingonberry juices were almost equal (42.30 ± 0.27 and 42.38 ± 0.39 mg/mL, respectively) and contributed up to 98.6% of total sugars, whereas amounts of sucrose were very low (1.17 ± 0.01 mg/mL). Assessed amounts of total sugars were slightly higher in lingonberry juices than in juices of bilberry, cloudberry, blackcurrant, and strawberry, and almost two times higher than those of redcurrant, cranberry, and black crowberry [23]. Recent studies have shown that sugars in lingonberry juices could be detected by a sensitive spectrophotometric method using enzymatic assay kits specific for these carbohydrates. It was proclaimed that squeezed lingonberry juices had 38.9 ± 0.43 mg/mL of fructose and 45.4 ± 0.71 mg/mL of glucose. Contents of sugars were similar to those of elderberry juices, but higher ($p < 0.05$) than in cornelian cherry juices [24]. One more report revealed that bioprocessing unaffected, fully riped Finnish lingonberries accumulated high amounts of fructose (260 ± 0.01 mg/g DW), glucose (248 ± 0.03 mg/g DW), and sucrose (23.0 ± 0.01 mg/g DW) [21].

Our determined sugar amounts might seem higher than in previous studies, except the latter one, in which observed sugar composition was consistent with the results of the present study. It can be explained that in all of the researches mentioned above, except the latter one, the results were expressed for fresh raw material, meanwhile in ours for dry raw material (lyophilized lingonberries). The differences in contents of sugars also can be attributed primarily to the morphotype of lingonberries, as well as geographical locations, prevailing climatic conditions, fruit ripeness, their collecting date, and diversity of processing, extraction, and sugar analysis.

Notwithstanding the distinctions between sugar concentrations, contributions of fructose, glucose, and sucrose of total sugars were partly consistent in previous studies, and a number of reports proved that the main sugars of lingonberries are fructose and glucose. The amounts of other sugar components could appear only after hydrolysis of polysaccharide fraction. Ross et al., by using gas–liquid chromatography with FID detector, found impressively high amounts of arabinose, xylose, and galactose, and lower amounts of mannose, fucose, and rhamnose in water-extractable polysaccharides fraction from Northern Manitoba lingonberries [25]. Some of these sugars were looked at in the present study as well, but results showed that they cannot be found in lingonberries as free sugars.

Results of the present study and literature data revealed that sugar concentration in lingonberries is higher than in the most popular berries, like bilberries, strawberries, and cranberries. However, the sweet taste is hidden because of the high organic acid content. Several studies have shown that lingonberries accumulate high amounts of citric, fumaric, and shikimic, and lower amounts of tartaric, benzoic and malic acids, which result in pH decreasing of lingonberries [8,21,23]. Bioprocessing of lingonberries with enzymes, lactic acid bacterias, yeast, or their combination has an important impact on sugars composition, and enzyme treatment could be a potential tool for decreasing the acidic flavor of lingonberries [21].

It is acknowledged that lingonberries are indigenous to the sandy, northern, temperate, boreal forests; they prefer light and well-drained, porous, acidic (pH range between 4.3 and 5.5) soils. However, lingonberries are not demanding—they are resistant to temperature fluctuations, require very little water, and can grow in very different habitats within its extensive natural range, from dry oligotrophic pinewoods to raised bogs [26–28]. Lithuanian boreal forests seem to be a suitable place for the growth of lingonberries. Considering the sugar amounts in lingonberries from different collecting locations of Lithuania, it was noticed that the amounts of sugars in medium humidity, very infertile, pine tree with full sun or partial shade forests (e.g., Varėna, Valkininkai, Aukštadvaris, Marcinkonys) were higher ($p < 0.05$) than in medium humidity, medium fertility, with large variety of tree species shaded forests (e.g., Gineitiškės, Jurašiškės). Thus, our results are in accordance with the literature data and indicate that lingonberries accumulate higher amounts of compounds in sunny, dry tree sites, and even very infertile land can be a great growth place for lingonberries. Detailed studies are needed on the accumulation of other bioactive compounds in different soils, determining the organic and mineral composition of the soil.

Our determined amounts of sugars in different cultivars of lingonberries were partly consistent with their description of the flavors and yield. Cultivars in which berries are characterized as weakly acidic or sweet-and-sour in taste were distinguished by the highest amounts of sugars ('Erntedank', 'Sussi', 'Kostromička', which were attributed to the same cluster, and 'Ertekrone', which was attributed to a separate cluster). Meanwhile, the cultivars in which berries are described as having a sour taste and producing poor fall crop accumulated the lowest amounts of fructose and glucose ('Sanna' and 'Rubin', which were attributed to the same cluster) [26,29].

The composition of bioactive compounds in cultivated lingonberries is the subject of numerous studies. Lee et al. analyzed five different cultivars, including Swedish cultivars 'Sanna' and 'Sussi', which were also examined in our study. They assessed that lingonberries of these cultivars accumulated the lowest ($p < 0.05$) amounts of amino acids and moderate amounts of anthocyanins, total phenolics, and total tannins [13]. The lowest sugar productivity by 'Sanna' and one of the highest by 'Sussi' was observed in the present material. Phenolic compounds from lingonberry leaves within the same cultivars and lower taxa as in the present study were investigated previously by us. The greatest amounts of phenolics were found in the leaf extracts from 'Rubin' and 'Kostromskaja rozovaja' cultivars, whereas the lowest ones in 'Erntedank', 'Erntesegen', and 'Sanna' cultivars. The cluster analysis revealed that, according to the composition of phenolic compounds, the clusters were related to the countries of origin, especially with German and Russian origin cultivars [30]. According to the present findings, 'Rubin' and 'Kostromskaja rozovaja' cultivars accumulated just moderate amounts of sugars in berries, 'Sanna' with the lowest ($p < 0.05$), and 'Erntedank', 'Erntesegen' with the highest ones. Furthermore, there was no link between the cultivar country of origin and the quantities of sugars in berries. Contents of sugars do not seem to correlate with the contents of other compounds in the same cultivars and lower taxa of lingonberries. The productivity of cultivars in terms of sugars and in terms of other compounds is probably different. However, it is hard to compare the results from the earlier and present study, because of the different studied cultivars or raw materials.

Taking into account the importance of genetic differences and control of cultivation conditions, it is anticipated that amounts of bioactive compounds should be different among wild clones and cultivated plants. Notwithstanding, we found that there were no statistically significant differences in sugar amounts between cultivated and wild lingonberries. Several researchers found higher levels of phenolic compounds in wild fruits, meanwhile, the concentration of total sugars was quite similar between cultivated and wild fruits, as in our study [8,31,32]. This information could be relevant for breeders that are interested in sugar levels in the development of new cultivars, and it indicates that they should look at some other cultivation techniques that may help affect the sugar content. The successful development of lingonberry cultivars would increase the market size.

Altitude and latitude of location have an impact on temperature and solar radiation. As the latitude of a location increases, it receives less sunlight, whereas increasing altitude results in a decrease in pressure and thus in temperature. It is anticipated that most plants may adapt to higher latitudes and altitudes. Harsh weather conditions could affect processes associated with plant development and significantly enhance the biosynthesis of bioactive compounds [33,34]. Vyas et al. determined that amounts of secondary metabolites—anthocyanins, proanthocyanidins, and total antioxidant activity—of wild lingonberries positively correlated with latitude and altitude of the berries' collecting locations [35]. Our study showed contrary results—higher altitude and latitude, less sunlight and lower temperature reduced sugar production in lingonberries. Consequently, we suggest that the synthesis of primary metabolites does not intensify under the harsh weather conditions.

The variability and contents of bioactive compounds in plants depend on many factors, such as the already discussed genetic and environmental factors, cultivation conditions, processing, extraction method, and also maturity stage [36]. Numerous studies have been conducted to determine the amounts of bioactive compounds in various berries during the growing season, thus finding out the optimal collecting time [36–38]. Hence, we figured out that the changes in the sugar levels during the growing season were apparent in lingonberries and the highest amounts accumulated at the end of the vegetation. So, late September would be the optimal collecting time for those who prefer sweeter berries. Analysis of the relationship of sugar amounts in lingonberries and consumer expectations would help to develop the best quality standards for collecting dates.

Although there are considerable amounts of sugars in lingonberries, there is no need to worry about high sugar intake with these berries leading to deleterious health effects. These effects may occur if only more than about 1.25 kg of fresh lingonberries would be eaten daily, and more than 2.5 kg/day of fresh lingonberries would contribute to weight gain [6]. Meanwhile, the moderate intake of lingonberries may trigger satiety and promote a positive energy balance due to sugars; also lingonberry inclusion in the diet predisposes prevention of various human chronic diseases, because of the richness of the phenolic antioxidants [39]. Published papers show the potential benefit of lingonberries against diabetes and hypertension. These berries can inhibit α-amylase, α-glucosidase, anti-diabetic agent acarbose, and significantly enhance glucose uptake in human liver cells, decreasing glycemia and insulin levels [40,41]. Kivimäki et al. reported that lingonberry juices at small concentrations affect plasma inflammatory markers, clinical chemistry variables, and may lower blood pressure in long-term treatment [42]. Furthermore, lingonberry extracts with strong antioxidant function consumed orally or topically can protect dermal collagen protein, reduce the production and activity of elastinase, relieve skin wrinkles and colored spots, and thus improve skin conditions [43,44]. Therefore, products of lingonberries are promising beauty and health therapeutic candidates in the cosmetic and pharmaceutical industries.

4. Materials and Methods

4.1. Chemicals and Solvents

Analytical and chromatographic grade reference compounds were used for this study: Xylose, arabinose, glucose, galactose, xylitol, mannitol, sorbitol, inositol, ribose, fructose, mannose, adonitol, sucrose, maltose, lactose, and maltitol were purchased from Sigma-Aldrich GmbH (Steinheim, Germany). HPLC grade acetonitrile was obtained from Sigma-Aldrich GmbH (Steinheim, Germany), and purified deionized water (18.2 mW/cm) was produced using the Millipore (Millipore, Bedford, MA, USA) water purification system.

4.2. Plant Material

4.2.1. Wild Lingonberries

The description of collecting locations of tested lingonberry wild clones is displayed in Table 2. These collecting locations of wild clones differed from each other by soil moisture and degree of yield, therefore by the quality of growing conditions. The soil of lingonberry collecting locations was medium humidity, very infertile, with predominant Scots pine (*Pinus sylvestris* L.) tree species in Varėna, Valkininkai, Aukštadvaris, Marcinkonys, and Juodlė forests; medium humidity, infertile, with predominant Silver birch (*Betula pendula* Roth) and European spruce (*Picea abies* (L.) H. Karst.) tree species in Rudnia and Gudžiai forests; and medium humidity, medium fertility, with a large variety of tree species in Gineitiškės, Varčia, and Jurašiškės forests.

Table 2. Collecting locations of wild lingonberries, with their latitudes, longitudes, and altitudes.

Forest	Latitude (°)	Longitude (°)	Altitude (m)
Rudnia	54.40	24.49	137
Gineitiškės	54.49	24.39	155
Marcinkonys	54.07	24.43	123
Varėna	54.29	24.44	136
Valkininkai	54.36	24.85	116
Gudžiai	54.36	24.43	136
Bingeliai	54.15	24.25	112
Šilainė	54.08	23.71	135
Varčia	54.32	24.21	148
Aukštadvaris	54.57	24.61	167
Juodlė	55.83	22.94	141
Jurašiškės	54.10	23.89	135

Samples of wild lingonberries were collected in berry formation stage (third decade of August, 2017) in the twelve forests mentioned above, and also during different vegetative phases: Massive blooming (2 August, 2017), summer blooming (12 August, 2017), berry formation (21 August, 2017), berry ripening (2 September, 2017), massive berry ripening (16 September, 2017), and at the end of the vegetation (26 September, 2017) in Rudnia forest. These collecting times were chosen according to the lingonberry vegetative phases in Lithuania [26].

Lithuania, a flat country overlooking the Baltic Sea, has a humid continental climate, which can be described as a typical European continental influenced climate with warm, dry summers and fairly severe winters. Agricultural land covers more than 50% of Lithuania; forested land consists of about 28%, with 1.8 million ha. Lithuania is situated within the so-called mixed forest belt, with a high percentage of broadleaves and mixed conifer–broadleaved stands. The average solar radiation during the lingonberries' growing season from April to September of 2017 was 490 MJ/m^2 and ranged between 259 MJ/m^2 in September and 710 MJ/m^2 in May; meanwhile, the average precipitation was 61 mm and ranged between 20 mm in May and 125 mm in September. Average temperatures varied from 5 °C in April to 17 °C in August. The lowest moisture (53%) during the lingonberries' growing season in 2017 was determined in May, meanwhile the highest ones—75% and 80%—in August and September, respectively, when berries were collected for this study. It should be noted that the duration of sunshine in 2017 in Lithuania was about 1600 h, and it is much lower compared with previous years; meanwhile, the average temperature of 2017 years was 7.6 °C, which is 0.7 °C above standard climate rate. The meteorological data were obtained from the archive of the Lithuanian Hydrometeorological Service under the Ministry of Environment.

4.2.2. Cultivated Lingonberries

The cultivated lingonberries were collected in the field collection of the Botanical Garden of Šiauliai University (55°55′57′′N, 23°16′59′′E (WGS)). The following seven cultivars of lingonberry were tested: Russian cultivars—'Kostromskaja rozovaja' (registered in 1995), 'Kostromička' (1995), and 'Rubin' (1995); Swedish cultivars—'Sanna' (1987) and 'Sussi' (1986); and German cultivars—'Erntedank' (1975) and 'Erntekrone' (1978). Also, one variety (taxonomic rank between subspecies and form) of lingonberries—*V. vitis-idaea* var. *leucocarpum* Asch. et Magnus —was included in the study. Lingonberries belonging to this variety distinguish themselves by white berries, and the first time they were found was in 1993 in the forest of Svencioneliai district, Lithuania [27,45].

Lingonberries were cultivated in a partially shaded place, with acidic and well-drained soil. According to meteorological situation, fertilization and irrigation were periodically applied. The dynamics of meteorological factors during the growing season of cultivated lingonberries corresponded to those of wild clones. Fruits of different cultivars and lower taxa of lingonberries were collected at the end of August 2017 (berry formation stage).

4.3. Sample Preparation and Extraction of Sugars

After collecting, lingonberries were immediately frozen and subjected to lyophilization in ZIRBUS sublimator 3 × 4 × 5/20 (ZIRBUS Technology, Bad Grund, Germany) at a pressure of 0.01 mbar (condenser temperature, –85 °C). To grind lyophilized berries to a fine powder, the Retsch 200 mill (Haan, Germany) was used. Lyophilizates of lingonberries were comprised of 0.5 kg berries of each cultivar, lower taxa or wild clones from different forests. All obtained results were re-calculated for dry raw plant material.

One gram of the ground lyophilized lingonberries was added to 15 mL of distilled water in the conical flask and extracted three times in an ultrasonic bath (Elmasonic P, Singen, Germany) for 10 min. After the extraction, the homogenates were centrifugated for 5 min at 8500 rpm in a Biofuge Stratos centrifuge, and obtained supernatants were filtered through a membrane filter with a pore size of 0.22 μm (Carl Roth GmbH, Karlsruhe, Germany).

4.4. Qualitative and Quantitative Analysis of Sugars by HPLC–ELSD Method

The determination of sugar contents was performed using the Waters 2695 Alliance system (Waters, Milford, MA, USA) equipped with a Waters 2424 evaporative light-scattering detector (ELSD). Separation of sugars was carried out using Shodex SUGAR SZ5532 (Showa Denko KK) column (150 × 6.0 mm), according to the methodology described by Zymone et al. [46]. The gradient consisted of eluent A (water) and B (acetonitrile) and followed: 0–5 min—81% B, 5–20 min—81–70% B,

20–22 min—70% B, 23 min—81% B, with the eluent flow rate—1 mL/min and injection volume—10 μL. As the ELSD nebulizer gas (25 psi), nitrogen was used and tube temperature was set to 60 °C. Chromatographic peak identification was carried out by comparing the retention times of the analyte and reference compounds. For sugar quantification, calibration curves were constructed.

4.5. Method Validation

The analytical HPLC–ELSD method was validated in terms of linearity, LOD, LOQ, precision accuracy, and system suitability according to the ICH Q2(R1) guidelines [47]. To find out the linearity, standard solutions of authentic samples of sugars were prepared. The standard curves were based on five concentrations, each analyzed in triplicate. LOD and LOQ were determined based on a signal-to-noise ratio (S/N). The detection limit was defined as the concentration that gave a signal-to-noise ratio (S/N) >3 and the quantification limit as the concentration that gave S/N >10. The precision of the method was evaluated by measurement in intra-day (for repeatability) and inter-day (for intermediate precision) variability tests, calculating the relative standard deviation (RSD) of peak areas or retention times. Accuracy of the method was expressed as percent recoveries, which were studied by adding known amounts of standards to the samples. System suitability parameters—resolution and selectivity—were calculated using Empower™ System Suitability software.

4.6. Statistical Analysis

Statistical analysis was conducted using SPSS 21.0 (SPSS Inc., Chicago, IL, USA) and Microsoft Office Excel 2010 (Microsoft, Redmond, WA, USA). The amounts of sugars were expressed as the mean (M) of three measurements ± standard deviation (SD). Analysis of variance (ANOVA) with Tukey's HSD post-hoc test and independent samples t-test were performed to determine the significant differences among the wild and cultivated lingonberries ($\alpha = 0.05$). Correlations were tested using Pearson's correlation test. Hierarchical cluster analysis was carried out using the centroid clustering method with squared Euclidean distances.

5. Conclusions

Observed sugar amounts in lingonberries are not dangerously high, and consequently, do not seem to be hazardous for consumers of food or health and wellness products of lingonberries. The same sugars with dominant fructose, glucose, and low amounts of sucrose were found in wild and cultivated lingonberries. As a lingonberry product authentication tool, these simple sugars could be searched to prevent adulterations. The presence of moderate levels of fructose in lingonberries reveals potential type 1 fimbriae inhibiting activity and relevance for further studies. Intraspecific variability was detected when comparing the content of sugars in wild clones or cultivated lingonberries, regarding to phenological growth stages. The highest contents of sugars were observed in berries collected at the end of the vegetation—full ripening stage, from sunny, well-drained soil locations with higher solar radiation and temperature. Consideration of these factors may result in lingonberry yields with preferred sugar levels. Naturally sweeter food products of lingonberries would reduce the need for added sugars, whereas reduced sugar levels in orally consumed pharmaceuticals or nutraceuticals would increase the acceptability of consumers.

Author Contributions: Conceptualization, L.R.; methodology, R.R.; investigation, G.V. and J.V.; resources, R.V. V.M. and D.B.; data curation, G.V. and R.R.; visualization, G.V.; writing—original draft preparation, G.V.; writing—review and editing, L.R. and V.M.; supervision, L.R.

Funding: This research received no external funding.

Conflicts of Interest: The authors declare no conflicts of interest.

References

1. World Health Organization. *Guideline: Sugars Intake for Adults and Children*; World Health Organization: Geneva, Switzerland, 2015; pp. 1–5.
2. Van Dam, R.M.; Seidell, J.C. Carbohydrate Intake and Obesity. *Eur. J. Clin. Nutr.* **2007**, *61*, 75–99. [CrossRef] [PubMed]
3. Johnson, R.K.; Appel, L.J.; Brands, M.; Howard, B.V.; Lefevre, M.; Lustig, R.H.; Sacks, F.; Steffen, L.M.; Wylie-Rosett, J. Dietary Sugars Intake and Cardiovascular Health a Scientific Statement from the American Heart Association. *Circulation* **2009**, *120*, 1011–1020. [CrossRef] [PubMed]
4. Cummings, J.H.; Stephen, A.M. Carbohydrate Terminology and Classification. *Eur. J. Clin. Nut.* **2007**, *61*, 5–18. [CrossRef] [PubMed]
5. Tuck, C.J.; Muir, J.G.; Barrett, J.S.; Gibson, P.R. Fermentable Oligosaccharides, Disaccharides, Monosaccharides and Polyols: Role in Irritable Bowel Syndrome. *Expert. Rev. Gastroent.* **2014**, *8*, 819–834. [CrossRef] [PubMed]
6. Rizkalla, S.W. Health Implications of Fructose Consumption: A Review of Recent Data. *Nutr. Metab. (Lond)* **2010**, *7*, 82. [CrossRef]
7. Rosa, M.; Prado, C.; Podazza, G.; Interdonato, R.; González, J.A.; Hilal, M.; Prado, F.E. Soluble Sugars-Metabolism, Sensing and Abiotic Stress a Complex Network in the Life of Plants. *Plant. Signal. Behav.* **2009**, *4*, 388–393. [CrossRef]
8. Mikulic-Petkovsek, M.; Schmitzer, V.; Slatnar, A.; Stampar, F.; Veberic, R. Composition of Sugars, Organic Acids, and Total Phenolics in 25 Wild or Cultivated Berry Species. *J. Food. Sci.* **2012**, *77*, 1064–1070. [CrossRef]
9. Hisano, M.; Bruschini, H.; Nicodemo, A.C.; Srougi, M. Cranberries and Lower Urinary Tract Infection Prevention. *Clinics (Sao Paulo)* **2012**, *67*, 661–667. [CrossRef]
10. Ofek, I.; Hasty, D.L.; Sharon, N. Anti-Adhesion Therapy of Bacterial Diseases: Prospects and Problems. *FEMS. Immunol. Med. Microbiol.* **2003**, *38*, 181–191. [CrossRef]
11. Foxman, B. The Epidemiology of Urinary Tract Infection. *Nat. Rev. Urol.* **2010**, *7*, 653–660. [CrossRef]
12. Dróżdż, P.; Seziene, V.; Wójcik, J.; Pyrzyńska, K. Evaluation of Bioactive Compounds, Minerals and Antioxidant Activity of Lingonberry (*Vaccinium vitis-idaea* L.) Fruits. *Molecules* **2018**, *23*, 53. [CrossRef] [PubMed]
13. Lee, J.; Finn, C.E. Lingonberry (*Vaccinium vitis-idaea* L.) Grown in the Pacific Northwest of North America: Anthocyanin and Free Amino Acid Composition. *J. Funct. Foods.* **2012**, *4*, 213–218. [CrossRef]
14. Suomela, J.P.; Vaarno, J.; Sandell, M.; Lehtonen, H.M.; Tahvonen, R.; Viikari, J.; Kallio, H. Children's Hedonic Response to Berry Products: Effect of Chemical Composition of Berries and HTAS2R38 Genotype on Liking. *Food. Chem.* **2012**, *135*, 1210–1219. [CrossRef] [PubMed]
15. Kylli, P.; Nohynek, L.; Puupponen-Pimiä, R.; Westerlund-Wikström, B.; Leppänen, T.; Welling, J.; Moilanen, E.; Heinonen, M. Lingonberry (*Vaccinium vitis-idaea*) and European Cranberry (*Vaccinium microcarpon*) Proanthocyanidins: Isolation, Identification, and Bioactivities. *J. Agric. Food. Chem.* **2011**, *59*, 3373–3384. [CrossRef] [PubMed]
16. Klavins, L.; Klavina, L.; Huna, A.; Klavins, M. Polyphenols, Carbohydrates and Lipids in Berries of *Vaccinium* Species. *Environ. Exp. Biol.* **2015**, *13*, 147–158, 2255-958.
17. Fan, Z.L.; Wang, Z.Y.; Liu, J.R. Cold-Field Fruit Extracts Exert Different Antioxidant and Antiproliferative Activities *in Vitro*. *Food. Chem.* **2011**, *129*, 402–407. [CrossRef]
18. Fan, Z.L.; Wang, Z.Y.; Zuo, L.L.; Tian, S.Q. Protective Effect of Anthocyanins from Lingonberry on Radiation-Induced Damages. *Inter. J. Env. Res. Pub. Heal.* **2012**, *9*, 4732–4743. [CrossRef]
19. Alam, Z.; Roncal, J.; Peña-Castillo, L. Genetic Variation Associated with Healthy Traits and Environmental Conditions in *Vaccinium Vitis-Idaea*. *BMC. Genomics.* **2018**, *19*. [CrossRef]
20. Gustavsson, B.A. Genetic Variation in Horticulturally Important Traits of Fifteen Wild Lingonberry *Vaccinium Vitis-Idaea* L. Populations. *Euphytica* **2001**, *120*, 173–182. [CrossRef]
21. Viljanen, K.; Heiniö, R.L.; Juvonen, R.; Kössö, T.; Puupponen-Pimiä, R. Relation of Sensory Perception with Chemical Composition of Bioprocessed Lingonberry. *Food. Chem.* **2014**, *157*, 148–156. [CrossRef]
22. Varo, P.; Laine, R.; Veijalainen, K.; Espo, A.; Wetterhoff, A.; Koivistoinen, P. Dietary Fibre and Available Carbohydrates in Finnish Vegetables and Fruits. *Agric. Food. Sci.* **1984**, *56*, 49–59. [CrossRef]
23. Viljakainen, S.; Visti, A.; Laakso, S. Concentrations of Organic Acids and Soluble Sugars in Juices from Nordic Berries. *Acta. Agric. Scand. Sect. B. Soil. Plant. Sci.* **2002**, *52*, 101–109. [CrossRef]

24. Antolak, H.; Czyzowska, A.; Sakač, M.; Mišan, A.; Đuragić, O.; Kregiel, D. Phenolic Compounds Contained in Little-Known Wild Fruits as Antiadhesive Agents Against the Beverage-Spoiling Bacteria Asaia Spp. *Molecules* **2017**, *22*, 1256. [CrossRef] [PubMed]
25. Ross, K.A.; Godfrey, D.; Fukumoto, L. The Chemical Composition, Antioxidant Activity and α-Glucosidase Inhibitory Activity of Water-Extractable Polysaccharide Conjugates from Northern Manitoba Lingonberry. *Cogent. Food. Agric.* **2015**, *1*. [CrossRef]
26. Bandzaitiene, Z.; Daubaras, R.; Labokas, J. *Brukne: Vaccinium vitis-idaea* L.; Botanikos instituto leidykla: Vilnius, Lithuania, 2007; pp. 25–133.
27. Paal, T. Lingonberry (*Vaccinium vitis-idaea* L.) Research in Estonia: An overview. *Acta. Hortic.* **2006**, *715*, 203–218. [CrossRef]
28. Haffner, K.E. Ecology of *Vaccinium* growing. *Acta. Hortic.* **1993**, *346*, 214–220. [CrossRef]
29. Penhallegon, R. Lingonberry Production Guide for the Pacific Northwest. Available online: https://catalog.extension.oregonstate.edu/pnw583 (accessed on 29 September 2019).
30. Raudone, L.; Vilkickyte, G.; Pitkauskaite, L.; Raudonis, R.; Vainoriene, R.; Motiekaityte, V. Antioxidant Activities of *Vaccinium vitis-idaea* L. Leaves within Cultivars and Their Phenolic Compounds. *Molecules* **2019**, *24*, 844. [CrossRef]
31. Ma, B.; Chen, J.; Zheng, H.; Fang, T.; Ogutu, C.; Li, S.; Han, Y.; Wu, B. Comparative Assessment of Sugar and Malic Acid Composition in Cultivated and Wild Apples. *Food. Chem.* **2015**, *172*, 86–91. [CrossRef]
32. Guerrero, C.J.; Ciampi, P.L.; Castilla, C.A.; Medel, S.F.; Schalchli, S.H.; Hormazabal, U.E.; Bensch, T.E.; Alberdi, L.M. Antioxidant Capacity, Anthocyanins, and Total Phenols of Wild and Cultivated Berries in Chile. *Chil. J. Agric. Res.* **2010**, *70*, 537–544. [CrossRef]
33. Yang, L.; Wen, K.S.; Ruan, X.; Zhao, Y.X.; Wei, F.; Wang, Q. Response of Plant Secondary Metabolites to Environmental Factors. *Molecules* **2018**, *23*, 762. [CrossRef]
34. Jaakola, L.; Hohtola, A. Effect of Latitude on Flavonoid Biosynthesis in Plants. *Plant. Cell. Environ.* **2010**, *33*, 1239–1247. [CrossRef] [PubMed]
35. Vyas, P.; Curran, N.H.; Igamberdiev, A.U.; Debnath, S.C. Antioxidant Properties of Lingonberry (*Vaccinium vitis-idaea* L.) Leaves within a Set of Wild Clones and Cultivars. *Can. J. Plant. Sci.* **2015**, *95*, 663–669. [CrossRef]
36. Skrovankova, S.; Sumczynski, D.; Mlcek, J.; Jurikova, T.; Sochor, J. Bioactive Compounds and Antioxidant Activity in Different Types of Berries. *Int. J. Mol. Sci.* **2015**, *16*, 24673–24706. [CrossRef] [PubMed]
37. Bujor, O.-C.; Le Bourvellec, C.; Volf, I.; Popa, V.I.; Dufour, C. Seasonal Variations of the Phenolic Constituents in Bilberry (*Vaccinium myrtillus* L.) Leaves, Stems and Fruits, and Their Antioxidant Activity. *Food. Chem.* **2016**, *213*, 58–68. [CrossRef] [PubMed]
38. Yao, L.; Caffin, N.; D'Arcy, B.; Jiang, Y.; Shi, J.; Singanusong, R.; Liu, X.; Datta, N.; Kakuda, Y.; Xu, Y. Seasonal Variations of Phenolic Compounds in Australia-Grown Tea (*Camellia sinensis*). *J. Agric. Food. Chem.* **2005**, *53*, 6477–6483. [CrossRef]
39. Dróżdż, P.; Seziene, V.; Pyrzynska, K. Phytochemical Properties and Antioxidant Activities of Extracts from Wild Blueberries and Lingonberries. *Plant. Foods. Hum. Nutr.* **2017**, *72*, 360–364. [CrossRef]
40. Eid, H.M.; Ouchfoun, M.; Brault, A.; Vallerand, D.; Musallam, L.; Arnason, J.T.; Haddad, P.S. Lingonberry (*Vaccinium Vitis-Idaea* L.) Exhibits Antidiabetic Activities in a Mouse Model of Diet-Induced Obesity. *Evid-Based. Compl. Alt.* **2014**, *645812*, 1–10. [CrossRef]
41. Ho, G.T.T.; Nguyen, T.K.Y.; Kase, E.T.; Tadesse, M.; Barsett, H.; Wangensteen, H. Enhanced Glucose Uptake in Human Liver Cells and Inhibition of Carbohydrate Hydrolyzing Enzymes by Nordic Berry Extracts. *Molecules* **2017**, *22*, 1806. [CrossRef]
42. Kivimäki, A.S.; Siltari, A.; Ehlers, P.I.; Korpela, R.; Vapaatalo, H. Lingonberry Juice Lowers Blood Pressure of Spontaneously Hypertensive Rats (SHR). *J. Funct. Foods.* **2013**, *5*, 1432–1440. [CrossRef]
43. Addor, F.A.S. Antioxidants in Dermatology. *An. Bras. Dermatol.* **2017**, *92*, 356–362. [CrossRef]
44. Pimple, B.P.; Badole, S.L. Polyphenols: A Remedy for Skin Wrinkles. In *Polyphenols in Human Health and Disease*; Academic Press: Cambridge, MA, USA, 2013; Volume 1, pp. 861–869.
45. Malciute, A.; Naujalis, J.R.; Vilkonis, K.K. Cowberry (*Vaccinium vitis-idaea*) Collection in the Botanical Garden of Siauliai University: Composition and General Condition. *Jaunųjų. Mokslininkų. darbai.* **2008**, *5*, 81–84, 1648-8776.

46. Zymone, K.; Raudone, L.; Raudonis, R.; Marksa, M.; Ivanauskas, L.; Janulis, V. Phytochemical Profiling of Fruit Powders of Twenty *Sorbus* L. Cultivars. *Molecules* **2018**, *23*, 2593. [CrossRef] [PubMed]
47. ICH Q2(R1). Validation of Analytical Procedures: Text and Methodology. Current Step 4 Version. 2005. Available online: https://pacificbiolabs.com/wp-content/uploads/2017/12/Q2_R1_Guideline-4.pdf (accessed on 27 October 1994).

Sample Availability: Samples of the compounds are available from the authors.

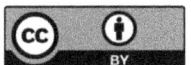

© 2019 by the authors. Licensee MDPI, Basel, Switzerland. This article is an open access article distributed under the terms and conditions of the Creative Commons Attribution (CC BY) license (http://creativecommons.org/licenses/by/4.0/).

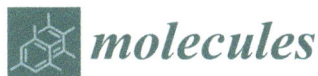

Article

NO$_x$-, IL-1β-, TNF-α-, and IL-6-Inhibiting Effects and Trypanocidal Activity of Banana (*Musa acuminata*) Bracts and Flowers: UPLC-HRESI-MS Detection of Phenylpropanoid Sucrose Esters

Louis P. Sandjo [1,*], Marcus V. P. dos Santos Nascimento [2], Milene de H. Moraes [3], Luiza Manaut Rodrigues [3], Eduardo M. Dalmarco [2], Maique W. Biavatti [4] and Mario Steindel [3,*]

[1] Department of Chemistry, Federal University of Santa Catarina, 88040-900 Florianópolis, Brazil
[2] Department of Clinical Analysis, Centre of Health Sciences, Federal University of Santa Catarina, 88 040 970 Florianópolis, Brazil; mmmarcusster@gmail.com (M.V.P.d.S.N.); eduardo.dalmarco@ufsc.br (E.M.D.)
[3] Laboratory of Protozoology, Department of Microbiology, Immunology and Parasitology Centre of biological sciences, Federal University of Santa Catarina, 88040-900 Florianópolis, Brazil; milenehoehr@gmail.com (M.d.H.M.); luizamanaut@gmail.com (L.M.R.)
[4] Department of Pharmaceutical Sciences, Centre of Health Sciences, Federal University of Santa Catarina, 88040-900 Florianópolis, Brazil; maique.biavatti@ufsc.br
* Correspondence: p.l.sandjo@ufsc.br (L.P.S); mario.steindel@ufsc.br (M.S.); Tel.: +55-483-721-3624 (L.P.S); +55-483-721-2958 (M.S.)

Academic Editor: Toshio Morikawa
Received: 14 November 2019; Accepted: 9 December 2019; Published: 13 December 2019

Abstract: Banana inflorescences are a byproduct of banana cultivation consumed in various regions of Brazil as a non-conventional food. This byproduct represents an alternative food supply that can contribute to the resolution of nutritional problems and hunger. This product is also used in Asia as a traditional remedy for the treatment of various illnesses such as bronchitis and dysentery. However, there is a lack of chemical and pharmacological data to support its consumption as a functional food. Therefore, this work aimed to study the anti-inflammatory action of *Musa acuminata* blossom by quantifying the cytokine levels (NO$_x$, IL-1β, TNF-α, and IL-6) in peritoneal neutrophils, and to study its antiparasitic activities using the intracellular forms of *T. cruzi*, *L. amazonensis*, and *L. infantum*. This work also aimed to establish the chemical profile of the inflorescence using UPLC-ESI-MS analysis. Flowers and the crude bract extracts were partitioned in dichloromethane and *n*-butanol to afford four fractions (FDCM, FNBU, BDCM, and BNBU). FDCM showed moderate trypanocidal activity and promising anti-inflammatory properties by inhibiting IL-1β, TNF-α, and IL-6. BDCM significantly inhibited the secretion of TNF-α, while BNBU was active against IL-6 and NO$_x$. LCMS data of these fractions revealed an unprecedented presence of arylpropanoid sucroses alongside flavonoids, triterpenes, benzofurans, stilbenes, and iridoids. The obtained results revealed that banana inflorescences could be used as an anti-inflammatory food ingredient to control inflammatory diseases.

Keywords: banana inflorescences; anti-inflammatory activity; antiparasitic activity; UPLC-ESI-MS; arylpropanoid sucroses

1. Introduction

Several nutritionists and food chemists have been working intensively with non-conventional food plants (NCFPs). Fruits, seeds, roots, flowers, leaves, or entire plants can constitute these foods and, in most cases, they represent a new cultural food value for various communities [1].

However, some NCFPs are only occasionally consumed, while others are actually daily dishes in rural localities. The intensification of the use of nonconventional food plants has been widely influenced by socioeconomic conditions (decrease of buying power), taste, and natural calamities such as unfavorable dry seasons and flood [2]. Therefore, these plants play a crucial role as an alternative food supply able to prevent nutritional problems and hunger [2]. The race to introduce NCFPs as food alternatives has sometimes meant that scientific investigations to support the safety of consumers have been lacking. Plants newly considered NCFPs must be chemically studied in order to rule out the presence of toxins, mutagenic, carcinogenic, and teratogenic substances, and other harmful metabolites. Chemical study can also bring to light substances with beneficial biological activity and good nutritional value. This last indication was the main focus of this work; the present study aimed to establish the chemical profile of *Musa acuminata* inflorescences, which are widely consumed in rural areas of Brazilian Amazonia, coast regions of Parana, and São Paulo [3]. "Salpição de mangará" and "amilácea", meaning, respectively, "salad of banana heart" and "starchy", are the two principal dishes made of *Musa* flower [1]. Apart from being consumed, *Musa* inflorescences and other parts of the plant are used popularly in Asia and Africa to cure dysentery, hypertension, diabetes, ulcers, and bronchitis [4]. In South Africa, a decoction of this flower is taken three times a day to normalize blood pressure [5]. Various biological investigations have been previously performed with banana flowers of different *Musa* species. Among these, the most studied are the inflorescences from *Musa paradicicus*, *Musa* sp var Nanjangud rasa bale, and *Musa acuminata*, which, respectively, have shown antioxidant, antihyperglycaemic, and anticholesterolaemic activities [6–8]. To date, chemical investigations conducted on *Musa acuminata* have focused intensively on rhizomes, unripe fruits, and tissues, from which phenalenones and phenylphenalenones have been identified as the predominant components [9–11]. These compounds have been described to have a phytoalexin role for *Musa* species against pathogenic crop microorganisms [9–11].

As the literature search on *Musa acuminata* inflorescences revealed few pharmacological and phytochemical studies, this work aimed to biologically and chemically investigate the abovementioned plant material. A part of our research goal was to search for and select non-conventional edible plants from Brazilian Amazonia that are potential anti-inflammatory and antiparasitic treatments. Diseases caused by parasites or leading to inflammation are a health problem in this area, which is why this work aimed to search in the crude extract of the banana inflorescence for natural products possessing an inhibitory effect against inflammatory mediators, including IL-1B, NO_x, IL-6, and TNF-α. More importantly, we evaluated their antiparasitic activities against the intracellular forms of *Leishmania amazonensis*, *L. infantum*, and *Trypanosoma cruzi* amastigotes grown in human monocytic THP-1 cells. The results obtained prompted us to establish the chemical profile of each fraction based on their UPLC-ESI-MS/MS dereplication.

2. Results

Flowers and bracts of *M. acuminata* blossom were separated and extracted with methanol. Because of the presence of insoluble precipitate whether in water or in polar organic solvents, both crude extracts were separately poured into water and were extracted successively with dichloromethane and *n*-butanol, affording four fractions (flower: FDCM and FNBU, respectively; bract: BDCM and BNBU, respectively).

2.1. Biological Activities

2.1.1. Anti-Inflammatory Activity

Cell Viability

The effects of the organic fractions on isolated mouse neutrophils were determined by trypan blue exclusion test of cell viability, as shown in Figure 1. FDCM and BNBU showed significant toxicity when tested from 10 to 1000 µg/mL ($p < 0.05$). The other two fractions, FNBU and BDCM, showed no effect on neutrophil viability at the tested concentrations ($p > 0.05$).

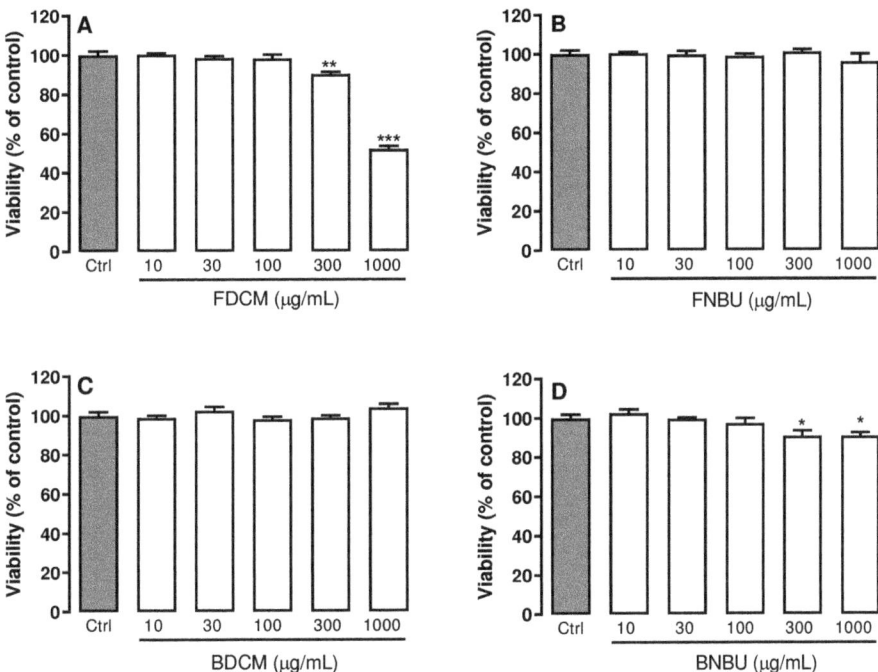

Figure 1. Effects of flower fraction from dichloromethane partition (FDCM) (**A**), flower fraction from *n*-butanol partition (FNBU) (**B**), bract fraction from dichloromethane partition (BDCM) (**C**), and bract fraction from *n*-butanol partition (BNBU) (**D**) on neutrophil viability. Control: peritoneal neutrophils isolated from mice treated only with vehicle; 10–1000: peritoneal neutrophils isolated from mice treated with concentrations of each specific extract ranging from 10 to 1000 µg/mL. Each group represents the mean ± standard error of the mean; $n = 3$/group. * $p < 0.05$, ** $p < 0.01$, and *** $p < 0.001$ compared to the control group (ctrl).

Inhibition Study on Cytokine Secretion (IL-1β, TNF-α, and IL-6)

On the basis of the results obtained from the cell viability assay, inhibition effects of the fractions were evaluated on pro-inflammatory mediators at non-cytotoxic concentrations. Only FDCM showed significant inhibition of IL-1β levels, reducing the levels of this inflammatory mediator by 51.9% ± 7.2% ($p < 0.001$) of when tested at 100 µg/mL (Figure 2A). Other fractions in turn weakly affected secretion of this inflammatory mediator ($p > 0.05$) (Figure 2B–D).

While the level of TNF-α was decreased by 46.1% ± 8.0% ($p < 0.05$) when neutrophils were treated with FDCM at 100 µg/mL (Figure 3A), BDCM at concentrations of 30 and 100 µg/mL inhibited the secretion of the same cytokine by 46.5% ± 8.6% and 50.7% ± 6.2%, respectively ($p < 0.01$) (Figure 3C). On the other hand, FNBU and BNBU did not reduce this inflammatory mediator ($p > 0.05$) (Figure 3B,D).

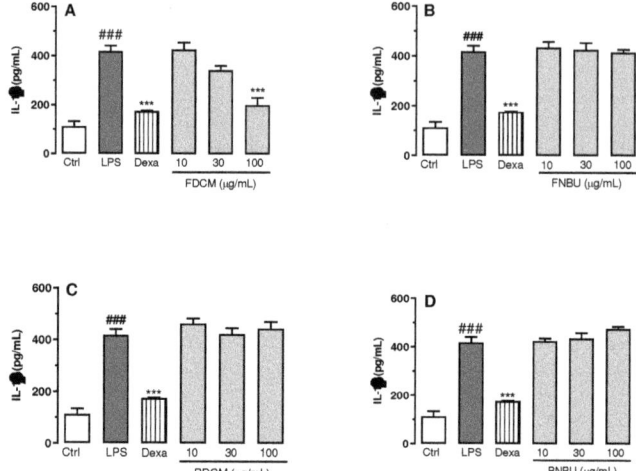

Figure 2. Effect of FDCM (**A**), FNBU (**B**), BDCM (**C**), and BNBU (**D**) on IL-1β secretion by LPS-stimulated peritoneal murine neutrophils. Control: peritoneal neutrophils isolated from mice treated only with vehicle; LPS: peritoneal neutrophils isolated from mice stimulated with LPS and treated with vehicle; 10–100: peritoneal neutrophils isolated from mice stimulated with LPS and treated with concentrations of each specific extract ranging from 10 to 100 μg/mL. Each group represents the mean ± standard error of the mean; $n = 3$/group. ### $p < 0.001$ compared to the Ctrl group. *** $p < 0.001$ compared to the Ctrl group.

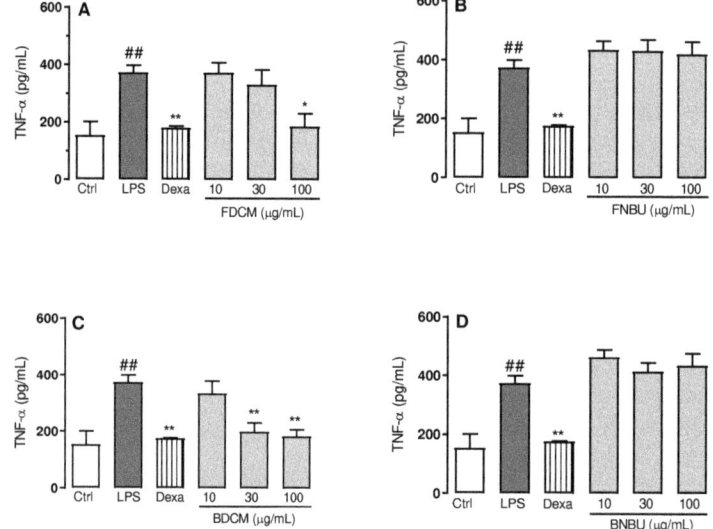

Figure 3. Effect of FDCM (**A**), FNBU (**B**), BDCM (**C**), and BNBU (**D**) on TNF-α secretion by LPS-stimulated peritoneal murine neutrophils. Control: peritoneal neutrophils isolated from mice treated only with vehicle; LPS: peritoneal neutrophils isolated from mice stimulated with LPS and treated with vehicle; 10–100: peritoneal neutrophils isolated from mice stimulated with LPS and treated with concentrations of each specific extract ranging from 10 to 100 μg/mL. Each group represents the mean ± standard error of the mean; $n = 3$/group. ## $p < 0.001$ compared to the Ctrl group. * $p < 0.01$ and ** $p < 0.001$ compared to the Ctrl group.

Weak reductions of the IL-6 level were observed with FDCM (22.3% ± 6.4%) ($p < 0.05$) at 100 µg/mL (Figure 4A), and with BNBU at 30 and 100 µg/mL (23.8% ± 5.0% and 43.2% ± 6.2%, respectively) ($p < 0.05$) (Figure 4A,D). FNBU and BDCM showed no inhibition effect against this inflammatory cytokine ($p > 0.05$) (Figure 4B,C).

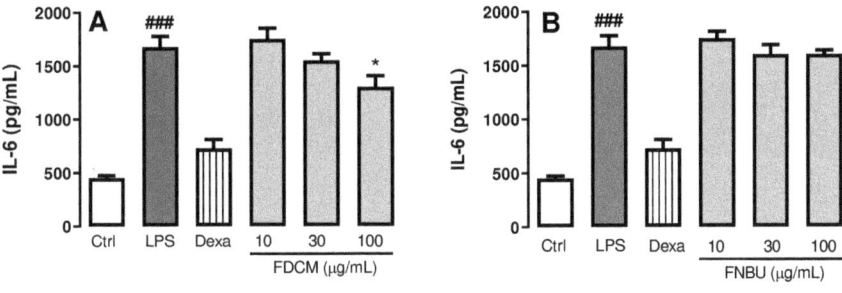

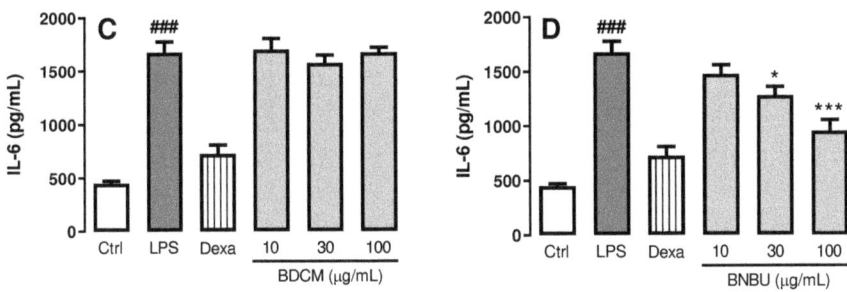

Figure 4. Effect of FDCM (**A**), FNBU (**B**), BDCM (**C**), and BNBU (**D**) on IL-6 secretion by LPS-stimulated peritoneal murine neutrophils. Control: peritoneal neutrophils isolated from mice treated only with vehicle; LPS: peritoneal neutrophils isolated from mice stimulated with LPS and treated with vehicle; 10–100: peritoneal neutrophils isolated from mice stimulated with LPS and treated with concentrations of each specific extract ranging from 10 to 100 µg/mL. Each group represents the mean ± standard error of the mean; $n = 3$/group. ### $p < 0.001$ compared to the Ctrl group. * $p < 0.01$ and *** $p < 0.001$ compared to the Ctrl group.

Measurement of NO_x Production by Mouse Neutrophils

FDCM, FNBU, and BDCM were unable to reduce the levels of NO_x secretion regardless of the concentrations tested ($p > 0.05$) (Figure 5A–C), whereas BNBU was able to reduce the production of this inflammatory mediator by 40.2% ± 7.6% and 46.5% ± 5.2%, respectively, ($p < 0.01$) when tested at 30 and 100 µg/mL (Figure 5D).

The relationship between the inflammatory cytokines produced by parasites during infection and their virulence [12–15] prompted us to evaluate all the fractions against the intracellular forms of *T. cruzi*, *L. amazonensis*, and *L. infantum* amastigotes, as well as the viability of the THP-1 cells (human monocytic cell line) used as host.

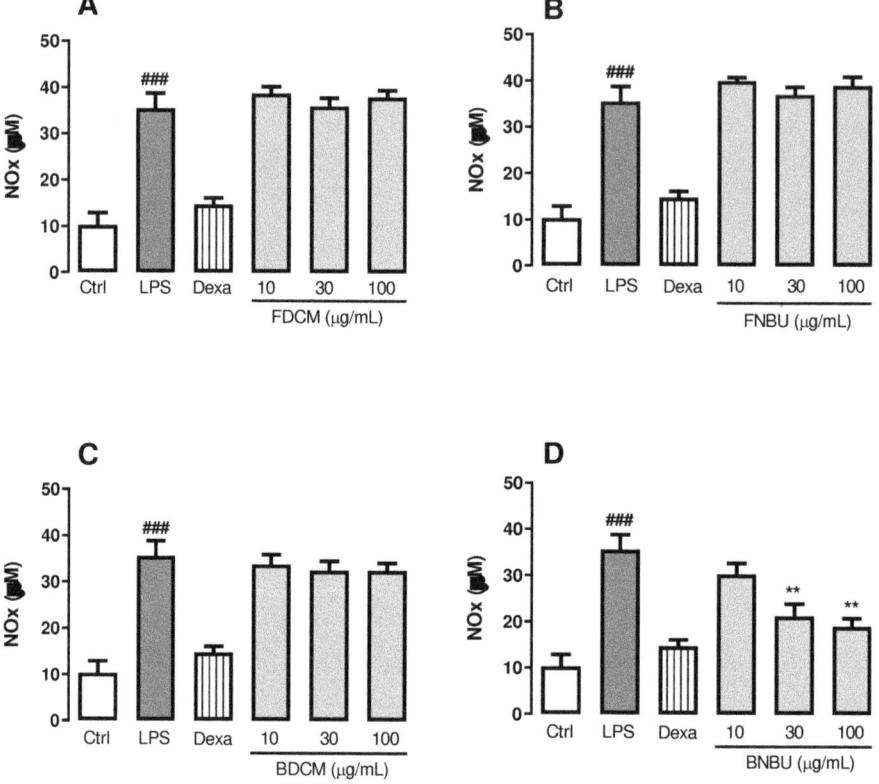

Figure 5. Effect of FDCM (**A**), FNBU (**B**), BDCM (**C**), and BNBU (**D**) on NO$_x$ secretion by LPS-stimulated peritoneal murine neutrophils. Control: peritoneal neutrophils isolated from mice treated only with vehicle; LPS: peritoneal neutrophils isolated from mice stimulated with LPS and treated with vehicle; 10–100: peritoneal neutrophils isolated from mice stimulated with LPS and treated with concentrations of each specific extract ranging from 10 to 100 μg/mL. Each group represents the mean ± standard error of the mean; $n = 3$/group. ### $p < 0.001$ compared to the Ctrl group. ** $p < 0.01$ compared to the Ctrl group.

2.1.2. Antitrypanosomal and Antileishmanial Activities

FDCM also revealed low toxicity to THP-1 cells with a CC$_{50}$ value of 341.5 μg/mL, leading to a selectivity index of 9.14 (Table 1). As the cytotoxicity of FDCM was nearly 300 μg/mL, a non-toxic concentration of 50 μg/mL was considered to preserve the viability of the macrophage, with the aim of observing significant antiparasitic activity.

FDCM inhibited 90.37% of *T. cruzi* growth, corresponding to an IC$_{50}$ value of 37.35 μg/mL. It also showed weak effects against *L. amazonensis*, and *L. infantum* amastigotes, with inhibition of 37.13% and 11.04%, respectively. The remaining fractions showed weak to no activity against *T. cruzi* and the studied *Leishmania* species.

Table 1. In vitro activity of the inflorescence fractions at concentrations of 50 µg/mL against *Trypanosoma cruzi*, *Leishmania amazonensis*, and *L. infantum* intracellular amastigotes.

Fractions	T. cruzi		L. amazonensis		L. infantum		THP-1 (Human Monocyte Cells)	SI
	% inhibition	IC$_{50}$ (µg/mL)	% inhibition	IC$_{50}$ (µg/mL)	% inhibition	IC$_{50}$ (µg/mL)	CC$_{50}$ (µg/mL)	
FDCM	90.37% ± 1.17%	37.35 ± 0.97	37.13% ± 3.15%	ND	11.04% ± 1.51%	ND	341.50 ± 17.20	9.14
FNBU	NA	ND	1.71% ± 0.62%	ND	NA	ND	ND	ND
BDCM	NA	ND	NI	ND	NA	ND	ND	ND
BNBU	5.37% ± 0.32%	ND	5.52% ± 2.30%	ND	NA	ND	ND	ND
Benznidazole	93.48% ± 1.04%	10.18 ± 0.3	-	-	-	-	>500	>49.11
Amphotericin B	-	-	84.14% ± 1.37%	0.09 ± 0.02	76.42% ± 4.24%	0.11 ± 0.03	-	-

NA: no activity; ND: not determined; SI: selectivity index. IC$_{50}$: the concentration of each sample that reduced parasite viability by 50% when compared to untreated control, estimated by non-linear regression of concentration–response curves.

2.2. Chemistry

The hyphenated techniques UPLC-ESIMS and UPLC-ESI-MS^2 were used to establish the chemical compositions of FDCM, FNBU, BDCM, and BNBU, as they showed promising biological activity against inflammation mediators. Their constituents were exclusively sensitive to the negative ionization mode, and the base peak ionization (BPI) was used as the acquisition parameter of the chromatograms (Figure 6). An error equal to or less than ±5 ppm was considered for the determination of the molecular formula. FDCM showed in its LC-ESI-MS chromatogram the presence of 15 metabolites, while 23 components were detected in FNBU (Tables S1 and S2).

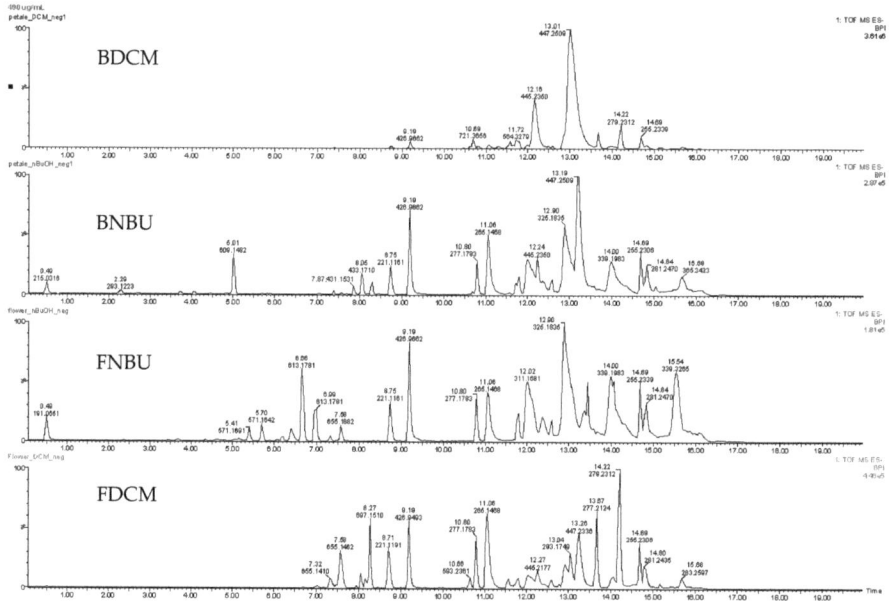

Figure 6. Spectra of the dichloromethane and *n*-butanol flower (FDCM and FNBU, respectively) and bract (BDCM and BNBU, respectively) fractions.

The first two metabolites of FDCM were detected at 6.66 and 6.99 min with the same mass value, *m/z* 613.1731, corresponding to the elemental composition $C_{27}H_{34}O_{16}$. Due to their low quantity in the extract, no fragment was obtained in the tandem mass analysis. However, on their MS spectra, a fragmentation pattern corresponding to a loss of ketene (42 Da) was observed. The obtained *m/z* 571.1544 fragment is a typical in-source-generated product, of which the mechanism has previously been studied and reported [16]. A literature search of this elemental composition led to the structure of four isomeric acetylated sucroses, namely mumeose G, mumeose S, mumeose H, and tomenside A. Up to now, these arylpropanoid sucroses have never been previously reported in banana species.

Two other metabolites appeared in the chromatogram at tR 7.32 and 7.58 min with the same mass value, *m/z* 655.1874, corresponding to $C_{29}H_{36}O_{17}$. Both were different from the precedents at 6.66 and 6.99 min by 42 Da, indicating their acetylated derivatives. The tandem mass data of *m/z* 655.1874 showed ions consistent with structures of coumaric acid (*m/z* 163.0352), monoglycosylated coumaric acid (*m/z* 349.0909), and triacetylated disaccharide (*m/z* 467.1384) (Figure S1). The metabolites at tR 7.32 and 7.58 min gave an almost similar fragmentation pattern, permitting their isomeric relationship to be deduced. A literature search of $C_{29}H_{36}O_{17}$ led to the structures mumeose I, mumeose L, mumeose Q, mumeose U, and mumeose T, previously obtained from the flower buds of *Prunus mume* [17,18]. The exact structures of the compounds could not be determined based on the mass spectrometric data. However, the m/z 349.0909 fragment (Figure S1), corresponding to the monoacetylated glycosyl coumaric acid ion, suggested muneose L and U as potential structures of the metabolite detected at 7.32 min. The isomer (tR 7.58 min) revealed in its MS^2 spectrum (Figure S1) a fragment at m/z 391.0948, leading to the structure of 4,6,2',6'-O-tetraacetyl-3-O-p-coumaroylsucrose. This compound was previously obtained from the fruits of *Prunus jamasakura* [19].

Four more compounds were detected with the same mass value, m/z 697.1997, at 7.84, 8.05, 8.16, and 8.27 min. The molecular formula was $C_{31}H_{38}O_{18}$, different from that of muneose L and U by 42 Da, corresponding to an acetyl group. This observation indicated m/z 697.1997 to be an acetylated derivative of 4,6,2',6'-O-tetraacetyl-3-O-p-coumaroylsucrose. These four metabolites showed almost similar features in their tandem mass spectra. However, the one at 7.94 min gave a fragment ion at m/z 391.0988 instead of m/z 349.0870, suggesting the presence of only an acetyl group on the pentose unit. The aforementioned information led to the structure of two positional isomers, mumeose V and mumeose D. Both compounds were previously identified from the flower buds of *Prunus mume* [17]. The remaining metabolites gave in their MS/MS spectra an m/z 391.0988 fragment ion alongside m/z 349.0870, both supporting the presence of two acetyl groups on the pentose, as found in 1,6,2',6'-O-tetraacetyl-3-O-trans-p-coumaroylsucrose. This elemental composition together with the obtained fragment ions led to the structures of four positional isomers, namely prunose I or mumeose N, or mumeose M or mumeose O. These metabolites were all previously obtained from the flower buds of *Prunus mume* [18].

Metabolites related to fatty acids were characterized from 14.22 to 15.68 min based only on their chemical compositions, because no fragments were observed in their tandem mass spectra.

LCMS analysis of FNBU showed the presence of 22 metabolites, among which quinic acid was detected at 0.49 min with an m/z 191.0551 $[C_7H_{12}O_6-H]^-$. Characterization of some components was made possible by the interpretation of their tandem mass data compared to those reported in the literature. Thus, the peak at 2.18 min showed a mass value of m/z 487.1465, corresponding to $[C_{21}H_{28}O_{13}-H]^-$. Its tandem mass data displayed ions at m/z 307.0706, 163.0431, and 145.0352, corresponding respectively to $[M-H-180]^-$, $[M-H-2\times162]^-$, and $[M-H-180-162]^-$. The diminution of the precursor mass value by 180 Da and 162 Da occurred when the m/z 487.1465 fragment lost a hexopyranose unit or a hexofuranose unit. The m/z 163.0431 and 145.0352 fragments corresponding to the coumaric acid ion were formed after the loss of sucrose [20]. A literature search led to the structure of three isomeric metabolites, among which 3-O-p-coumaroylsucrose was assigned as the structure. This metabolite was previously identified in dried fruits of *Prunus domestica* [21].

Another metabolite was found at 2.37 min with m/z 487.1465 $[C_{21}H_{28}O_{13}-H]^-$, suggesting an isomer of 3-O-p-coumaroylsucrose. Tandem mass of the m/z 487.1465 data showed fragment ions at m/z 341.0868 and 179.0580, which were formed after the loss of a deoxyhexose (146 Da) and a disaccharide (deoxyhexose + hexose, 308 Da), respectively. The m/z 179.0580 aglycone was characterized as caffeic acid, and the structure of this metabolite was assigned as cistanoside F. Its fragmentation behavior was similar to that previously reported [22].

The metabolite at 3.43 min with m/z 529.1561 $[C_{23}H_{30}O_{14}-H]^-$ gave in its MS/MS spectrum ions at m/z 487.1449, 469.1057, and 341.0905, formed after the precursor lost an acetyl group (42 Da), acetic acid (60 Da), and acetyldeoxyhexose (188 Da), respectively. The m/z 341.0905 fragment ion suggested this metabolite to be related to cistanoside F. Based on the aforementioned information, the structure of m/z 529.1561 was assigned to be a derivative of acetyl cistanoside F.

Two other isomers were observed at 3.69 and 4.35 min with the mass value m/z 529.1561 $[C_{23}H_{30}O_{14}-H]^-$. These compounds differed from 3-O-p-coumaroylsucrose by 42 Da, suggesting an acetyl derivative. Both isomers also showed a fragmentation pattern similar to 3-O-p-coumaroylsucrose with fragment ions at m/z 487.1330 [M-H-ketene (42 Da)]$^-$, 307.0742 [M-H-acetylhexose (222 Da)]$^-$, 163.0405 [M-H-sucrose]$^-$, and 145.0352 [M-H-sucrose-H_2O]$^-$. The abovementioned data led to the structure being related to mumeose A and acetyl 3-O-p-coumaroylsucrose.

Four peaks at 4.60, 5.15, 5.41, and 5.70 min showed the same mass value, m/z 571.1642 $[C_{25}H_{32}O_{15}-H]^-$. Their molecular formulas differed from that of muneose A by 42 Da, consistent with an acetylated derivative. These compounds gave similar fragment ions at m/z 529.1467, 511.1470, 307.0814, 163.0405, and 145.0352 in their tandem mass spectra. The m/z 529.1467 and 511.1470 ions were formed from the loss of an acetyl group (42 and 60 Da). The m/z 307.0814 ion was produced from the precursor after the loss of a diacetylhexose (264 Da). The structure of the aglycone was also assigned as coumaric acid based on the presence of the m/z 163.0405 and 145.0352 ions [20]. On the basis of the abovementioned information, the structures of these metabolites were assigned as positional isomers of mumeose B, P, or R, previously isolated from the flower buds of Prunus mune [17].

Four other positional isomers were also found in this fraction at 6.18, 6.40, 6.66, and 6.99 min (m/z 613.1731 $[C_{25}H_{32}O_{15}-H]^-$). These compounds contained three acetyl groups as their mass value differed from m/z 571.1642 by 42 Da, indicating a triacetyl 3-O-p-coumaroylsucrose derivative. All the m/z 613.1731 precursors gave in their MS/MS spectra similar fragments at m/z 571.1592, 553.1507, 529.1467, 511.1423, 349.0909, 307.0814, 163.0378, and 145.0278, while the m/z 571.1592 and 553.1507 fragments corresponded respectively to [M-ketene (42 Da)-H]$^-$ and [M-acetic acid (60 Da)-H]$^-$. The m/z 529.1467 and 511.1423 fragments were consistent with [M-H-2xketene(84 Da)]$^-$ and [M-H-2xacetic acid (120 Da)]$^-$. The m/z 349.0909 [M-264 (diacetylhexose)-H]$^-$ ion suggested the presence of an acetyl group on the sugar directly attached to the aglycone. Furthermore, this fragment lost a ketene (42 Da) to afford an m/z of 307.0814. As observed in the MS spectrum of the abovementioned metabolites, the aglycone was coumaric acid, consistent with an m/z 163.0378 and its dehydrated m/z 145.0278 fragment ion [20]. Because the position of the acetyl groups could not be determined using MS data, these four metabolite structures were deduced to be related to tomenside B based on the aforementioned information. Tomenside B is a triacetylated phenylpropanoid sucrose previously obtained from Prunus tomentosa leaves [23].

LCMS data of FNBU also showed two metabolites at 7.32 and 7.58 min with the same mass value, m/z 655.1882 $[C_{29}H_{36}O_{17}-H]^-$. Their structures were found to be related to muneose L and U for the metabolite at 7.32 min, while its isomer at tR 7.58 min was characterized as 4,6,2′,6′-O-tetraacetyl-3-O-p-coumaroylsucrose. A procyanidin derivative and a glycosylated flavonoid were found at m/z 1197.2529 $[2xC_{32}H_{24}O_{12}+HCO_2]^-$ and 637.1405 $[C_{27}H_{28}O_{15}+HCO_2]^-$, respectively. The lack of fragmentation was presumably due to their low quantities in the fraction. A pentacyclic triterpenic acid and a caffeate of betuline were also detected at 13.45 and 14.07 min with the mass values of m/z 455.3515 $[C_{30}H_{48}O_3-H]^-$ and 609.4099 $[C_{39}H_{56}O_5-H]^-$, respectively.

LCMS analysis of these BDCM fraction showed the presence of nine compounds, among which four were characterized (Table S2). The structure of the first metabolite at 7.36 min with an m/z 177.0550 $[C_{10}H_{10}O_3-H]^-$ was assigned as coumaric acid methyl ester or 4-methoxycinnamic acid. No fragment was found to completely elucidate its structure.

The compound at 10.69 min showed ions at m/z 721.3635 $[M+HCO_2]^-$ and m/z 675.3600 $[M-H]^-$, corresponding to $C_{33}H_{56}O_{14}$. This compound afforded on its MS/MS spectrum a fragment ion at m/z 593.3170, consistent with the loss of 2-methylbuta-1,3-dien-1-one (82 Da). The m/z 723.3801 $[C_{33}H_{58}O_{14}+HCO_2]^-$ precursor ion did not provide a fragment ion; however, the structures of 3′-O-isobutyryl-3-O-isovaleryl-2-O-lauroylsucrose and 2,3,4-tri(5-methylhexanoyl)-α-D-glucopyranosyl-β-D-fructofuranoside were suggested. The metabolites between 11.76 and 13.78 min did not furnish any fragment ions, but the literature indicated a structural relationship with stilbene. This group of metabolites has already been reported in Musaceae [24].

BNBU's LCMS data (Table S2) showed a peak at 2.29 min with m/z 293.1223, corresponding to $[C_{12}H_{22}O_8-H]^-$. A literature search provided γ-methyl-δ-hydroxy-pentanoic acid β-D-glucopyranoside as a reliable structure [25].

The m/z 609.1482 peak at 5.01 min $[C_{27}H_{30}O_{16}-H]^-$ gave fragment ions at m/z 581.1510 and 461.1089. The m/z 581.1510 fragment was formed when the precursor lost CO (28 Da); this fragment in turn dehydrated and afforded m/z 461.1089 after a retro-Diels–Alder rearrangement (Figure S2).

The structure of this metabolite was deduced to be 6,8-di-C-β-D-glucopyranosyl-luteoline, previously detected in *Citrus* peels [26].

The peak at 7.87 min with m/z 431.1531 $[C_{19}H_{28}O_{11}-H]^-$ showed on its tandem mass spectrum ions at m/z 349.0985 $[M-CH_3CH_2OH-2H_2O-H]^-$, 331.0892 $[M-CH_3CH_2OH-3H_2O-H]^-$, and 113.0320 $[M-aglycone-H_2O-H_2CO-H]^-$ (Figure S3). This information led to the structure of diffusosides A or B, two diastereomeric iridoids previously obtained from *Hedyotis diffusa* [27].

The peak at 8.05 min with an m/z of 433.1710 $[C_{19}H_{30}O_{11}-H]^-$ showed in its MS/MS spectrum a fragmentation pattern similar to that of the precedent metabolite, indicating another iridoid derivative. The m/z 351.1140 ion was obtained after the precursor eliminated CH_3CH_2OH (46 Da) and $2H_2O$ (36 Da). The m/z 333.1045 ion was formed after the removal of CH_3CH_2OH (46 Da) and three molecules of H_2O (54 Da), while the m/z 113.0298 ion was produced from the loss of the aglycone (272 Da), H_2O (18 Da), and CH_2CO (30 Da).

This information, together with that presented in Figure S4, indicated the structure of 7-O-ethylmorroniside. Another iridoid was found at 8.31 min with an m/z of 435.1851 $[C_{19}H_{32}O_{11}-H]^-$. This metabolite was heavier than 7-O-ethylmorroniside by a double bond equivalence. No structure matched the tandem mass data; however, the similarity between its fragment ions and those of 7-O-ethylmorroniside enabled the deduction that this metabolite was an iridoid derivative.

Two other metabolites were found at 8.75 and 13.23 min with m/z values of 221.1178 and 447.2509, respectively. The lack of fragmentation limited their structural assignment; however, a literature search indicated that these compound structures were related to those of an alkylated phenol and a stilbene, respectively.

2.3. Discussion

The cytotoxic effect of the studied extracts on the isolated mouse neutrophils showed that FDCM and BNBU reduced these cells' viability at concentrations equal to or greater than 300 μM. Alongside acetylated arylpropanoid sucroses, FDCM was also composed of fatty acids and other phenolics, while FNBU was formed of flavonoids, triterpenes, cyclohexanetetrol, and a low quantity of acetylated arylpropanoid sucroses (Table 2). The most concentrated sucrose, at 8.27 min (m/z 697.1997), and its positional isomers were presumably responsible for the cytotoxicity observed against neutrophil cells. However, their weak concentration in FNBU might support why this fraction lacked cytotoxic activity. Interestingly, compounds related to 3-phenylpropanoid-triacetyl sucrose esters, such as tomensides A–D and numeose C, demonstrated cytotoxicity against four human cancer cell lines in a previous study, although no information was provided about their selectivity towards normal cells [23].

Table 2. The chemical constituents characterized in banana inflorescence fractions.

Group of Characterized Metabolites	Fractions			
	FDCM	FNBU	BDCM	BNBU
Arylpropanoid sucroses	X	X		
Phenolics	X	X		X
Fatty acids	X		X	
Cyclohexanetetrol		X		
Flavonoids		X		X
Triterpenes		X		
Arylpropanoids			X	
Glycolipids			X	X
Stilbenes			X	X
Arylbenzofurans			X	X
Iridoids				X

The LCMS data of BDCM showed the presence of arylpropanoids, glycolipids, arylbenzofurans, fatty acids, and stilbenes; among them, an m/z 447.2509 stilbene derivative was the major component. No cytotoxicity was observed for this fraction. However, neutrophil cells responded slightly to BNBU, which was rich in glycolipids, stilbenes, flavonoids, arylbenzofurans, other phenolics, and iridoids, among which 6,8-di-C-glycosylated luteolin and an O-acyl glycoside were the main components. A previous study revealed that 6,8-di-C-β-D-glucopyranosyl-luteolin (lucenin-2) is weakly or not cytotoxic against five cancer cell lines [28]. Therefore, iridoids might be responsible for the cytotoxic effect on neutrophils, since some of these metabolites have been described as antiproliferative agents [29]. No toxicity study was found in the literature on banana inflorescences; however, previous bioassays have shown that its incorporation in rat diets might modulate serum cholesterol and glucose [8].

The anti-inflammatory effect of these fractions was evaluated at concentrations ranging from 10 to 100 µM. A different inhibitory profile was observed when these fractions were tested on the anti-inflammatory mediators IL-1β, TNF-α, NO_x, and IL-6. FDCM, rich in phenylpropanoid sucroses (m/z 613.1731, 655.1882, and 697.1997), fatty acids, and other phenolic compounds, inhibited the mediators IL-1β, TNF-α, and IL-6; its anti-inflammatory activity was presumably related to the presence of these phenolic glycosides. This conclusion is supported by former studies reporting similar metabolites with the same pharmacological property [30]. These arylpropanoid sucroses have also been described as inhibitors of aldose reductase, which is involved in various inflammatory disorders [17,18]. In fact, inhibition of aldose reductase might reduce reactive oxygen species and, therefore, prevent the inflammatory signals induced by cytokines and other factors [17,18]. Despite the presence of these metabolites in FNBU, no inhibition effect was observed on IL-1β, TNF-α, IL-6, and NO_x levels. FNBU showed traces of metabolites at m/z 613.1731, 655.1882, and 697.1997 in its LCMS data, alongside other arylpropanoid sucroses (3-O-p-coumaroylsucrose, cistanoside F, and acetyl cistanoside F derivative), flavonoid derivatives, and pentacyclic triterpenes. These classes of metabolites are recognized to possess anti-inflammatory properties [31,32]. Therefore, the lack of anti-inflammatory activity of FNBU might have been due to the low concentrations of these components, which were not sufficient to produce the expected effect.

BDCM contained a stilbene derivative which, among other metabolites, inhibited only TNF-α. This fraction displayed a chemical profile different from those of FDCM and FNBU, and the lack of sucroses might be why this fraction showed a different inhibition profile. On the other hand, its effect on TNF-α level could have been associated with the presence of a stilbene, of which the analogues, such as resveratrol, are known to be inhibitors of TNF-α [33]. In addition, the presence in BDCM of coumaric acid methyl ester (7.36 min, m/z 177.0550) related to the aglycone of the arylpropanoid sucroses could also have contributed to the inhibition of TNF-α levels. The similarity of BNBU and FDCM relied on an unidentified phenolic, although BNBU was able to inhibit the increase of NO_x and IL-6 levels. Considering the chemical profiles and the inhibition effects of FNBU and BDCM, iridoids and the phenolic derivative might have been responsible for the anti-inflammatory activity of BNBU. Iridoids structurally related to those found in BNBU, such as morroniside and geniposide, have been described as anti-inflammatory agents, and morroniside in particular is a NO_x inhibitor [34]. The presence of a diffusoside derivative and 7-O-ethylmorroniside might support the observed anti-inflammatory activity of this fraction. Lucenin-2, a 6,8-di-C-glycosylated flavone, could also have contributed to this activity based on previous results describing its anti-inflammatory properties [35].

Since inflammatory cytokines are produced during parasite infections and these cytokines are also manifestly related to their virulence [12–15], this study also aimed to investigate whether fractions from banana blossom could exert antiparasitic effects against intracellular *T. cruzi*, *L. amazonensis*, and *L. infantum* amastigotes.

As human monocyte THP-1 cells were used as the macrophage, their viability when treated with the only active fraction (FDCM) was evaluated. This fraction was weakly cytotoxic to the THP-1 cell line. As observed with the neutrophil cells, FDCM, composed essentially of phenylpropanoid sucroses, required a high concentration to affect cell viability.

Only FDCM showed antitrypanosomal activity against the intracellular form of *T. cruzi* with a good selectivity index. It has been reported in the literature that human macrophages infected with *T. cruzi* display an increased level of MMP-9, which has a strong relationship with the production of inflammatory cytokines such as IL-1β, TNF-α, and IL-6 [14]. Therefore, the trypanocidal activity observed for FDCM might have had a relationship with its anti-inflammatory effect by inhibiting these three cytokines. In contrast to FDCM, which concomitantly inhibited three cytokines, BDCM solely inhibited the cytokine TNF-α and showed no effect against *T. cruzi*. This observation led to the conclusion that FDCM displayed antitrypanosomal activity, because it could reduce the levels of these three cytokines without inhibiting the level of NO_x. It has been reported that nitrogen-derived species (NO_x) have a crucial role for the immune system by protecting cells against intracellular *T. cruzi* infection [36]. Therefore, the selective effect on the cytokines but not NO_x is important for antitrypanosomal activity. Nitrogen oxide species chemically specifically modify cysteine-containing proteins in *T. cruzi*, and can potentially interact with the metalloproteins that mediate crucial metabolic processes [36]. This might support why BNBU did not show any trypanocidal activity. None of the fractions were active against the studied *Leishmania* species, indicating that the inhibition of IL-1β, TNF-α, and IL-6 cytokines and NO_x species might affect the growth of *Leishmania*.

As this non-conventional food showed various biological benefits, it can be classified as a functional food, although more studies including toxicology and balanced diet studies need to be performed.

3. Materials and Methods

3.1. Plant Identification

The inflorescences of *Musa acuminata* were collected in Itacorubi/Florianópolis in March 2017. A voucher was deposited under the number RB 02574A in the Jardim Botanico (Botanical Garden) of Rio de Janeiro Herbarium (RB).

3.2. Anti-Inflammatory Assays

3.2.1. Mouse Neutrophil Isolation and Primary Culture

Mouse neutrophils were collected from mouse peritoneal leakage and maintained in Dulbecco's Modified Eagle Medium (DMEM) (Gibco, Grand Island, NY, USA) with 10% fetal bovine serum, 100 U/mL of penicillin, and 100 mg/mL of streptomycin incubated at 37 °C in a humidified CO_2 incubator. The peritoneal neutrophils were obtained after injection of oyster glycogen into the peritoneal mouse cavity, as described by Silva and co-workers with some modifications [37]. A total 3 mL of oyster glycogen at 1% (w/v) dissolved in sterile phosphate-buffered saline (PBS) was injected into the peritoneal mouse cavity, and after 4 h the animals were euthanized by overdose of xylazine and ketamine administered intravenously (i.v.). After euthanasia, 3 mL of sterile PBS was injected into the peritoneal cavity and the cavity was massaged for 10 s to suspend the neutrophils. An incision was made using sterile surgical material and the peritoneal leakage was collected in 50 mL sterile tubes and stored immediately in an ice bath. Furthermore, a pool of peritoneally collected neutrophils was made in order to obtain 1×10^6 neutrophils/well. A reduced number of animals were used with respect to the 3Rs (Replacement, Reduction and Refinement) principle [38]. The procedures were approved by the Committee for Ethics in Animal Research from UFSC (Protocol 8665141117) and were in accordance with the National Institutes of Health (NIH) Guide for the Care and Use of Laboratory Animals.

3.2.2. Lipopolysaccharide Stimulation of Isolated Neutrophils

The neutrophils were preincubated after plate distribution with or without different concentrations (10, 30, and 100 μg/mL) of the studied fractions for 1 h, and then the medium was exchanged with fresh DMEM mixed with lipopolysaccharide (LPS) at a final concentration of 5 μg/mL and incubated for 16 h at 37 °C in a CO_2 incubator (5%).

3.2.3. Cell Viability Assay Using the Isolated Neutrophilis

The extracts were added to each well at different final concentrations (10, 30, 100, 300, and 1000 µM) and incubated for 16 h at 37 °C in a CO_2 incubator (5%). This procedure was performed after the neutrophils were plated in a 96 well plate with DMEM culture medium enriched with 10% fetal bovine serum and 1% (w/w) penicillin/streptomycin. The entire experiment was conducted in triplicate and repeated on two different days of experimentation. The viability of the neutrophils after treating with the blossom fractions was evaluated using the colorimetric (3-(4,5-dimethylthiazol-2-yl)-2,5-diphenyltetrazolium bromide) MTT assay. The supernatant was discarded after incubation for 16 h and MTT solution (5 mg/mL) was added to each well, followed by incubation for a further 3 h at 37 °C in a CO_2 incubator (5%). The medium was then discarded again and dimethylsufoxide (DMSO) was added to dissolve the formazan dye. The optical density was checked at 540 nm using an ELISA reader (Infinite M200, Tecan, Männedorf, Switzerland).

3.2.4. Cell Inflammation Assay on Isolated Neutropils

In order to evaluate the effect of the standards and the fractions on inflamed ex vivo mouse neutrophils, cells were designated to different groups (n = 4/group) consisting of the following: (a) blank control (Ctrl, uninflamed neutrophils), cells treated only with vehicle; (b) negative control (LPS, lipopolysaccharide-inflamed neutrophils), cells stimulated only with LPS (5 µg/mL); (c) positive controls (dexamethasone: Dexa, reference anti-inflammatory drug treatment), cells pre-treated with Dexa (10 µM) and after 0.5 h stimulated with LPS (5 µg/mL); and (d) experimental groups (studied extracts), cells pre-treated with the extracts at 10, 30, and 100 µg/mL and stimulated after 0.5 h with LPS (5 µg/mL). All experimental groups were incubated for 16 h at 37 °C in a CO_2 atmosphere (5%). The supernatant was collected for further inflammatory analysis and comparisons (NO_x, IL-1β, TNF-α, and IL-6).

3.2.5. Measurement of NO_x Production in Neutrophils

The production of NO metabolites by mouse neutrophils (n = 10 per experiment) was determined using Griess reagent. Measures of 100 µL of the Griess reagent were mixed with 50 µL of cell supernatant and incubated for 40 min at 37 °C. Absorbance at 540 nm was measured with interpolation from the nitrite standard curve (0–20 µM), and the results are expressed in µM.

3.2.6. Quantification of Pro-Inflammatory Cytokines Levels (IL-1β, TNF-α, and IL-6) in Neutrophils

The interleukin-1β (IL-1β), tumoral necrosis factor alpha (TNF-α), and interleukin 6 (IL-6) levels in the neutrophil supernatants were quantified as follows. The supernatant was removed and submitted to determination of the concentrations of IL-1β, TNF-α, and IL-6 using a commercially available enzyme-linked immunosorbent assay kit (Peprotech, Rocky Hill, NJ, USA) according to the manufacturer's instructions. Cytokine level was estimated by interpolation from the standard curve and the results are expressed in pg/mL.

3.3. Antiparasitic Assays

3.3.1. In Vitro Antitrypanosomal and Antileishmanial Assays

The human macrophage cell line THP-1 (ATCC TIB202) was grown in RPMI-1640 without phenol red (Sigma-Aldrich, St Louis, MO, USA), supplemented with 10% FBS (Life Technologies, Carlsbad, CA), 12.5 mM HEPES, penicillin (100 U/mL), streptomycin (100 µg/mL), and Glutamax (2 mM), at 37 °C in a 5% CO_2 incubator. Schneider's insect medium (Sigma Chemical Co., St Louis, MO, USA) supplemented with 5% heat-inactivated FBS and 2% human urine at 26 °C was used to grow *L. amazonensis* MHOM/BR/77/LTB0016 and *L. infantum* (MHOM/BR/74/PP75) promastigotes, expressing β-galactosidase. THP-1 cells (4.0×10^4 per well) were cultivated in 96 well microplates with complete

RPMI-1640 medium supplemented with 100 ng/mL of phorbol 12-myristate 13-acetate (PMA) (Sigma Chemical Co.) for 72 h at 37 °C in 5% CO_2, to allow THP-1 cell differentiation into non-dividing macrophages [39]. Four day old culture promastigotes (4.0×10^6 parasites/mL) were washed twice with phosphate-buffered saline (PBS), pH 7.4, and incubated in RPMI-1640 supplemented with 10% heat-inactivated human B+ serum for 1 h at 34 °C for parasite opsonization. Macrophages were incubated with a parasite/cell ratio of 10:1 for 4 h at 34 °C and 5% CO_2. Thereafter, non-adherent parasites were removed by washing with PBS solution. Infected cells were incubated with 180 μL of fully supplemented RPMI-1640 medium for another 24 h to allow the transformation of promastigotes into intracellular amastigotes. The β-galactosidase *T. cruzi*, Tulahuén strain was obtained from the Laboratory of Cellular and Molecular Parasitology, Centro de Pesquisas René Rachou, FIOCRUZ, Belo Horizonte. Culture-derived trypomastigotes raised from an infected L929 cell line were used to infect differentiated THP-1 cells (4.0×10^4 cells/well) in 96 well microplates in a parasite/cell ratio of 2:1, and were then incubated overnight at 37 °C in a 5% CO_2 atmosphere. The medium containing non-internalized parasites was removed and replaced with 180 μL of fresh medium [40]. Samples were solubilized in dimethylsulfoxide (DMSO) Merck® and serially diluted (500 μg/mL to 2 μg/mL). The infected cell monolayer was treated with 50 μg/μL of each sample, in triplicate, followed by incubation for 48 h at 34 °C or 37 °C, 5% CO_2. After treatment, cells were carefully washed with PBS and incubated for 16 h at 37 °C with 250 μL of chlorophenol red-β-D-galactopyranoside (CPRG) (Sigma-Aldrich Co.) at 100 μM and Nonidet P-40 (NP-40) (Amresco Inc, Solon, OH, USA) 0.1%. Optical density was read at 570/630 nm in an Infinite M200 (Tecan, Grödig, Austria) [41,42]. The concentration of each sample that reduced parasite viability by 50% when compared to untreated control (IC_{50}) was estimated by non-linear regression of concentration–response curves. Amphotericin B (Sigma-Aldrich) and benznidazole (Sigma-Aldrich) were used as positive controls for antileishmanial and antitrypanosomal activities, respectively, and DMSO 1% as negative control. The concentrations able to inhibit 50% (IC_{50}) of the parasites and the proliferation of THP-1 cells (CC_{50}) were used to express the antiparasitic activity and cytotoxicity, respectively. Selectivity index (SI) of each sample was determined by the ratio of CC_{50}/IC_{50}.

3.3.2. Cell Viability Assay (MTT)

THP-1 cells were grown and cultivated in 96 well microplates (4.0×10^4 cells/well), treated with the compounds serially diluted in concentrations ranging from 2 μg/mL to 500 μg/mL, and incubated for 72 h at 37 °C, 5% CO_2. The plates were centrifuged ($3700 \times g$/7 min), the supernatant was removed, and the cells were resuspended in 50 μL of a solution of MTT (Amresco) at 3 mg/mL in saline buffer and incubated for 4 h at 37 °C, 5% CO_2 before being centrifuged ($3700 \times g$/7 min), and the formazan salt was solubilized in 100 μL DMSO. Optical density was determined at 540 nm in a Tecan® Infinite M200 spectrophotometer. DMSO 1% (*v/v*) and DMSO 50% (*v/v*) were the negative and positive controls, respectively. The IC_{50} values were calculated by non-linear regression using the GraphPad Prism program [40].

3.4. LCMS analysis

3.4.1. Chemicals

Acetonitrile and formic acid were purchased from Tedia (São Paulo, Brazil). A Milli-Q system (18.2MΩ, Millipore, Simplipak, France) was used to prepare ultrapure water. Syringe filters (13 mm, 0.22 μm) were bought from Analítica (São Paulo, Brazil).

3.4.2. Extraction, Fractionation, and Sample Preparation

The banana inflorescences were separated into bracts (228 g) and flowers (60 g), which were extracted in methanol (500 and 100 mL respectively). Both extractions furnished crude extracts of 70 mg from the petals and 40 mg from flowers. Each crude extract was diluted in water and separated by liquid-liquid non-miscible extraction process with dichloromethane and n-butanol. FDCM (5 mg) and FNBU (7 mg) were obtained from the flowers, whereas BDCM (4.8 mg) and BNBU (10 mg) were obtained from the bracts. An total 3 mg of each sample was diluted with 4 mL of acetonitrile and methanol (1:1, v/v) to afford solutions with concentrations of 750 µg/mL, which were filtered using a 0.22 µm syringe filter.

3.4.3. LC-MS Method

An Acquity UPLC system class H (Waters, Milford, MA, USA) equipped with a photodiode array (PDA) detector, sample manager, and a quaternary solvent manager as well as a BEH C18 column (50 mm, 1.0 mm, particle size 1.7 µm (Waters)) was used for the separation. The column and the sample tray were maintained at temperatures of 40 °C and 20 °C, respectively. A sample volume of 3 µL was subjected to a gradient condition at flow rate of 0.3 mL/min: 95% A (water/formic acid, 99.9/0.1 (v/v)) and 5% B (acetonitrile); 0–2 min, 95% of A; 2–10 min, 55% of A; 10–15 min, 5% of A; 15–20 min, 95% of A.

A Xevo G2-S QTof (Waters) bearing an electrospray ionization (ESI) probe operating in positive and negative ionization modes was coupled to the UPLC device and used to detect the chemical components of each extract. Nebuliser gas: nitrogen; cone gas flow: 100 L/h; desolvation gas flow: 900 L/h; sampling cone 40 V; source offset 80 V; collision gas: argon; lockspray reference sample was leucine encephalin with reference masses at m/z 554.2615 (ESI−). The desolvation and the ionization source were maintained during the analyses at 250 °C and 90 °C, respectively, while the capillary voltage was 3 kV. A range of 25 to 35 eV was used as the collision energy. Data were acquired in a range of 100–1500 Da, at a scan time of 1.0 s over 20 min, and were processed with MassLynx V4.1 (Waters).

Molecular formulas were determined by calculation using MassLynx's elemental composition tool. The choice of each molecular formula was restricted by a tolerance of 5 ppm between the calculated and the measured mass values.

4. Conclusions

This work focused on the anti-inflammatory activities of the fractions from banana flower and bracts against NO_x and cytokines, including IL-1β, TNF-α, and IL-6. Their effects on intracellular forms of T. cruzi, L. amazonensis, and L. infantum amastigote were also investigated. Only the flower fraction from the dichloromethane partition showed simultaneous anti-inflammatory and antitrypanosomal activities. None of these fractions displayed antileishmanial activites against L. amazonensis and L. infantum. Interestingly, the fraction from the dichloromethane partition (FDCM), rich in arylpropanoid sucroses, was the most prominent with respect to the investigated biological activities. Fractions showed different anti-inflammatory activities on the tested cytokines. All fractions showed anti-inflammatory activity against at least one cytokine except FNBU. The chemical profiles established by UPLC-ESI-QTOFMS of FDCM, FNBU, BDCM, and BNBU showed the presence of 15, 22, 8, and 9 metabolites, respectively. LCMS data of FDCM revealed the presence of eight arylpropanoid sucroses alongside one phenolic metabolite, four fatty acids, and two unidentified metabolites. FNBU, on the other hand showed the presence of 16 arylpropanoid sucroses in its LCMS data, together with 1 cyclohexanetetrol acid, 1 phenolic compound, 2 flavonoids, and 2 triterpenes. While the LCMS data of BDCM displayed an arylpropanoid, two glycolipids, two stilbenes, one arylbenzofuran, and two fatty acids, those of BNBU showed the presence of one fatty acid, one glycolipid, one arylbenzofuran, one flavonoid, three iridoids, one stilbene, one phenolic derivative, and one unidentified metabolite. The abovementioned results emphasized the health benefit of this non-conventional food and its chemical composition. Therefore, banana blossom may have applications as a dietary food supplement or as a potential functional ingredient to control inflammation.

Supplementary Materials: The following are available online, Figure S1: Fragmentation pattern of the metabolites m/z 655.1874 with retention times 7.32 min (left) and 7.58 min (right), Figure S2: Fragmentation pattern of the metabolite m/z 609.1482, Figure S3: Fragmentation pattern of m/z 431.1553, Figure S4: Fragmentation pattern of *m/z* 433.1710, Table S1: Chemical constituents of the flower fractions, Table S2: Chemical constituents of the bract fractions.

Author Contributions: Conception of the project, L.P.S. and M.S.; biological assays, M.V.P.d.S.N., M.d.H.M. and L.M.R.; LCMS analysis, L.P.S.; Original draft preparation, L.P.S, M.S. and E.M.D.; manuscript reading and supervision of the LCMS analysis, M.W.B.

Funding: The authors would like to thank CAPES-PNPD and CNPq for the post-doctoral scholarship and the financial support, respectively.

Acknowledgments: L.P.S., M.W.B. and M.S. would also like to thank Resnet NPND to facilitate a collaborative network group.

Conflicts of Interest: All the authors declare no conflict of interest.

References

1. Nunes, H. *PANC gourmet: Ensaios culinários*; Instituto Plantarum: São Paulo, Brazil, 2017; pp. 88–89.
2. Azam, F.M.S.; Biswas, A.; Mannan, A.; Afsana, N.A.; Jahan, R.; Rahmatullah, M. Are Famine Food Plants Also Ethnomedicinal Plants? An Ethnomedicinal Appraisal of Famine Food Plants of Two Districts of Bangladesh. *Evid Based Complement. Altern. Med.* **2014**, *2014*. [CrossRef] [PubMed]
3. Kinupp, V.F.; Lorenzi, H. *Plantas Alimentícias Não Convencionais (PANC) no Brasil: Guia de identificação, aspectos nutricionais e receitas ilustradas*; Instituto de Plantarum de Estudos de Flora: São Paulo, Brasil, 2014; pp. 538–542.
4. Mathew, N.S.; Negi, P.S. Traditional uses, phytochemistry and pharmacology of wild banana (*Musaacuminata* Colla). A Review. *J. Ethnopharmacol.* **2017**, *196*, 124–140. [CrossRef] [PubMed]
5. Chintamunnee, V.; Mahomoodally, M.F. Herbal medicine commonly used against non-communicable diseases in the tropical island of Mauritius. *J. Herb Med.* **2012**, *2*, 113–125. [CrossRef]
6. China, R.; Dutta, S.; Sen, S.; Chakrabarti, R.; Bhowmik, D.; Ghosh, S.; Dhar, P. In vitro Antioxidant Activity of Different Cultivars of Banana Flower (*Musa paradicicus* L.) Extracts Available in India. *J Food Sci.* **2011**, *76*, C1292–C1299. [CrossRef] [PubMed]
7. Ramu, R.; Shirahatti, P.S.; Dhanabal, S.P.; Zameer, F.; Dhananjaya, B.L.; Prasad, M.N.N. Investigation of Antihyperglycaemic Activity of Banana (*Musa* sp. Var. Nanjangud rasa bale) Flower in Normal and Diabetic Rats. *Pharm. Mag.* **2017**, *13*, S417–S423. [CrossRef]
8. Liyanage, R.; Gunasegaram, S.; Visvanathan, R.; Jayathilake, C.; Weththasinghe, P.; Jayawardana, B.C.; Vidanarachchi, J.K. Banana Blossom (*Musa acuminate* Colla) Incorporated Experimental Diets Modulate Serum Cholesterol and Serum Glucose Level in Wistar Rats Fed with Cholesterol. *Cholesterol*. **2016**. [CrossRef]
9. Otálvaro, F.; Nanclares, J.; Vásquez, L.E.; Quiñones, W.; Echeverri, F.; Arango, R.; Schneider, B. Phenalenone-type compounds from *Musa acuminata* var. "Yangambi km 5" (AAA) and their activity against *Mycosphaerella fijiensis*. *J. Nat. Prod.* **2007**, *70*, 887–890.
10. Hölscher, D.; Buerkert, A.; Schneider, B. Phenylphenalenones Accumulate in Plant Tissues of Two Banana Cultivars in Response to Herbivory by the Banana Weevil and Banana Stem Weevil. *Plants* **2016**, *5*. [CrossRef]
11. Kamo, T.; Kato, N.; Hirai, N.; Tsuda, M.; Fujioka, D.; Ohigashi, H. Phenylphenalenone-type Phytoalexins from Unripe Buñgulan Banana Fruit. *Biosci Biotechnol Biochem.* **1998**, *62*, 95–101. [CrossRef]
12. Oliveira, W.N.; Ribeiro, L.E.; Schrieffer, A.; Machado, P.; Carvalho, E.M.; Bacellar, O. The role of inflammatory and anti-inflammatory cytokines inthe pathogenesis of human tegumentary leishmaniasis. *Cytokine* **2014**, *66*, 127–132. [CrossRef]
13. Morgado, F.N.; de Carvalho, L.M.V.; Leite-Silva, J.; Seba, A.J.; Pimentel, M.I.F.; Fagundes, A.; Madeira, M.F.; Lyra, M.R.; Oliveira, M.M.; Schubach, A.O.; et al. Unbalanced inflammatory reaction could increase tissue destruction and worsen skin infectious diseases—a comparative study of leishmaniasis and sporotrichosis. *Sci. Rep.* **2018**, *8*. [CrossRef] [PubMed]
14. Vazquez, B.P.; Vazquez, T.P.; Miguel, C.B.; Rodrigues, W.F.; Mendes, M.T.; de Oliveira, C.J.F.; Javier Chica, E.L. Inflammatory responses and intestinal injury development during acute Trypanosoma cruzi infection are associated with the parasite load. *Parasites Vectors* **2015**, *8*. [CrossRef] [PubMed]
15. de Pinho, R.T.; da Silva, W.S.; de Castro Cortes, L.M.; da Silva Vasconcelos Sousa, P.; de Araujo Soares, R.O.; Alve, C.R. Production of MMP-9 and inflammatory cytokines by *Trypanosoma cruzi*-infected macrophages. *Exp. Parasitol.* **2014**, *147*, 72–80. [CrossRef] [PubMed]

16. Abrankó, L.; García-Reyes, J.F.; Molina-Díaz, A. In-source fragmentation and accurate mass analysis of multiclass flavonoid conjugates by electrospray ionization time-of-flight mass spectrometry. *J. Mass Spectrom.* **2011**, *46*, 478–488. [CrossRef]
17. Fujimoto, K.; Nakamura, S.; Matsumoto, T.; Ohta, T.; Yoshikawa, M.; Ogawa, K.; Kashiwazaki, E.; Matsuda, H. Structures of acylated sucroses from the flower buds of *Prunus Mume*. *J. Nat. Med.* **2014**, *68*, 481–487. [CrossRef]
18. Nakamura, S.; Fujimoto, K.; Matsumoto, T.; Ohta, T.; Ogawa, K.; Tamura, H.; Matsuda, H.; Yoshikawa, M. Structures of acylated sucroses and an acylated flavonol glycoside and inhibitory effects of constituents on aldose reductase from the flower buds of *Prunus mume*. *J. Nat. Med.* **2013**, *67*, 799–806. [CrossRef]
19. Shimazaki, N.; Mimaki, Y.; Sashida, Y. Prunasin and acetylated phenylpropanoic acid sucrose esters, bitter principles from the fruits of *Prunus jamasakura* and *P. Maximowiczii*. *Phytochemistry* **1991**, *30*, 1475–1480. [CrossRef]
20. Bonta, R.K. Application of HPLC and ESI-MS techniques in the analysis of phenolic acids and flavonoids from green leafy vegetables (GLVs). *J. Pharm. Anal.* **2017**, *7*, 349–364. [CrossRef]
21. Kayano, S.; Kikuzaki, H.; Hashimoto, S.; Kasamatsu, K.; Ikami, T.; Nakatani, N. Glucosyl terpenates from the dried fruits of *Prunus domestica* L. *Phytochem. Lett.* **2014**, *8*, 132–136. [CrossRef]
22. Sanz, M.; de Simón, B.F.; Cadahía, E.; Esteruelas, E.; Muñoz, A.M.; Hernández, T.; Estrella, I.; Pinto, E. LC-DAD/ESI-MS/MS study of phenolic compounds in ash (*Fraxinus excelsior* L. and *F. americana* L.) heartwood. Effect of toasting intensity at cooperage. *J. Mass Spectrom.* **2012**, *47*, 905–918. [CrossRef]
23. Zhao, W.; Huang, X.-X.; Yu, L.-H.; Liu, Q.-B.; Li, L.-Z.; Sun, Q.; Song, S.-J. Tomensides A–D, new antiproliferative phenylpropanoid sucrose esters from *Prunus tomentosa* leaves. *Bioorg. Med. Chem. Lett.* **2014**, *24*, 2459–2462. [CrossRef] [PubMed]
24. Hölscher, D.; Schneider, B. A resveratrol dimer from *Anigozanthos preissii* and *Musa Cavendish*. *Phytochemistry* **1996**, *43*, 471–473. [CrossRef]
25. Ono, M.; Uenosono, Y.; Umaoka, H.; Shiono, Y.; Ikeda, T.; Okawa, M.; Kinjo, J.; Yoshimitsu, H.; Nohara, T. Five New Steroidal Glycosides from the Stems of *Solanum sodomaeum*. *Chem Pharm Bull.* **2009**, *57*, 759–763. [CrossRef] [PubMed]
26. Guccione, C.; Bergonzi, M.C.; Piazzini, V.; Bilia, A.R. A Simple and Rapid HPLC-PDA MS Method for the Profiling of *Citrus* Peels and Traditional Italian Liquors*. *Planta Med.* **2016**, *82*, 1039–1045. [CrossRef] [PubMed]
27. Zhang, Y.; Chen, Y.; Fan, C.; Ye, W.; Luo, J. Two new iridoid glucosides from *Hedyotis diffusa*. *Fitoterapia* **2010**, *81*, 515–517. [CrossRef]
28. Hussein, S.R.; Latif, R.R.A.; Marzouk, M.M.; Elkhateeb, A.; Mohammed, R.S.; Soliman, A.A.F.; Abdel-Hameed, E.-S.S. Spectrometric analysis, phenolics isolation and cytotoxic activity of *Stipagrostis plumosa* (Family Poaceae). *Chem Pap.* **2018**, *72*, 29–37. [CrossRef]
29. Shan, M.; Yu, S.; Yan, H.; Guo, S.; Xiao, W.; Wang, Z.; Zhang, L.; Ding, A.; Wu, Q.; Li, S.F.Y. A Review on the Phytochemistry, Pharmacology, Pharmacokinetics and Toxicology of Geniposide, a Natural Product. *Molecules* **2017**, *22*. [CrossRef]
30. Chang, C.L.; Zhang, L.J.; Chen, R.Y.; Kuo, L.M.; Huang, J.P.; Huang, H.C.; Lee, K.H.; Wu, Y.C.; Kuo, Y.H. Antioxidant and anti-inflammatory phenylpropanoid derivatives from *Calamus quiquesetinervius*. *J. Nat. Prod.* **2010**, *73*, 1482–1488. [CrossRef]
31. Dawé, A.; Mbiantcha, M.; Yakai, F.; Jabeen, A.; Ali, M.S.; Lateef, M.; Ngadjui, B.T. Flavonoids and triterpenes from *Combretum fragrans* with anti-inflammatory, antioxidant and antidiabetic potential. *Z Nat. C.* **2018**, *73*, 211–219. [CrossRef]
32. Rao, Y.K.; Fang, S.H.; Tzeng, Y.M. Anti-inflammatory activities of flavonoids and a triterpene caffeate isolated from *Bauhinia variegata*. *Phytother Res.* **2008**, *22*, 957–962. [CrossRef]
33. Deng, Y.H.; Alex, D.; Huang, H.Q.; Wang, N.; Yu, N.; Wang, Y.T.; Leung, G.P.; Lee, S.M. Inhibition of TNF-α-mediated endothelial cell-monocyte cell adhesion and adhesion molecules expression by the resveratrol derivative, trans-3,5,4′-trimethoxystilbene. *Phytother Res.* **2011**, *25*, 451–457. [CrossRef] [PubMed]
34. An, S.J.; Pae, H.O.; Oh, G.S.; Choi, B.M.; Jeong, S.; Jang, S.I.; Oh, H.; Kwon, T.O.; Song, C.E.; Chung, H.T. Inhibition of TNF-alpha, IL-1beta, and IL-6 productions and NF-kappa B activation in lipopolysaccharide-activated RAW 264.7 macrophages by catalposide, an iridoid glycoside isolated from *Catalpa ovata* G. Don (Bignoniaceae). *Int. Immunopharmacol.* **2002**, *2*, 1137–1181. [CrossRef]

35. Kim, M.K.; Yun, K.J.; Lim, D.H.; Kim, J.; Jang, Y.P. Anti-Inflammatory Properties of Flavone di-C-Glycosides as Active Principles of *Camellia Mistletoe, Korthalsella japonica*. *Biomol.* **2016**, *24*, 630–637. [CrossRef] [PubMed]
36. Gutierrez, F.R.S.; Mineo, T.W.P.; Pavanelli, W.R.; Guedes, P.M.M.; Silva, J.S. The effects of nitric oxide on the immune system during *Trypanosoma cruzi* infection. *Mem. Inst. Oswaldo Cruzrio De Jan.* **2009**, *104*, 236–245. [CrossRef] [PubMed]
37. Silva, A.M.; Machado, I.D.; Santin, J.R.; de Melo, I.L.; Pedrosa, G.V.; Genovese, M.I.; Farsky, S.H.; Mancini-Filho, J. Aqueous extract of *Rosmarinus officinalis* L. inhibits neutrophil influx and cytokine secretion. *Phytother Res.* **2015**, *29*, 125–133. [CrossRef] [PubMed]
38. Flecknell, P. Replacement, reduction and refinement. *ALTEX* **2002**, *19*, 73–78. [CrossRef]
39. Schwende, H.; Fitzke, E.; Ambs, P.; Dieter, P. Differences in the state of differentiation of THP-1 cells induced by phorbol ester and 1,25-dihydroxyvitamin D3. *J. Leukoc Biol.* **1996**, *59*, 555–561. [CrossRef]
40. Buckner, F.S.; Verlinde, C.L.; La Flamme, A.C.; Van Voorhis, W.C. Efficient technique for screening drugs for activity against *Trypanosoma cruzi* using parasites expressing β-galactoside. *Antimicrob. Agents Chemother* **1996**, *40*, 2592–2597. [CrossRef]
41. Sieuwerts, A.M.; Klijn, J.G.M.; Peters, H.A.; Foekens, J.A. The MTT tetrazolium salt assay scrutinized: How to use this assay reliably to measure metabolic activity of cell cultures in vitro for the assessment of growth characteristics, IC_{50}-values and cell survival. *Clin. Chem. Lab. Med.* **1995**, *33*, 813–824. [CrossRef]
42. Van de Loosdrecht, A.; Nennie, E.; Ossenkoppele, G.; Beelen, R.; Langenhuijsen, M. Cell mediated cytotoxicity against U 937 cells by human monocytes and macrophages in a modified colorimetric MTT assay. A Methodol. Study. *J. Immunol. Methods* **1991**, *141*, 15–22. [CrossRef]

Sample Availability: Samples of the compounds are not available from the authors.

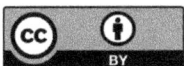

© 2019 by the authors. Licensee MDPI, Basel, Switzerland. This article is an open access article distributed under the terms and conditions of the Creative Commons Attribution (CC BY) license (http://creativecommons.org/licenses/by/4.0/).

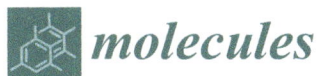

Article

A New Eucalyptol-Rich Lavender (*Lavandula stoechas* L.) Essential Oil: Emerging Potential for Therapy against Inflammation and Cancer

Mohamed Nadjib Boukhatem [1,2,*], Thangirala Sudha [1], Noureldien H.E. Darwish [1,3], Henni Chader [4,5], Asma Belkadi [6], Mehdi Rajabi [1], Aicha Houche [2], Fatma Benkebailli [2], Faiza Oudjida [7] and Shaker A. Mousa [1]

1. The Pharmaceutical Research Institute, Albany College of Pharmacy and Health Sciences, Rensselaer, New York, NY 12144, USA; sudha.thangirala@acphs.edu (T.S.); nour_darwish83@yahoo.com (N.H.E.D.); m.rajabi.s@gmail.com (M.R.); shaker.mousa@acphs.edu (S.A.M.)
2. Département de Biologie et Physiologie Celulaire, Faculté des Sciences de la Nature et de la Vie, Université-Saad Dahlab-Blida 1, Blida 09000, Algeria; hoch.snv@gmail.com (A.H.); benkpharma@gmail.com (F.B.)
3. Hematology Unit, Clinical Pathology Department, Mansoura Faculty of Medicine, Mansoura University, Mansoura 35516, Egypt
4. Laboratoire de Pharmaco-Toxicologie, Laboratoire National de Contrôle des Produits Pharmaceutiques (LNCPP), Dely-Ibrahim, Algiers 16047, Algeria; hennichader@hotmail.fr
5. Faculté de Médecine-Université Ben Youcef Ben Khedda-Alger I, Algiers 16000, Algeria
6. Laboratoire Pharmaco-Toxicologie, Centre de Recherche & Développement Saidal, Algiers 16004, Algeria; santepharmacrd@gmail.com
7. Laboratoire d'Anatomie Pathologique, Centre Hospitalo-Universitiare de Beni-Messous, Algiers 16206, Algeria; medchem2020@gmail.com
* Correspondence: mn.boukhatem@yahoo.fr; Tel.: +213-664-983-174

Academic Editor: Toshio Morikawa
Received: 5 May 2020; Accepted: 18 May 2020; Published: 12 August 2020

Abstract: Background/Aim: natural products are a potential source for drug discovery and development of cancer chemoprevention. Considering that drugs currently available for the treatment of inflammatory and cancer conditions show undesirable side effects, this research was designed to evaluate, for the first time, the in vitro anticancer activity of Algerian *Lavandula stoechas* essential oil (LSEO) against different cancer cell lines, as well as its in vitro and in vivo topical and acute anti-inflammatory properties. Materials and Methods: the LSEO was extracted by steam distillation, and chemical composition analysis was performed using gas chromatography. The main compounds identified in LSEO were oxygenated monoterpenes, such as 1,8-Cineole (61.36%). LSEO exhibited a potent anti-inflammatory activity using the xylene-induced mouse ear edema model. Results: LSEO (200 and 20 mg/kg) was able to significantly reduce ($p < 0.05$) the carrageenan-induced paw edema with a similar effect to that observed for the positive control. Topical application of LSEO at doses of 82 and 410 mg/kg significantly reduced acute ear edema in 51.4% and 80.1% of the mice, respectively. Histological analysis confirmed that LSEO inhibited the skin inflammatory response. Moreover, LSEO was tested for its antitumor activity against different cancer cell lines. LSEO was found to be significantly active against human gastric adenocarcinoma (AGS), Melanoma MV3, and breast carcinoma MDA-MB-231 cells, with median inhibitory concentration (IC_{50}) values of 0.035 ± 0.018, 0.06 ± 0.022 and 0.259 ± 0.089 µL/mL, respectively. Altogether, these results open a new field of investigation into the characterization of the molecules involved in anti-proliferative processes. Conclusion: We suggest that LSEO, with 1,8-Cineole as the major active component, is a promising candidate for use in skin care products with anti-inflammatory and anticancer properties.

The results of this study may provide an experimental basis for further systematic research, rational development, and clinical utilization of lavender resources.

Keywords: *Lavandula stoechas* essential oil; topical anti-inflammatory effect; anticancer activity; melanoma cell lines; 1,8-Cineole

1. Introduction

Inflammation is regarded as an important baseline reaction responsible for manifestations of various chronic diseases such as cancer, septic shock, diabetes, atherosclerosis, and obesity. Tissue damage determines the development of inflammation by mechanisms that include the production of chemical mediators, the recruitment of specific cells and an increased rate of cell division. These inflammatory mediators, when present in excess, inhibit apoptosis [1] and lead to the loss of tissue homeostasis, which favors the onset of mutations that could lead to cancer development [1–4].

Recent findings have expanded the concept that inflammation is a serious component of cancer growth and progression. Chronic inflammation has been associated to several steps involved in carcinogenesis, comprising cellular alteration, promotion, proliferation, invasion, angiogenesis, and metastasis [3]. Many cancers arise from sites of infection, chronic irritation, and inflammation. It is now becoming clear that the tumor microenvironment, which is largely orchestrated by inflammatory cells, is an indispensable participant in the neoplastic process, fostering proliferation, survival, and migration [3]. In some types of cancer, the inflammatory process is present before a malignant change occurs; however, in other types of cancer, an oncogenic change induces an inflammatory micro-environment that promotes the development of tumors [1,2].

In this context, drug discoveries of new agents with anti-inflammatory and anticancer properties have a unique interest for medical care. Several in vivo and in vitro models of inflammation and cancer have been used for the discovery of new therapeutic agents. The identification of antitumor or anticancer properties could test the drug in different cancer cell lines with a principal objective of separating features associated with cytotoxic effect toward many cell lines from those that affect only a specific cell type [5–7].

Many traditional medicines, phytochemical extracts, essential oils (EOs), and volatile constituents extracted from aromatic herbs and medicinal plants have been widely used as anti-inflammatory, antitumor, antioxidant, and antimicrobial agents for the prevention and treatment of different human diseases [2,5,8]. Several studies have demonstrated the anti-inflammatory and anticancer activities of products derived from plants, such as EOs. Many cytotoxic molecules that are of plant origin are widely used in chemotherapy [2,9]. EOs from some Lamiaceae species, such as lavender, have shown effectiveness in these processes [5,10].

Algeria is a country with many unknown plants whose compounds could be used in medicine [8]. Among the various plants with putative pharmacological properties, lavender species are common in Algeria. The genus *Lavandula* consists of approximately 20 species with more than 100 varieties of lavender. *Lavandula stoechas*, locally known as "El Halhal", is an evergreen shrub, and it usually grows up to one meter high with spike violet flowers. *L. stoechas*, or wild lavender, is one of the plants with aromatic leaves and attractive bracts at the top of the flowers. It grows in western Mediterranean countries, Algeria, Tunisia, Italy, France, Spain, Turkey, and India [8,11–13].

Lavandula is an important genus of the Lamiaceae family that comprises EO-producing plants relevant to the food, cosmetic, perfumery, and pharmaceutical industries. *Lavandula stoechas* essential oils (LSEO) from lavender plants have been used for the first aid cure of wounds, abscesses, and burns [11,13]. Recently, Rahmati et al. [14] and Rafiee et al. [15] demonstrated anxiolytic, sedative, and antispasmodic activities. The chemical composition and antimicrobial evaluation of LSEO have been the subject of several studies over the years [12,16,17]. However, there are very few detailed publications on its anti-inflammatory and anticancer properties. To our knowledge, the EO of *L. stoechas* grown in the Cherchell region (North-Center of Algeria) has not yet been reported in the literature. Taking this into account, the present research was designed to evaluate, for the first time, the in vitro anticancer activity of Algerian LSEO against different cancer cell lines as well as its in vitro and in vivo topical and acute anti-inflammatory properties.

2. Results and Discussion

2.1. Chemical Composition of Lavandula stoechas Essential Oil

We used EO extracted from the aerial parts of *Lavandula stoechas*. Determination of the chemical composition of LSEO was done using gas chromatography-mass spectrometry (GC-MS), and quantitative and qualitative compositions are shown in Table 1 and Figure 1.

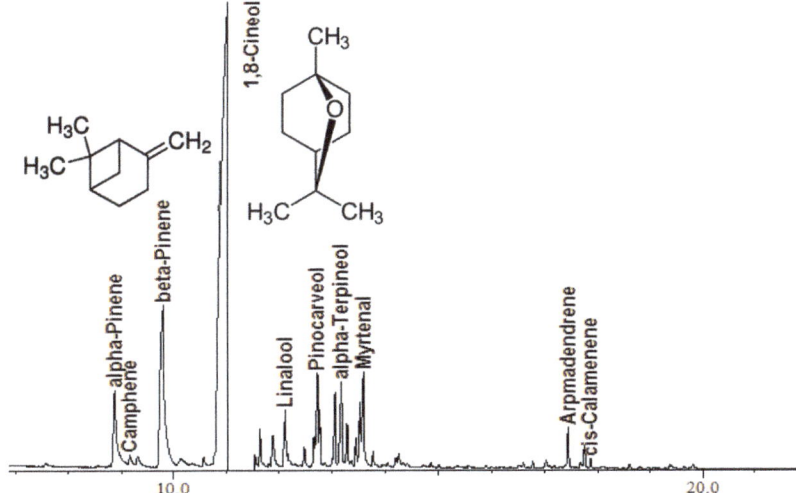

Figure 1. The chemical profile of *Lavandula stoechas* essential oil extracted using steam distillation. (X-axis in minutes).

Different constituents were detected and quantified, and 21 compounds were identified. The LSEO consisted mainly of oxygenated monoterpenes (79.23%) and low amounts of hydrocarbons (1.84%). Eucalyptol (1,8-cineole) was found to be the major component (61.36%), followed by β-pinene (13.83%) and α-pinene (4.75%). Other compounds were detected but were less than 3% (Table 1). Thus, LSEO from Algeria extracted by steam distillation may be classified as a "Eucalyptol Chemotype".

L. stoechas has been the object of several phytochemical studies that have pointed out a high chemical variability, allowing the establishment of several chemotypes. LSEO is characterized by significant variations in the amounts of fenchone, camphor, and 1,8-cineole, and the fenchone/camphor chemotype is the most commonly identified [8,17,18].

Our findings are in discordance with others carried out on *Lavandula stoechas* collected from other regions worldwide [16,17,19]. Indeed, others studies reported the richness of LSEO in fenchone and camphor as the major constituents. Vokou et al. [16] reported that *L. stoechas* is rich in EO, and the principal compounds were fenchone (41%), 1,8-cineole (29%), and α-pinene (1.6%). Ristorcelli et al. [20] reported the chemical composition of the EOs from 50 samples of *L. stoechas* from different areas of Corsica (France) during the flowering stage; they found important variations in the major constituents: fenchone, 15–75%; camphor, 2–56%; and 1,8-cineole, 1–8%. The variations detected in LSEO between our research and others are surely related to the disparity in the area of collection. This may be explained by the influence of the external environment on the synthesis and regulation of secondary metabolism pathways in medicinal plants. In fact, the chemical composition of medicinal flora differs with phenological transformations, harvestings area, collected parts, and methods of distillation [13,19].

Table 1. Chemical composition of the volatile oil extracted from *Lavandula stoechas* using a steam distillation method.

Retention Time (min)	Name	%
8.874	α-Pinene	4.75
9.155	Camphene	0.35
9.808	β-Pinene	13.83
11.031	1,8-Cineole	61.36
11.640	*cis*-Linalool oxide	0.92
11.887	*trans*-Linalool oxide	1.39
12.114	Linalool	1.63
12.475	α-Campholenal	0.44
12.734	Pinocarveol	2.12
12.778	Camphor	0.63
13.067	Pinocarvone	2.04
13.181	α-Terpineol	3.15
13.288	Terpineol-4	0.96
13.453	Cryptone	0.59
13.532	α-Terpineol	1.14
13.598	Myrtenal	2.36
13.781	Verbenone	0.29
14.261	Carvone	0.21
17.442	Aromadendrene	0.98
17.749	δ-Elemene	0.66
17.863	*cis*-Calamenene	0.20
	Oxygenated Monoterpenes	79.23
	Monoterene Hydrocarbons	18.93
	Sesquiterpene Hydrocarbons	1.84

2.2. Anti-Inflammatory Activity In Vitro

2.2.1. Irritation Test in Red Blood Cell System Cellular Model

The results of in vitro anti-inflammatory activity determined by the human red blood cell membrane stabilization method were shown in Table 2. The LSEO showed a concentration dependent anti-inflammatory activity, and the protection percent increased with an increase in the concentration of the samples. At a concentration of 3 µL/mL, the LSEO produced 74.471 ± 0.465% inhibition of human red blood cells (HRBC) hemolysis ($p < 0.05$) as compared with 27.552 ± 3.354% produced by standard NSAID sodium diclofenac. However, when comparing IC_{50} values, it is clear from the data that sodium diclofenac showed greater response than LSEO.

The LSEO exhibited a membrane stabilization effect by inhibiting hypotonicity-induced lysis of HRBC membrane. This membrane is analogous to the lysosomal membrane and its stabilization implies that the LSEO may stabilize lysosomal membranes as well. Stabilization of lysosomal membrane is essential in decreasing the inflammatory reaction by stopping the discharge of lysosomal components of activated neutrophil such as bactericidal enzymes and proteases, which cause further tissue inflammation and destruction upon extracellular release [21,22]. Although the exact mechanism of the membrane stabilization by the LSEO extract is not known yet, hypotonicity-induced hemolysis may arise from shrinkage of the cells due to osmotic loss of intracellular electrolyte and fluid components. The LSEO may inhibit the processes, which may stimulate or enhance the efflux of these intracellular components [23]. Karthik et al. [24] have reported that the lavender EO presented RBC membrane stabilization action by preventing hypotonicity-induced lysis of erythrocyte membrane. Both the lavender EO and the positive control (NSAID) displayed anti-inflammatory activity, but the NSAID being more effective. Erythrocyte membrane stabilization is an important mechanism to inhibit the leakage of cellular constituents (protein and fluids) into the tissues during a time of increased penetrability initiated by inflammatory mediators.

Table 2. Effect of LSEO on stabilization of HRBC membrane in vitro.

Treatment	Concentration	Absorbance (560 nm)	% Inhibition of Hemolysis	IC_{50} [#]
Control (PBS)		0.568	-	-
LSEO (µL/mL)	6	0.370	34.917 ± 1.939 [D]	6.214 ± 0.776 [B]
	3	0.145	74.471 ± 0.465 [C]	
	1.5	0.064	88.791 ± 0.101 [B]	
	0.8	0.042	92.605 ± 0.000 [A]	
	0.4	0.042	92.605 ± 0.465 [A]	
Sodium diclofenac (mg/mL)	30	0.46	19.014 ± 12.707 [F]	1.198 ± 0.735 [A]
	3	0.411	27.552 ± 3.354 [E]	
	0.3	0.045	92.165 ± 0.419 [A]	
	0.03	0.041	92.693 ± 0.227 [A]	
	0.003	0.04	92.913 ± 0.221 [A]	

Each value represents the mean ± SD. LSEO: *Lavandula stoechas* Essential Oil. IC_{50}: Median Inhibitory Concentration; HRBC: Human Red Blood Cells; PBS: phosphate-buffered saline. [#] Means within the same column followed by the same letter are not significantly different ($p > 0.05$) according to ANOVA analysis followed by Tukey's post hoc multiple comparison tests.

2.2.2. Inhibition of Denaturation of Bovine Serum Albumin

Denaturation of protein is a recognized source of inflammation. Therefore, as part of the examination to assess the anti-inflammatory mechanism of LSEO, its aptitude to inhibit BSA denaturation was calculated. The inhibitory action of different concentration of LSEO on BSA denaturation is shown in Table 3. It has been found that denaturation of BSA is inhibited by several NSAIDs such as indomethacin and salicylic acid, proving this assay to be useful in the detection of other anti-inflammatory compounds. It was detected from this assay that eucalyptol rich fraction of LSEO presented a dose-dependent maximum inhibition of denaturation of BSA of 72.625 ± 2.56% at 0.4 µL/mL and a standard NSAID (sodium diclofenac) revealed maximum inhibition of 76.117 ± 0.534% at the 0.01 mg/mL. On the basis of these results, LSEO showed significant anti-inflammatory activity (IC_{50} = 2.447 ± 0.873 µL/mL, $p < 0.05$) as compared to NSAID control (IC_{50} = 8.260 ± 0.943 µL/mL), and suggests that LSEO has potential anti-inflammatory activity.

The most commonly used drugs for management of inflammatory conditions are NSAIDs and steroids, which have several adverse effects, especially gastric irritation leading to formation of gastric ulcers [21–23]. Denaturation of tissue proteins is one of the well-documented causes of inflammation. The preliminary screening with the BSA assay indicated that LSEO has significant levels of protection against heat denaturation of the protein. Therefore, protection against protein denaturation, which was the central mechanism of action of NSAIDs, could play an important part in anti-rheumatic and anti-inflammatory actions. The anti-inflammatory effect of EOs may be due to the presence of oxygenated monoterpenes such as eucalyptol and linalool either singly or in combination [23,25].

Table 3. Effect of LSEO on heat-induced protein denaturation.

Treatment	Concentration	Absorbance (560 nm)	% Inhibition of BSA	IC_{50} [#]
Control (PBS)		1.288	-	-
LSEO (µL/mL)	6	0.067	62.569 ± 0.967 [E]	2.447 ± 0.873 [A]
	3	0.061	65.735 ± 0.853 [D]	
	1.5	0.054	69.832 ± 0.558 [C]	
	0.8	0.048	73.184 ± 0.558 [B]	
	0.4	0.049	72.625 ± 2.560 [B]	
Sodium diclofenac (mg/mL)	10	0.165	7.960 ± 7.741 [F]	8.260 ± 0.943 [B]
	1	0.04	77.932 ± 0.721 [A]	
	0.1	0.044	75.279 ± 2.555 [A]	
	0.01	0.043	76.117 ± 0.534 [A]	
	0.001	0.045	74.720 ± 0.279 [AB]	

Each value represents the mean ± SD. LSEO: *Lavandula stoechas* Essential Oil. IC_{50}: Median Inhibitory Concentration; BSA: Bovine Serum Albumin. [#] Means within the same column followed by the same letter are not significantly different ($p > 0.05$) according to ANOVA analysis followed by Tukey's post hoc multiple comparison tests.

2.3. In Vivo Anti-Inflammatory Activity Assay

2.3.1. Carrageenan-Induced Paw Edema

Carrageenan-induced mice paw edema is often used to evaluate the anti-inflammatory effect of diverse natural bioactive compounds such as phytochemical extracts and EO. The anti-inflammatory activity of orally administered LSEO (2, 20, and 200 mg/kg) was determined using the same paw edema model. As shown in Table 4, in comparison with the NSAID indomethacin, LSEO exhibited a significantly high anti-inflammatory activity in a dose-dependent manner.

Table 4. In vivo anti-inflammatory effect of LSEO using carrageenan induced-paw edema.

Treatment (Dose µg/kg)	Weight (mean, mg) ± SD			% Inhibition of Edema
	Left Hind Paw	Right Hind Paw	Edema Weight [#]	
LSEO (200)	126.10 ± 8.00	110.12 ± 7.12	15.975 ± 7.31 [A]	47.0588
LSEO (20)	138.48 ± 10.1	121.00 ± 6.72	17.480 ± 8.71 [A]	42.0712
LSEO (2)	146.08 ± 8.61	122.35 ± 6.00	23.733 ± 9.22 [A,B]	21.3476
Positive control (Indomethacin)	161.25 ± 6.12	144.50 ± 6.18	16.750 ± 7.50 [A]	44.4904
Negative control	154.30 ± 7.65	124.12 ± 10.0	30.175 ± 13.41 [B]	/

Groups of animals ($n = 5$ mice per group) were pretreated with vehicle, Indomethacin (25 mg/kg, p.o.) or LSEO at doses of 2, 20, and 200 mg/kg *per os* (p.o.) 30 min before carrageenan-induced paw edema. LSEO: *Lavandula stoechas* Essential Oil. [#] Means within the same column followed by the same capital letter are not significantly different ($p > 0.05$) according to ANOVA analysis followed by Tukey's post hoc multiple comparison test.

At 4 h after oral administration of LSEO, the degree of edema inhibition was similar for 20 mg/kg and 200 mg/kg (42.07% and 47.06%, respectively). This level of edema inhibition was comparable to the level observed using 25 mg/kg of the standard reference NSAID (44.5%).

Inflammatory illnesses are presently treated with steroidal and NSAIDs. Unfortunately, both of these widely prescribed treatment classes have important harmful side effects and fail in certain segments of the population [23]. Therefore, there is a need to develop and produce new treatments with novel mechanisms of action that do not generate significant side effects. It has been reported that a variety of EOs exhibit noticeable anti-inflammatory properties in numerous diverse models of inflammation. Investigations on the anti-inflammatory action of LSEO are limited. Only one research report suggested the aptitude of *Lavandula angustifolia* EO to reduce the carrageenan-induced paw edema in animals at doses of 200 mg/kg, even though the mode of action was not addressed in this publication [12]. The precise mechanism of the anti-inflammatory activity of the LSEO is unclear. Nevertheless, it has been reported that a number of constituents contribute to the incomplete reduction of the release of inflammation mediators. In recent years, numerous studies have reported oxygenated mono- and sesquiterpenes and their hydrocarbon derivatives as the main compounds of EOs, which have effective anti-inflammatory activity [5,26]. In our study, 1,8-cineole (eucalyptol) has been found to be the major compound in LSEO. It appears that 1,8-cineole can be partially linked with the observed pharmacological activity, but it is not apparent if the other oxygenated monoterpenes (fenchone, pinene) can also potentiate this effect. Our results are in agreement with those published for other EOs rich in 1,8-cineole that demonstrated a potent and strong anti-edematogenic effect [12,26,27]. They revealed that the EOs, which are rich in 1,8-cineole, showed analgesic and anti-inflammatory properties. Eucalyptol also exhibits an inhibitory effect in a number of tests of experimental inflammation in animals, using the carrageenan-induced paw edema test [26]. These activities may be linked with the aptitude of eucalyptol to suppress the arachidonic acid metabolism and cytokine production in human monocytes [27].

2.3.2. Xylene-Induced Ear Edema

Because the LSEO demonstrated an anti-inflammatory effect in the carrageenan-induced paw edema assay, the anti-inflammatory activity of LSEO was further evaluated by the inhibition of xylene-induced ear edema in mice. Topical application of xylene on the left ears caused noticeable edema as indicated by the augmentation in the earplug weight of the left ear compared with the untreated right ear (Table 5).

Table 5. *Lavandula stoechas* aromatic oil prevents xylene-induced ear edema in mice.

Treatment (Dose mg/kg)	Weight (mean, mg) ± SD			% Inhibition of Edema
	Left Ear	Right Ear	Edema Weight [#]	
LSEO (820)	22.97 ± 4.13	16.52 ± 0.73	6.45 ± 2.80 [B]	25.8620
LSEO (410)	16.37 ± 1.92	14.65 ± 2.22	1.72 ± 1.20 [A]	80.1724
LSEO (82)	22.72 ± 5.16	18.50 ± 1.99	4.22 ± 2.88 [B]	51.4367
Betasone® 0.5%	18.08 ± 2.79	15.50 ± 1.50	2.58 ± 1.49 [A,B]	70.3448
Voltarene Emulgel® 1%	20.70 ± 4.94	13.32 ± 1.35	7.38 ± 3.17 [B]	15.1724
Negative control (Vehicle)	28.10 ± 6.12	19.40 ± 4.13	8.70 ± 3.55 [C]	/

Data are presented as Mean (mg) ± Standard Deviation (SD) ($n = 5$ mice per group). LSEO: *Lavandula stoechas* Essential Oil. [#] Means within the same column followed by the same capital letter are not significantly different ($p > 0.05$) according to ANOVA one way analysis followed by Tukey's post hoc multiple comparison test.

In comparison with positive control (diclofenac topical gel), LSEO exhibited a powerful and effective anti-inflammatory activity in our experimental animal model. Diclofenac gel (Voltarène emulgène® 1%) produced 15.17% inhibition of xylene-induced edema, and this effect was statistically different and lower ($p < 0.05$) than that observed with all tested doses of LSEO. Further, LSEO reduced the inflammatory response by 80.1% for 410 mg/kg, which is higher than the positive control (Betasone) (70.3%). To the best of our knowledge, this is the first study to prove that LSEO has a significant topical anti-inflammatory activity in vivo. Consistent with current data, our previous report [28] showed that topical application of EOs can limit the inflammatory symptoms of edema and neutrophil accumulation. In phytotherapy, dermal application of EOs in a full body massage or to limited parts of the body is greatly pleasing. Many EOs are used as curative ingredients for inflammatory indications with lesional neutrophil accumulation: aphthous stomatitis, rheumatoid arthritis, and lesional fungal or bacterial contagions [8,11,29].

2.3.3. Mouse Ear Tissue Morphology

We investigated H&E-stained ear sections from xylene-induced animals (Figure 2). Xylene is a highly irritating substance that stimulated an inflammatory response in the epidermis. Xylene application resulted in a noticeable increase in ear thickness with obvious confirmation of edema, epidermal hyperplasia, and inflammatory cell infiltration in the dermis with associated connective tissue disruption (Figure 2D1,D2).

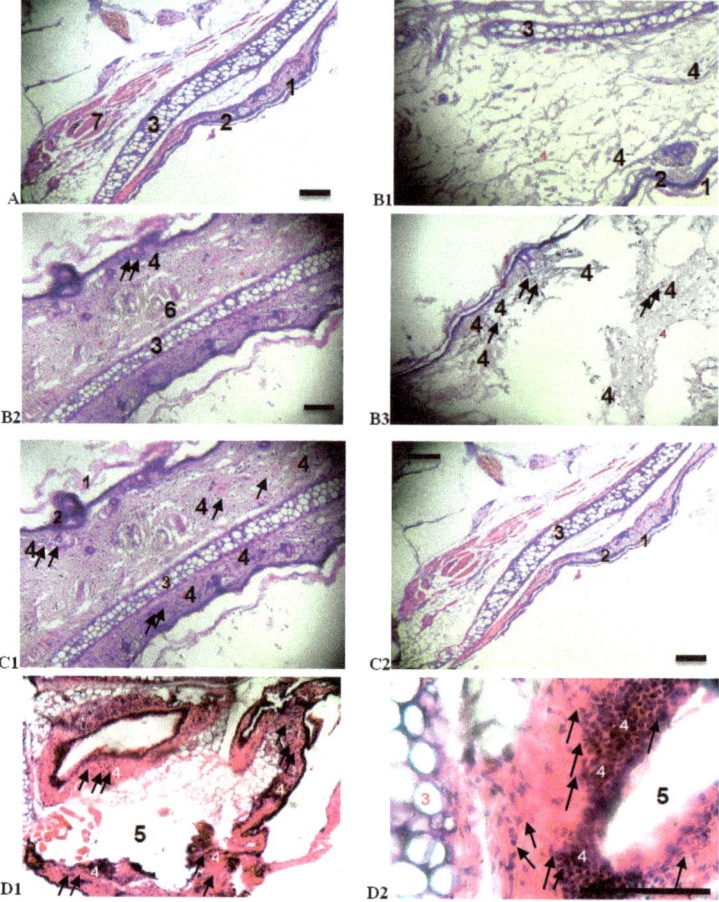

Figure 2. Sections of mice ear biopsies showing keratin, epidermal, dermal, muscle, and cartilage layers. Hematoxylin & Eosin stained sections were scored as mild (+), modest (++), and severe (+++) for edema and substantial inflammatory polymorphonuclear (PMN) cell infiltration in the dermis inflammation phase. (1) Keratin; (2) epidermal layer; (3) cartilage layer; (4) PMN; (5) edema; (6) muscle. (**A**) Right ear without treatment (×10). (**B**) *Lavandula stoechas* Essential Oil (LSEO) treatment with different doses (**B1**): LSEO 82 mg/kg (G × 10), (**B2**): LSEO 410 mg/kg (G × 10), (**B3**): LSEO 810 mg/kg (G × 10)) = edema (±); inflammatory cell infiltration (+), inflammation phase (±). (**C**) Positive control treatment (**C1**): Voltarène Emulgel (G × 10); (**C2**): betamethasone (G × 40) = edema (±); inflammatory cell infiltration (+), inflammation phase (±). (**D1**) Negative control (×10) = edema (++); inflammation phase (+++); inflammatory cell infiltration (+++) in epidermal and dermal layers, muscle, and cartilage. (**D2**) Negative control (×40). Scale − bar = 25 µm; black arrow indicates inflammatory polymorphonuclear cell infiltration.

By histological comparison, topical application of LSEO decreased ear thickness and associated pathological indicators to an extent comparable to the positive controls (sodium diclofenac and betamethasone gels) (Figure 2B,C). These findings directly demonstrate the properties of LSEO within the target tissue, providing additional confirmation that LSEO ameliorates xylene-induced contact dermatitis. Microscopic investigation showed the valuable anti-inflammatory activity of the topical application with LSEO. Compared to the control groups, edema was dramatically reduced by the previous topical treatment with LSEO (Figure 2A vs. Figure 2B). To the best of our knowledge, this is the first study to reveal that LSEO has a significant topical anti-inflammatory activity, which is confirmed by histology examination.

Current results are consistent with previous publications about other EOs using the carrageenan and xylene-induced edema methods [29–31]. In addition, the current results are in agreement with our previous research [32], in which histological analysis revealed that rose-scented geranium oil inhibited the skin inflammatory process in vivo. In conclusion, the results of our investigation support the traditional usage of LSEO as an anti-inflammatory agent, although there is a need for further investigations to better estimate its pharmaceutical potential and understand its mode of action.

2.4. Effects of LSEO on Cytotoxicity of Three Human Tumor Cell Lines

Because anti-proliferative screening models in vitro provide important preliminary data to help select compounds with potential antineoplastic properties for further study, the LSEO was tested in vitro for its potential human tumor cell growth inhibitory effect on human breast carcinoma MDA-MB-231, human gastric cancer AGS, and human melanoma MV3, using MTT assay. This is a non-radioactive, fast, and economical assay widely used to quantify cell viability and proliferation. As shown in Figure 3, LSEO had selective cytotoxicity on different tumor cells, and a potent anti-proliferative effect on AGS cells with IC_{50} value of 0.035 ± 0.018 µL/mL. This potent in vitro antitumor effect was also shown in MV3 and MDA-MB-231 cell assays, with IC_{50}s of 0.06 ± 0.022 µL/mL and 0.259 ± 0.089 µL/mL, respectively. To the best of our knowledge, this is the first report on the anti-proliferative activity of LSEO.

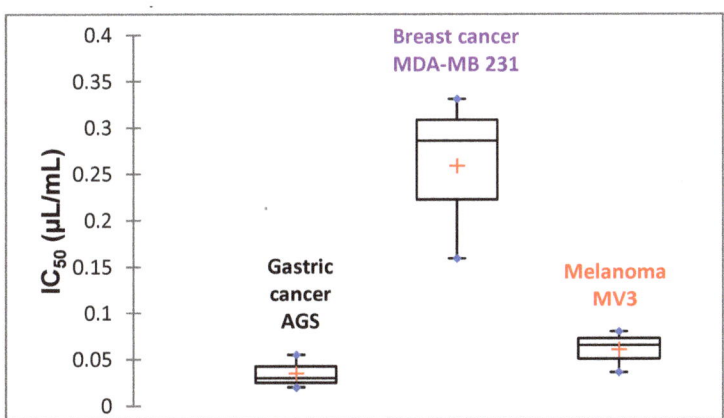

Figure 3. In vitro cytotoxic effect of LSEO against different cancer cell lines using MTT assay. IC_{50}: Median inhibitory concentration. Experiments were performed three times in octuplets.

It is shown in Figure 4 that LSEO has an important dose-dependent cytotoxic effect against all cancer cell lines tested. At higher concentration (4 µL/mL *v/v*), LSEO was more cytotoxic against AGS cells (88.1% lysis) than MV3 cells ((86.4% lysis) and MDA-MB-231 cells (79.5% lysis). At low concentration (0.032 µL/mL *v/v*) of LSEO, this same order of sensitivity was also obtained. AGS was the most sensitive cancer cells (80.8%) at the low concentration.

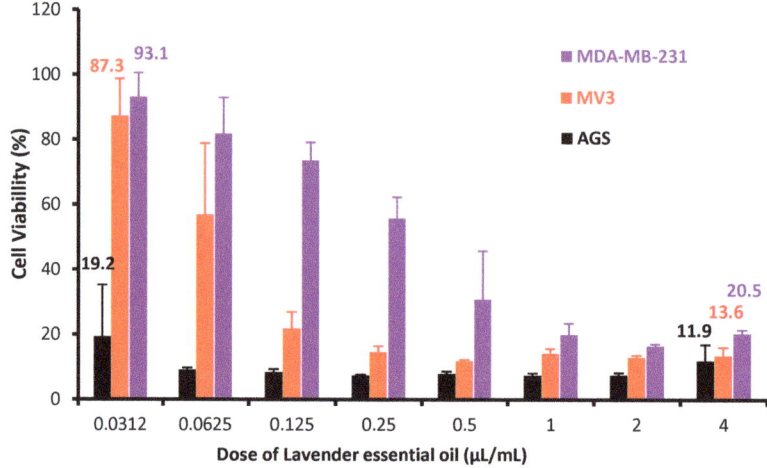

Figure 4. Anti-proliferative activity of LSEO after 24 h of exposure in the MTT assay. MDA-MB-231: human breast carcinoma cells; MV3: human melanoma; AGS: human gastric cancer. Experiments were performed three times in octuplets.

A previous investigation of another lavender species (*L. angustifolia*) EO showed cytotoxicity to human skin cells in vitro at a concentration of 0.25% (*v/v*) [10]. As we did not evaluate the cytotoxic effect of all chemicals present in LSEO against the three cancer cell lines, it is not possible to identify which of these compounds are responsible for the observed results. It appears from this analysis that EOs containing a high amount of eucalyptol are more cytotoxic than the others [33]. These results are in agreement with those of other authors who reported that the eucalyptol (1,8-cineole) has an important antitumor effect against tumor cell lines like hormone-refractory prostate cancer [7] and drug-resistant human lung cancer [6]. Specific induction of apoptosis, not necrosis, was observed in human colon cancer cell lines HCT116 and RKO by 1,8-cineole. The treatment with 1,8-cineole was associated with inactivation of survivin and Akt and activation of p38. These molecules induced cleaved poly(ADP-ribose) polymerase (PARP) and caspase-3, finally causing apoptosis. In xeno-transplanted SCID mice, the 1,8-cineole group showed significantly inhibited tumor progression compared to a control group [33,34]. On the other hand, Tayarani-Najaran et al. [35] studied the cytotoxicity and the mechanisms of cell death induced by the EO of *Lavandula angustifolia*, and were compared with both normal (human fibroblast cells) and malignant cancerous human cells (HeLa Human cervix carcinoma and MCF-7 lung adenocarcinoma cell lines). They found that the IC_{50} for normal cells was higher (>500 µg/mL) than that reported with cancer cell lines (IC_{50} HeLa = 31.92 µg/mL; IC_{50} HeLa = 31.92 µg/mL); thus, confirming a higher sensitivity of tumor cells as compared to normal cells.

LSEO with an anti-proliferative activity shows also in vitro and in vivo anti-inflammatory properties. Even though there is a relationship between these two activities, the various mechanisms involved for each EO could explain why there is variability of these effects. A link between inflammation and cancer has long been suspected, but its molecular nature remains to be defined. Chronic inflammation may directly affect the cells that eventually become transformed as well as exert indirect effects on the tumor cell through surrounding cells [4,36,37]. In summary, the cytotoxic activity of LSEO might be due to the synergic effects of different terpenes in the oil, or perhaps there are some other active compounds responsible for the cytotoxic activity of the essential oil, which deserves attention in the future.

3. Materials and Methods

3.1. Material

3.1.1. Extraction of *Lavandula stoechas* Essential Oil

Lavandula stoechas (Lamiaceae family) aerial parts were collected in 2016 in the region of Cherchell (Tipaza, Algeria). This area is located in the western region of Algiers and is situated at 36°34′3.014″ N and 12′14.376″ E in the central north of the country. LSEO was distilled from the leaves, stems, and flowers using alembic steam distillation. The process consists of passing water vapor at a high-pressure through an alembic (tank) filled with aromatic plants. The steam captures the volatile compounds that are confined in the secretory glands of the aromatic herb, which then pass through a cold-water frozen serpentine and condense into a liquid. Upon exit, phases of diverse densities are separated with the help of a "Florentine vase" and floral water and EO (also named "aromatic water") are obtained.

3.1.2. Solvents, Drugs and Chemicals

The following drugs and chemicals purchased from Sigma Chemical Co. (St. Louis, MO, USA) were used: dimethyl sulfoxide (DMSO), bovine serum albumin (BSA), sodium diclofenac, phosphate-buffered saline (PBS, 10 mM, pH 7.4), sterile saline solution (0.9% w/v NaCl), Alsever solution (2% dextrose, 0.8% sodium citrate, 0.5% citric acid, and 0.42% NaCl), 3-(4,5-dimethylthiazol-2yl)-2,5-diphenyl-tetrazolium bromide (MTT), xylene, Tween 80, acetone, and formaldehyde solutions. Voltarène emulgène® 1% (diethylamine diclofenac, Novartis, Algeria), Betasone® 0.05% (Betamethasone, Saidal Pharmaceuticals, Algiers, Algeria), and Indomet® 25 mg (Indomethacin, Saidal Pharmaceuticals, Algiers, Algeria) were also used. Roswell Park Memorial Institute (RPMI)-1640 medium and other cell-culture reagents including fetal bovine serum (FBS), penicillin, streptomycin, and amphotericin B were obtained from Gibco Inc. (Grand Island, NY, USA).

3.1.3. Animals

Swiss albino NMRI (The Naval Medical Research Institute, Institut Pasteur d'Algérie, Algiers, Algeria) mice of both sexes, weighing from 24–28 g and pathogen free, were obtained from animal breeding of the R&D Center of Saidal Pharmaceuticals and from the "Laboratoire National de Contrôle des Produits Pharmaceutiques" (Algiers, Algeria), respectively. The animals were left for 3 days at room conditions for acclimatization. A minimum of 5 animals were used in each group, and were kept at room temperature with a 12 h light/dark cycle. They were maintained on a standard pellet diet and water *ad libitum* throughout the experiment. The pellets for mice have been purchased from a commercial producer (National Livestock Food Office, Algiers, Algeria). Below is the composition of the pellets: Carbohydrates: 49.8%; Crude Protein: 23.5%; Crude Fat: 5.0%; Crude Fiber: 5.5%; Acid Insoluble Ash: 6.5%; Calcium: 1.1%; Phosphorus: 0.8%; Moisture: 12%; Vitamin A (UI/kg): 22,000; Vitamin D (UI/kg): 2000; Vitamin E (UI/kg): 100. All animal experiments have been conducted in accordance with directives approved by current institutional guidelines (Saidal Pharmaceuticals, Algiers, Algeria) for animal treatment (88-08/1988) and approved by the Council of the European Union (2010/63/EU) on the Protection of Animals Used for Scientific Purposes.

3.1.4. Cancer Cell Lines

Three human cancer cell lines were used. MDA-MB-231 cells, which are estrogen receptor-negative human breast cancer; human melanoma MV3 cells derived from lymph node with a high metastatic potential; and human gastric adenocarcinoma (AGS) cells. Cell lines were obtained from the American Type Culture Collection (ATCC, Manassas, VA, USA). Cells were maintained as a monolayer culture in the RPMI-1640 nutrient medium and were grown at 37 °C in a humidified chamber with 5% CO_2 as monolayer adherent cultures in 75 cm² tissue culture flasks, in a medium supplemented with 10% FBS, 1% penicillin, and 1% streptomycin.

3.2. Methods

3.2.1. Determination of the Chemical Composition of Essential Oil

Analysis and identification of the volatile compounds were performed using a Shimadzu GC-17A Gas Chromatograph coupled with a Shimadzu QP-5050A Mass Spectrometer detector (Shimadzu Corporation, Kyoto, Japan). The GC-MS system was equipped with a Tracsil Meta.X5 (95% dimethylpolysiloxane and 5% diphenylpolysiloxane) column (60 m × 0.25 mm, 0.25 µm film thickness). Analyses were carried out using helium as the carrier gas at a column flow rate of 0.3 mL/min and a total flow of 3.9 mL/min in a split ratio of 1:200 and the following program: (a) 80 °C for 0 min; (b) increase of 3 °C/min from 80 °C to 210 °C and hold for 1 min; (c) increase of 25 °C/min from 210 °C to 300 °C and hold for 3 min. The temperatures of the injector and detector were 230 °C and 300 °C, respectively. All compounds were identified using two different analytical methods: (1) comparison of experimental retention indexes (RI) with those of the literature; (2) mass spectra (authentic chemicals and National Institute of Standards and Technology (NIST05) spectral library collection). Only fully identified compounds are reported in this study.

3.2.2. In Vitro and In Vivo Anti-Inflammatory Activities

Anti-Inflammatory Test Using Erythrocyte System Cellular Model In Vitro

Preparation of blood samples for membrane stabilization assays: the human red blood cells (HRBC) membrane stabilization method has been used as a method to study the in vitro anti-inflammatory activity [23]. Human venous blood samples were freshly collected under informed consent from a healthy human volunteer, and put into test tubes containing anticoagulant (EDTA-Na_2 10%) and mixed with equal volume of Alsever solution. Blood samples were centrifuged at 2500 rpm for 5 min and the supernatant was removed. The cell suspension was washed with sterile saline solution and centrifuged at 2500 rpm for 5 min. This was repeated three times until the supernatant was clear and colorless and the packed cell volume was measured. The cellular component was reconstituted to a 40% suspension (v/v) with PBS (10 mM, pH 7.4) and was used in the assays.

Hypotonicity-induced hemolysis: Different concentrations of LSEO (6–0.4 µL/mL) were prepared using distilled water, and to each concentration 1 mL of PBS, 2 mL hyposaline and 0.5 mL of HRBC suspension were added. It was incubated at 37 °C for 30 min and centrifuged at 3000 rpm for 20 min. The hemoglobin content of the supernatant solution was estimated spectrophotometrically at 560 nm. Sodium diclofenac as a non-steroidal anti-inflammatory drug (NSAID) was used as a reference standard and a control was prepared by omitting the LSEO. The percentage inhibition of hemolysis or membrane stabilization was calculated according to the method described by Parvin et al. [21].

$$\text{Inhibition of hemolysis (\%)} = \left(\frac{A1 - A2 \text{ sample}}{A1} \right) \times 100$$

where: A1 = optical density of hypotonic-buffered saline solution alone and A2 = optical density of test sample in hypotonic solution.

Anti-Inflammatory Activity Using the Inhibition of Denaturation of Albumin In Vitro

The capability of LSEO to inhibit the denaturation of BSA was investigated by a method as reported by Rahman et al. [22]. Typically, different concentrations (6–0.4 µL/mL) of LSEO were prepared and the volumes were adjusted to 2.5 mL with 0.85% NaCl. Then 0.5 mL of BSA (5 mg/mL) was added. The mixture was incubated at 37 °C for 20 min and further incubated at 55 °C for 30 min. The tubes were cooled and 2.5 mL of 0.5 M PBS (pH 6.3) was added. The turbidity was measured spectrophotometrically at 560 nm. The assay was carried out in triplicates and the standard (sodium diclofenac) was used in place of the LSEO. Percentage inhibition of BSA denaturation was evaluated as follow:

$$\% \text{ Inhibition} = \left(\frac{\text{Abs Control} - \text{Abs Test}}{\text{Abs Control}}\right) \times 100$$

In Vivo Anti-Inflammatory Assay Using Carrageenan-Induced Paw Edema

This technique is based on a report by Bouhlali et al. [23]. Carrageenan is known to result in at least neutrophil-linked edematous inflammation. LSEO was diluted in 0.5% Tween 80 and administered 30 min prior to carrageenan injection. The control group received an equivalent volume of the vehicle (0.5% Tween 80 in 0.9% NaCl solution). LSEO at doses of 2, 20, or 200 mg/kg and vehicle were administrated *per os* (*p.o.*) 30 min before injecting the carrageenan. Paw edema was induced with a single 0.1 mL sub-plantar injection of carrageenan (0.1 mL) into the left hind paw of conscious mice. Indomethacin (25 mg/kg, *p.o.*) was used as positive control (NSAID). The mice were sacrificed 4 h later. The difference in weight between right untreated and left treated hind paws was calculated and results are expressed as the increase in paw weight (mg). The percentage inhibition of the inflammatory response was calculated for each mouse by comparison to the negative control, and calculated using the following formula:

$$\% \text{ Inhibition of edema} = \left(1 - \frac{\Delta Pt}{\Delta Pc}\right) \times 100$$

where ΔPt is the difference in paw weight in the drug-treated group, and ΔPc is the difference in paw weight in the control group.

In Vivo Anti-Inflammatory Activity Using Xylene-Induced Ear Edema

Topical anti-inflammatory activity was assessed as inhibition of xylene-induced ear edema in mice [23]. Male Swiss mice were divided into groups of 5 mice each. Thirty min after the dermal application of LSEO, 10 μL acetone solution containing 10% xylene was carefully applied to the anterior and posterior surfaces of the left ear. The right ear remained untreated. Vehicle (sweet almond oil), doses of LSEO diluted in almond oil (82, 410, and 820 mg/kg), and positive controls (Voltaren® Emulgel 1% and Betasone® 0.05%) were applied topically to the left ear about 30 min before the xylene application. At the maximum of the edematous response (4 h later), mice were sacrificed and a plug (5 mm in diameter) was removed from both treated (left) and untreated (right) ears. The edema response was calculated as the weight difference between the two plugs. LSEO anti-inflammatory potential was expressed as percentage of the edema weight reduction in treated mice in comparison to the control group, and calculated using the following formula:

$$\% \text{ Inhibition of edema} = \left(1 - \frac{\Delta Wt}{\Delta Wc}\right) \times 100$$

where ΔWt is the change in weight of ear tissue in the treated mice, and ΔWc is the change in weight of ear tissue in the control mice.

Morphological Analysis of Ear Tissue

The resulting inflammatory response was checked and monitored by measurement of edema formation and by microscopic observation. For morphological examination of cutaneous inflammation, biopsies from control and treated ears of animals were collected at the end of the experiment. Samples were fixed using 10% neutral buffered formalin, routinely processed, and sectioned at 6 μm using a microtome (Leica RM 2125RT, Nussloch, Germany). Sections were stained with Hematoxylin and Eosin (H&E) and the tissues were observed with a light microscope (Olympus CX41, Olympus, Tokyo, Japan) and graded as mild (+), moderate (++), and severe (+++) for inflammation phase. Infiltration and polymorphonuclear (PMN) cells' accumulations were also assessed [29].

3.2.3. Cytotoxic Activity Using MTT Test

MDA-MB-231, AGS, and MV3 cells were grown in RPMI-1640 medium supplemented with 10% FBS, penicillin (100 U/mL) and streptomycin (100 µg/mL). Cells were maintained at 37 °C in a humidified incubator with 5% CO_2 and regularly examined using an inverted microscope. The medium was replaced every two days and cells were sub-cultured at 70%–80% confluence. Cells in 96-well plates (100 µL/well) were exposed to different concentrations of LSEO (4 to 0.0312 µL/mL) in DMSO/RPMI (0.1% v/v) at 37 °C and 5% CO_2 for 24 h. Final DMSO concentration did not affect cell viability. The MTT colorimetric assay was used to evaluate the cytotoxic effect of LSEO [5]. MDA-MB-231, AGS, and MV3 cells were placed into 96-well culture plates (10×10^3 cells per well) and incubated for 24 h. Then, 100 µL of culture medium containing the specified concentration of the LSEO was added to each well. After exposure to serial concentrations of LSEO for 24 h at 37 °C and 5% CO_2, 100 µL of medium were carefully aspirated from each well and replaced by 100 µL of MTT solution (5 mg/mL in PBS). After addition of 100 µL PBS containing 0.5 mg/mL MTT, cells were incubated at 37 °C for 4 h. Formed formazan crystals were dissolved in 50 µL DMSO. Absorbances in the control and LSEO-treated wells were measured at 490 nm with an ELISA reader (BioTek, Winooski, VT, USA). Growth inhibition was calculated as follows:

$$\% \text{ cell viability} = \left(\frac{\text{Abs Test}}{\text{Abs Control}}\right) \times 100$$

Concentration median inhibitory concentration (IC_{50}) (µL/mL) was defined as the concentration of LSEO producing 50% inhibition of cell survival. It was determined from the cell survival diagrams.

3.2.4. Statistical Analysis

Mean values of treated groups were compared with those of a control group and analyzed using statistical methods. Data are reported as mean ± standard deviation (SD). Comparison between different groups was conducted with one-way analysis of variance (ANOVA) followed by Tukey's post hoc multiple comparison test. Differences with $p < 0.05$ between experimental groups were considered statistically significant. IC_{50} (median inhibitory concentration) was calculated from the dose response curve obtained by plotting percentage inhibition versus concentrations. Statistical data analysis was performed using XLStat 2014 software (Pro statistical software, Addinsoft, Paris, France).

4. Conclusions

In conclusion, we describe for the first time the anti-inflammatory and anticancer effects of LSEO and its chemical composition. Our results show that LSEO has important in vitro and in vivo anti-inflammatory and cytotoxic effects against melanoma, breast cancer, and gastric cancer cells. These data may serve as valuable research references for clinical research of medicines for treatment of inflammation and cancer in the future and also a tool promoting the use of therapeutic benefits of EOs. Considering that drugs currently available for the treatment of inflammatory and cancer conditions show undesirable side effects, the present results may have clinical relevance and open new possibilities for the development of novel anti-inflammatory and anticancer drugs. Further studies to elucidate the mechanisms of action, and the possible compounds involved in these activities, will be undertaken.

Author Contributions: Conception and design: M.N.B., T.S., N.H.E.D., H.C., S.A.M.; Financial support: H.C., A.B., F.O., S.A.M.; Administrative support: S.A.M., Formal analysis: M.N.B., T.S., N.H.E.D., H.C., A.H., F.B., F.O.; Provision of study materials and animals: H.C., A.B., F.O., S.A.M.; Collection and assembly of data: M.N.B., M.R., A.H., F.B.; GC-MS data analysis and interpretation: M.N.B., M.R.; Manuscript writing: M.N.B., S.A.M. Final approval of manuscript: all Authors. All authors have read and agreed to the published version of the manuscript.

Funding: This study was supported in part by the Fulbright Program Grant to Mohamed Nadjib Boukhatem, and administered by the United States Department of State, Bureau of Educational and Cultural Affairs with the cooperation of the Institute of International Education (USA).

Acknowledgments: The authors would like to thank Kelly Keating (The Pharmaceutical Research Institute, Albany College of Pharmacy and Health Sciences, Rensselaer, New York, USA) for proofreading, constructive criticism, and English editing of the manuscript. The authors would acknowledge the guidance of Dmitri

Zagorevski (Rensselaer Polytechnic Institute, Troy, New York, USA) for help with GC-MS analysis. The authors are profoundly grateful to the CRD Saidal Pharmaceutical and the "Labratoire National de Contrôle des Produits Pharmaceutiques" (Algiers, Algeria) for their technical assistance and support.

Conflicts of Interest: The authors declare no conflict of interest.

Abbreviations

ANOVA	analysis of variance
BSA	bovine serum albumin
DMSO	dimethyl sulfoxide
EO	essential oil
FBS	fetal bovine serum
GC-MS	gas chromatography-mass spectrometry
H&E	hematoxylin-eosin
HRBC	human red blood cells
IC_{50}	median inhibitory concentration
LE	left ear
LHP	left hind paw
LNCPP	Laboratoire National de Contrôle des Produits Pharmaceutiques
LSEO	*Lavandula stoechas* essential oil
MTT	3-(4,5-dimethylthiazol-2yl)-2,5-diphenyl-tetrazolium bromide
NIST	National Institute of Standards and Technology
NMRI	Naval Medical Research Institute
NSAID	non-steroidal anti-inflammatory drugs
PBS	phosphate-buffered saline
p.o.	*per os*
PARP	poly(ADP-ribose) polymerase
PMN	polymorphonuclear cells
R&D	Research and Development Center
RE	right ear
RHP	right hind paw
RI	retention index
rpm	rotation per minute
RPMI	Roswell Park Memorial Institute
RT	retention times

References

1. Monteleone, G.; Pallone, F.; Stolfi, C. The dual role of inflammation in colon carcinogenesis. *Int. J. Mol. Sci.* **2012**, *13*, 11071–11084. [CrossRef] [PubMed]
2. Bayala, B.; Bassole, I.H.N.; Gnoula, C.; Nebie, R.; Yonli, A.; Morel, L.; Simpore, J. Chemical composition, antioxidant, anti-inflammatory and anti-proliferative activities of essential oils of plants from Burkina Faso. *PLoS ONE* **2014**, *9*, e0092122. [CrossRef] [PubMed]
3. Coussens, L.M.; Werb, Z. Inflammation and cancer. *Nature* **2002**, *420*, 860–867. [CrossRef] [PubMed]
4. Greten, F.R.; Eckmann, L.; Greten, T.F.; Park, J.M.; Li, Z.W.; Egan, L.J.; Karin, M. IKKβ links inflammation and tumorigenesis in a mouse model of colitis-associated cancer. *Cell* **2004**, *118*, 285–296. [CrossRef] [PubMed]
5. Sun, Z.; Wang, H.; Wang, J.; Zhou, L.; Yang, P. Chemical composition and anti-inflammatory, cytotoxic and antioxidant activities of essential oil from leaves of *Mentha piperita* grown in China. *PLoS ONE* **2014**, *9*, e0114767. [CrossRef] [PubMed]
6. Özkan, A.; Erdoğan, A. Membrane and DNA damaging/protective effects of eugenol, eucalyptol, terpinen-4-ol, and camphor at various concentrations on parental and drug-resistant H1299 cells. *Turk. J. Biol.* **2013**, *37*, 405–413. [CrossRef]
7. Leighton, X.; Bera, A.; Eidelman, O.; Eklund, M.; Puthillathu, N.; Pollard, H.B.; Srivastava, M. High ANXA7 Potentiates eucalyptol toxicity in hormone-refractory prostate cancer. *Anticancer Res.* **2018**, *38*, 3831–3842. [CrossRef]

8. Boukhatem, M.N.; Ferhat, M.A.; Benassel, N.; Kameli, A. Lavande papillon (*Lavandula stoechas* L.): Une plante à parfum aux multiples vertus. *Phytothérapie* **2019**, in press. [CrossRef]
9. Bhalla, Y.; Gupta, V.K.; Jaitak, V. Anticancer activity of essential oils: A review. *J. Sci. Food Agric.* **2013**, *93*, 3643–3653. [CrossRef]
10. Prashar, A.; Locke, I.C.; Evans, C.S. Cytotoxicity of lavender oil and its major components to human skin cells. *Cell Prolifer.* **2004**, *37*, 221–229. [CrossRef]
11. Cavanagh, H.M.A.; Wilkinson, J.M. Biological activities of lavender essential oil. *Phytother. Res.* **2002**, *16*, 301–308. [CrossRef] [PubMed]
12. Hajhashemi, V.; Ghannadi, A.; Sharif, B. Anti-inflammatory and analgesic properties of the leaf extracts and essential oil of *Lavandula angustifolia* Mill. *J. Ethnopharmacol.* **2003**, *89*, 67–71. [CrossRef]
13. Bousta, D.; Farah, A. A Phytopharmacological review of a Mediterranean plant: *Lavandula stoechas* L. *Clin. Phytosci.* **2020**, *6*, 9. [CrossRef]
14. Rahmati, B.; Kiasalari, Z.; Roghani, M.; Khalili, M.; Ansari, F. Antidepressant and anxiolytic activity of Lavandula officinalis aerial parts hydroalcoholic extract in scopolamine-treated rats. *Pharmac. Biol.* **2017**, *55*, 958–965. [CrossRef]
15. Rafiee, M.; Kiani, Z.; Moezi, S.A.; Rad, G.H.M. The effects of lavender, valerian, and oxazepam on anxiety among hospitalized patients with coronary artery disease. *Mod. Care J.* **2018**, *15*. [CrossRef]
16. Vokou, D.; Chalkos, D.; Karamanlidou, G.; Yiangou, M. Activation of soil respiration and shift of the microbial population balance in soil as a response to *Lavandula stoechas* essential oil. *J. Chem. Ecol.* **2002**, *28*, 755–768. [CrossRef]
17. Amara, N.; Boukhatem, M.N.; Ferhat, M.A.; Kaibouche, N.; Laissaoui, O.; Boufridi, A. Applications potentielles de l'huile essentielle de lavande papillon (*Lavandula stoechas* L.) comme conservateur alimentaire naturel. *Phytothérapie* **2017**, 1–9. [CrossRef]
18. Wells, R.; Truong, F.; Adal, A.M.; Sarker, L.S.; Mahmoud, S.S. *Lavandula* Essential oils: A current review of applications in medicinal, food, and cosmetic industries of Lavender. *Nat. Prod. Comm.* **2018**, *13*. [CrossRef]
19. Benabdelkader, T.; Zitouni, A.; Guitton, Y.; Jullien, F.; Maitre, D.; Casabianca, H.; Kameli, A. Essential oils from wild populations of Algerian *Lavandula stoechas* L.: Composition, chemical variability, and in vitro biological properties. *Chem. Biodiv.* **2011**, *8*, 937–953. [CrossRef]
20. Ristorcelli, D.; Tomi, F.; Casanova, J. 13C-NMR as a tool for identification and enantiomeric differentiation of major terpenes exemplified by the essential oil of *Lavandula stoechas* L. ssp. *stoechas*. *Flav. Fragr. J.* **1998**, *13*, 154–158. [CrossRef]
21. Parvin, M.S.; Das, N.; Jahan, N.; Akhter, M.A.; Nahar, L.; Islam, M.E. Evaluation of in vitro anti-inflammatory and antibacterial potential of *Crescentia cujete* leaves and stem bark. *BMC Res. Notes* **2015**, *8*, 412. [CrossRef] [PubMed]
22. Rahman, H.; Eswaraiah, M.C.; Dutta, A.M. In-vitro anti-inflammatory and anti-arthritic activity of *Oryza Sativa* Var. *joha* rice (an aromatic indigenous rice of Assam). *Am. Eurasian J. Agric. Environ. Sci.* **2015**, *15*, 115–121. [CrossRef]
23. Bouhlali, E.D.T.; El Hilaly, J.; Ennassir, J.; Benlyas, M.; Alem, C.; Amarouch, M.Y.; Filali-Zegzouti, Y. Anti-inflammatory properties and phenolic profile of six Moroccan date fruit (*Phoenix dactylifera* L.) varieties. *J. King Saud Univ.-Sci.* **2018**, *30*, 519–526. [CrossRef]
24. Karthik, E.V.; Vishnu, V.; Gayathri Priya, R. Anti-inflammatory activity of lavender oil using HRBC membrane stabilising method. *Int. J. Pharm. Sci. Rev. Res.* **2016**, *2016*. 40, 254–258.
25. Williams, L.A.D.; O'Connar, A.; Latore, L.; Dennis, O.; Ringer, S.; Whittaker, J.A.; Kraus, W. The in vitro anti-denaturation effects induced by natural products and non-steroidal compounds in heat treated (immunogenic) bovine serum albumin is proposed as a screening assay for the detection of anti-inflammatory compounds, without the use of animals, in the early stages of the drug discovery process. *West Indian Med. J.* **2008**, *57*, 327–331.
26. Santos, F.A.; Rao, V.S.N. Anti-inflammatory and antinociceptive effects of 1,8-cineole a terpenoid oxide present in many plant essential oils. *Phytother. Res.* **2000**, *14*, 240–244. [CrossRef]
27. Juergens, U.R. Anti-inflammatory properties of the monoterpene 1,8-cineole: Current evidence for co-medication in inflammatory airway diseases. *Drug Res.* **2014**, *64*, 638–646. [CrossRef]
28. Boukhatem, M.N.; Ferhat, M.A.; Kameli, A.; Saidi, F.; Kebir, H.T. Lemon grass (*Cymbopogon citratus*) essential oil as a potent anti-inflammatory and antifungal drugs. *Libyan J. Med.* **2014**, *9*, 25431. [CrossRef]

29. Al-Reza, S.M.; Yoon, J.I.; Kim, H.J.; Kim, J.S.; Kang, S.C. Anti-inflammatory activity of seed essential oil from *Zizyphus jujuba*. *Food Chem. Toxicol.* **2010**, *48*, 639–643. [CrossRef]
30. Silva, G.L.; Luft, C.; Lunardelli, A.; Amaral, R.H.; Melo, D.A.; Donadio, M.V.; Mello, R.O. Antioxidant, analgesic and anti-inflammatory effects of lavender essential oil. *An. Acad. Bras. Ciênc.* **2015**, *87*, 1397–1408. [CrossRef]
31. Cardia, G.F.E.; Silva-Filho, S.E.; Silva, E.L.; Uchida, N.S.; Cavalcante, H.A.O.; Cassarotti, L.L.; Cuman, R.K.N. Effect of lavender (*Lavandula angustifolia*) essential oil on acute inflammatory response. *Evid.-Based Complem. Altern. Med.* **2018**. [CrossRef] [PubMed]
32. Boukhatem, M.N.; Kameli, A.; Ferhat, M.A.; Saidi, F.; Mekarnia, M. Rose geranium essential oil as a source of new and safe anti-inflammatory drugs. *Libyan J. Med.* **2013**, *8*, 22520. [CrossRef] [PubMed]
33. Murata, S.; Shiragami, R.; Kosugi, C.; Tezuka, T.; Yamazaki, M.; Hirano, A.; Koda, K. Antitumor effect of 1,8-cineole against colon cancer. *Oncol. Rep.* **2013**, *30*, 2647–2652. [CrossRef] [PubMed]
34. Cha, J.D.; Kim, Y.H.; Kim, J.Y. Essential oil and 1,8-cineole from *Artemisia lavandulae* folia induces apoptosis in KB cells via mitochondrial stress and caspase activation. *Food Sci. Biotechnol.* **2010**, *19*, 185–191. [CrossRef]
35. Tayarani-Najaran, Z.; Amiri, A.; Karimi, G.; Emami, S.A.; Asili, J.; Mousavi, S.H. Comparative studies of cytotoxic and apoptotic properties of different extracts and the essential oil of *Lavandula angustifolia* on malignant and normal cells. *Nutr. Cancer* **2014**, *66*, 424–434. [CrossRef]
36. Graham, J.G.; Quinn, M.L.; Fabricant, D.S.; Farnsworth, N.R. Plants used against cancer—An extension of the work of Jonathan Hartwell. *J. Ethnopharmacol.* **2000**, *73*, 347–377. [CrossRef]
37. Gezici, S. Promising anticancer activity of lavender (*Lavandula angustifolia* Mill.) essential oil through induction of both apoptosis and necrosis. *Ann. Phytomed.* **2018**, *7*, 38–45. [CrossRef]

Sample Availability: Samples of the compounds *Lavandula stoechas* Essential Oil are available from the authors.

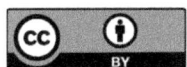

© 2020 by the authors. Licensee MDPI, Basel, Switzerland. This article is an open access article distributed under the terms and conditions of the Creative Commons Attribution (CC BY) license (http://creativecommons.org/licenses/by/4.0/).

Natural Herbal Estrogen-Mimetics (Phytoestrogens) Promote the Differentiation of Fallopian Tube Epithelium into Multi-Ciliated Cells via Estrogen Receptor Beta

Maobi Zhu, Sen Takeda and Tomohiko Iwano *

Department of Anatomy and Cell Biology, Graduate School of Medicine, University of Yamanashi, 1110 Shimo-Kateau, Chuo, Yamanashi 409-3898, Japan; mzhu-as@yamanashi.ac.jp (M.Z.); stakeda@yamanashi.ac.jp (S.T.)
* Correspondence: tiwano@yamanashi.ac.jp; Tel.: +81-55-273-9471

Abstract: Phytoestrogens are herbal polyphenolic compounds that exert various estrogen-like effects in animals and can be taken in easily from a foodstuff in daily life. The fallopian tube lumen, where transportation of the oocyte occurs, is lined with secretory cells and multi-ciliated epithelial cells. Recently, we showed that estrogen induces multi-ciliogenesis in the porcine fallopian tube epithelial cells (FTECs) through the activation of the estrogen receptor beta (ERβ) pathway and simultaneous inhibition of the Notch pathway. Thus, ingested phytoestrogens may induce FTEC ciliogenesis and thereby affect the fecundity. To address this issue, we added isoflavones (genistein, daidzein, or glycitin) and coumestan (coumestrol) to primary culture FTECs under air–liquid interface conditions and assessed the effects of each compound. All phytoestrogens except glycitin induced multi-ciliated cell differentiation, which followed Notch signal downregulation. On the contrary, the differentiation of secretory cells decreased slightly. Furthermore, genistein and daidzein had a slight effect on the proportion of proliferating cells exhibited by Ki67 expression. Ciliated-cell differentiation is inhibited by the ERβ antagonist, PHTPP. Thus, this study suggests that phytoestrogens can improve the fallopian tube epithelial sheet homeostasis by facilitating the genesis of multi-ciliated cells and this effect depends on the ERβ-mediated pathway.

Keywords: fallopian tube; phytoestrogen; ciliated cell; secretory cell; Notch

1. Introduction

The fallopian tube (FT) shares a developmental origin (Müllarian duct) with the uterus and serves as a route for bidirectional gamete transportation. The FT luminal wall is composed of secretory cells, multi-ciliated cells, and basal cells. Basal cells are a type of multipotent stem cell that gives rise to each specific cell type in the epithelium [1]. Secretory cells secrete mostly mucus materials that contain a series of compounds such as glycoproteins and growth factors [2]. Multi-ciliated cells have motile cilia on the apical surface to facilitate the flow of the mucous fluid [3]. Therefore, the FT cytohistological architecture is functionally adapted to cope with the physiology of the reproductive tract in vivo.

To modulate the FT environment, two major steroids, estrogen and progesterone, play important roles [4]. Previous studies suggested that estrogen can facilitate glycoprotein expression and secretion by secretory cells [2,5] and ciliogenesis in multi-ciliated cells [6], and the molecular mechanisms underlying this regulation remain unknown. Estrogen triggers the downstream pathway through the activation of estrogen receptors (ERs). Authentic estrogen receptors, ERα and ERβ, translocate from the cytoplasm to the nucleus when stimulated by estrogen, and they act as transcription factors to regulate downstream gene expression [7]. They are known to have specific targets depending on the coactivators. Knockout mouse studies showed that ERα is required for fertilization and embryonic development, and ERβ is essential for efficient ovulation [8]. However, the specific roles of ERs in conditioning the FT epithelial sheet remains unclear. Our previous study demonstrated that ERβ, but not ERα, promotes multi-ciliogenesis of FT epithelial cells by downregulating the Notch pathway [9].

Additionally, natural herbal hormone-like compounds affect the homeostasis of female reproductive tissues as an endocrine disruptor. Because all living things necessarily liaise with the external environment, they would be easily affected by ingested foodstuff. Phytoestrogen is an organic compound with estrogen-mimetic effects, and it is produced and stored in some plants such as soybeans, sprouts, and seeds [10]. Taking advantage of their effects, these plants are prescribed as unauthorized medicinal natural supplements to treat some diseases [10,11]. Conversely, a higher dosage of phytoestrogens has been suggested to stimulate the proliferation of ER-dependent breast cancer cells [12]. Among phytoestrogens, genistein, daidzein, and glycitin are categorized as isoflavones and coumestrol is a coumestan, and all of these are contained in beans and sprouts [13]. Previous studies have shown that they have a relatively higher affinity for ERβ rather than ERα [14–16]. Although several studies reported the effects of phytoestrogen on cancer cells [17–19], their actual roles in epithelial cell differentiation in the reproductive system remain unknown.

In this study, we examined the effects of phytoestrogens on the porcine FT epithelial cell differentiation using the air–liquid interface (ALI) culture system that we previously established [20]. Immunostaining of treated cells showed that phytoestrogens were able to preferentially promote multi-ciliated cell differentiation over that of secretory cells. This correlated well with downregulation of Delta-like protein 1 (DLL1), a Notch ligand, and reduced cleavage of Notch. In conclusion, the present study suggests the potential application of phytoestrogens to modulate the luminal homeostasis of the oviduct by promoting multi-ciliated epithelial cell differentiation.

2. Results
2.1. Phytoestrogens Promote Multi-Ciliated Cell Differentiation

In the previous study, we demonstrated that estrogen promoted multi-ciliated cell differentiation through ERβ [9]. Estrogen (estradiol, E2) and diarylpropionitrile (DPN), which is an ERβ agonist, promoted the multi-ciliogenesis in approximately 30% of FTECs in the ALI culture for 10 days as shown using anti-acetylated α-tubulin antibody, whereas the negative control showed ciliogenesis in less than 10% of the cells (Figure 1a–c). To evaluate the effect of the phytoestrogens on the differentiation of FTECs, we administered coumestrol, daidzein, genistein, or glycitin in the medium (Supplementary Figure S1). All, with the exception of glycitin, promoted the multi-ciliogenesis (Figure 1d). The efficiency of coumestrol, daidzein, and genistein for inducing multi-ciliogenesis was almost 30%, which is comparable with that of E2 and DPN. Dose dependency was observed between 1 and 10 µM, where each compound showed differential dose dependency (Figure 1e). Coumestrol shared a similar pattern with genistein and showed an inverse proportion of multi-ciliated cells by increasing the concentration from 1 to 10 µM. Conversely, daidzein increased the number of multi-ciliated cells in a concentration-dependent manner. Glycitin showed no significant induction of multi-ciliated cells at any concentration. Consistently, the upregulated phosphorylation of ERβ, which is related to its activation, was observed in the nuclei of cells treated with DPN, coumestrol, daidzein, and genistein, but less with glycitin (Supplementary Figure S2). Therefore, phytoestrogens, with the exception of glycitin, can promote ciliated cell differentiation, which is similar to the cases of E2 and DPN.

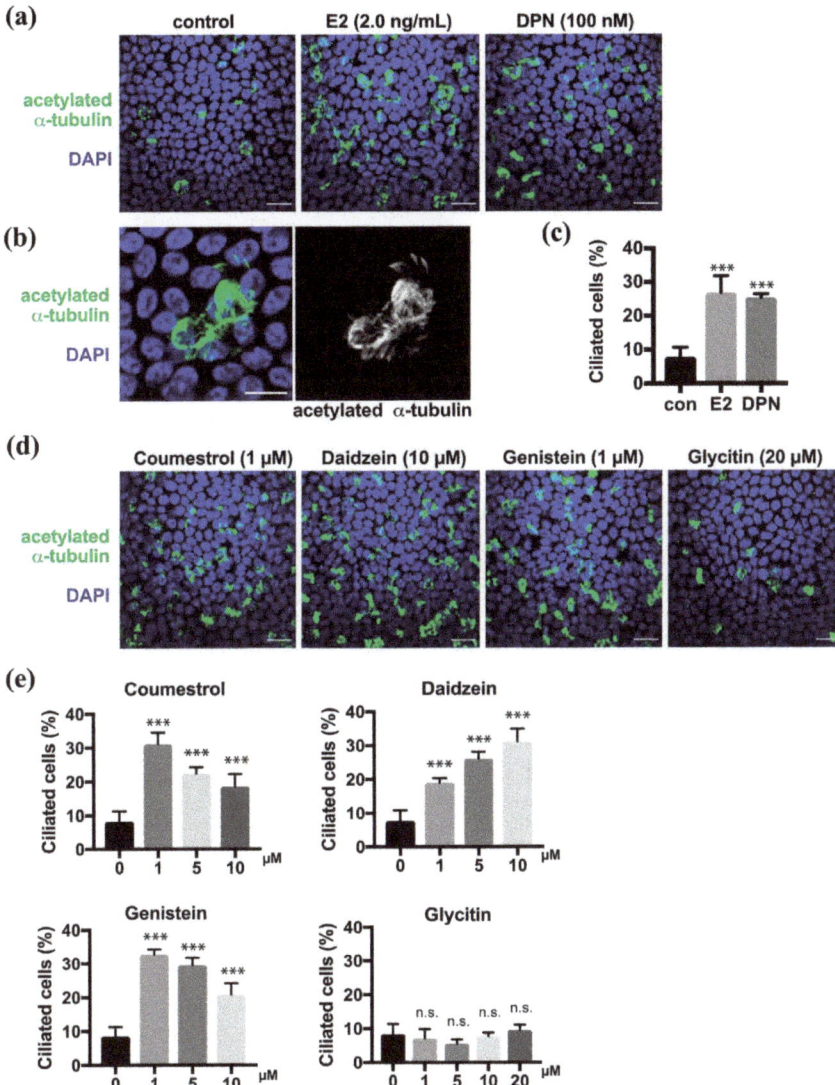

Figure 1. Coumestrol, daidzein, and genistein induce ciliated cell differentiation in fallopian tube epithelial cells (FTECs). (**a**) Staining for acetylated α-tubulin (green) and nuclei (blue) in porcine FTECs that were cultured for 10 days under air–liquid interface (ALI) conditions with E2 or diarylpropionitrile (DPN). (**b**) Magnified view of typical ac-tubulin-positive ciliated cells with multiple cilia. (**c**) The proportion of ciliated cells under each condition in (**a**) is presented. Data are presented as the mean ± SD (n = 5 fields). (**d**) Staining for acetylated α-tubulin (green) and nuclei counterstained with DAPI (blue) of cells cultured in the medium containing coumestrol, daidzein, genistein, or glycitin. (**e**) The proportion of ciliated cells under each condition in (**d**) is presented. Data are presented as the mean ± SD (n = 5 fields). n.s.: not significant; SD, standard deviation; DPN, diarylpropionitrile; con, control. Scale bars: 20 μm in (**a**) and (**d**); 10 μm in (**b**). Statistical significance was assigned as *** $p < 0.001$.

2.2. Phytoestrogens Slightly Affect the Proportion of Secretory Cells and Basal Cells

Because phytoestrogens promote differentiation into ciliated cells, we next focused on secretory cell differentiation. Pax8 is a lineage-specific transcription factor that is expressed in FT secretory cells. Multi-ciliated cells that were revealed by anti-acetylated α-tubulin antibody showed no or background levels of Pax8 in ALI culture at 10 days after induction (DAI) (Figure 2a). Upon treatment with DPN or phytoestrogens, the proportion of Pax8-positive secretory cells in the epithelial sheet varied depending on the species of compounds (Figure 2b). Coumestrol, daidzein, and glycitin did not show any significant changes in the proportion of the secretory cells compared with the control, whereas DPN and genistein slightly reduced the proportion of secretory cells compared with controls (Figure 2c). Finally, we examined the effects of phytoestrogens on basal cells because they are still present, and they replenish the epithelial sheet with differentiated cells in vivo. The proportion of basal cells that were positive for Ki67, which is a proliferation marker, did not change significantly in the presence of DPN, coumestrol, or glycitin, whereas this proportion significantly decreased and increased in response to daidzein and genistein, respectively, compared with controls (Figure 2d). Thus, several compounds affected the cell fate of secretory cells from basal cells.

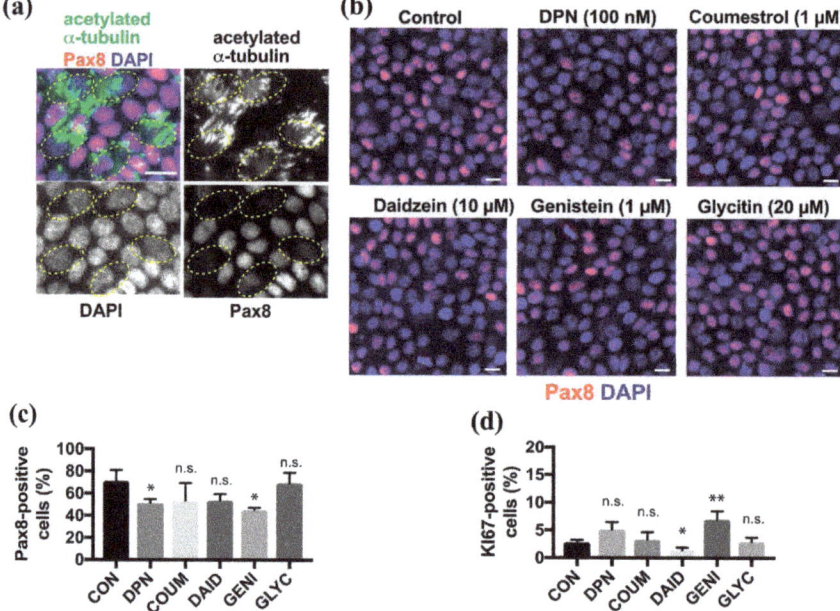

Figure 2. Genistein affects secretory cell differentiation and basal cell maintenance. (**a**) Staining for acetylated α-tubulin (green), Pax8 (red), and nuclei (blue) in FTECs cultured for 10 days under ALI conditions. Yellow circles indicate the ac-tubulin-positive ciliated cells with a lower Pax8 expression. (**b**) Staining for Pax8 (red) and nuclei (blue) of cells cultured in the medium containing DPN, coumestrol, daidzein, genistein, or glycitin. (**c**) The proportion of Pax8-positive in cells cultured under each condition in (**b**) is presented. Data are presented as the mean ± SD (n = 3 fields). (**d**) The proportion of Ki67-positive in cells that were cultured under each condition in (**b**) is presented. Data are presented as the mean ± SD (n = 3 fields). COUM, coumestrol; DAID, daidzein; GENI, genistein; GLYC, glycitin. n.s.: not significant; SD, standard deviation. Scale bars: 10 μm in (**b**). Statistical significance was assigned as * $p < 0.05$ and ** $p < 0.01$.

2.3. Induction of Multi-Ciliated Cell Differentiation Depends on the ERβ Pathway

We previously reported that E2 promoted multi-ciliated cell differentiation through ERβ. To analyze whether phytoestrogens share this molecular pathway, we examined their effect in the presence of the ERβ antagonist, PHTPP. FTECs under ALI-culture conditions at 7 DAI were treated with DPN, coumestrol, daidzein, or genistein at their optimal concentration to induce ciliogenesis (Figure 3a). In all cases, co-administration of PHTPP significantly inhibited ciliogenesis whereas the control group without PHTPP continued to undergo ciliogenesis (Figure 3b). This indicates that ERβ is involved in the mechanism of action for phytoestrogens.

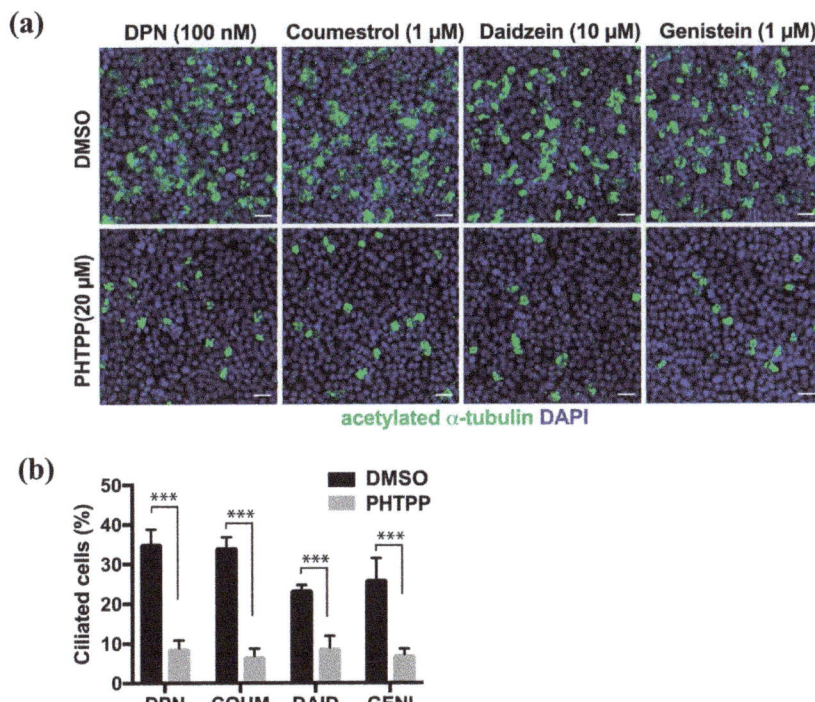

Figure 3. The induction of ciliated cells by phytoestrogens is suppressed by PHTPP, an ERβ antagonist. (**a**) Staining for acetylated α-tubulin (green) and nuclei (blue) of the FTECs that were cultured for 7 days in medium containing DPN, coumestrol, daidzein, and genistein with DMSO or PHTPP. (**b**) The proportion of ciliated cells that were cultured under each condition in (**a**) is presented. Data are presented as the mean ± SD (n = 5 fields). COUM, coumestrol; DAID, daidzein; GENI, genistein; GLYC, glycitin. SD, standard deviation; DPN, diarylpropionitrile; DMSO, dimethyl sulfoxide. Statistical significance was assigned as *** $p < 0.001$.

2.4. Coumestrol, Daidzein, and Genistein Suppress Notch Signaling

As we and another group have previously reported [9,21], the Notch signaling pathway plays an important role in regulating multi-ciliogenesis in the FT. Moreover, E2 and DPN antagonize the effect of Notch during multi-ciliogenesis. To examine the effects of phytoestrogens on Notch signaling, we quantified the level of Notch intracellular domain (NICD), which is a molecular marker of the activated Notch pathway. Twenty-four hours after treatment with coumestrol, daidzein, or genistein, the NICD level was reduced to half of the control value. This effect was attenuated by PHTPP treatment, confirming the involvement of ERβ pathway to suppress Notch signaling (Supplementary Fguire S3). We further investigated the expression of Notch ligands 24 h after treatment with phytoestrogens (Figure 4a). Coumestrol, daidzein, and genistein significantly suppressed DLL1 mRNA expression but had little effect on Delta-like protein 4 (DLL4), Jagged 1 (JAG1), or Jagged 2 (JAG2) mRNA expression, and the results were consistent with those of E2 and DPN (Figure 4b–e). These data indicate that coumestrol, daidzein, and genistein suppress Notch signaling by reducing DLL1 mRNA levels during the ciliogenesis. Thus, phytoestrogens can mimic the roles of endogenous estrogen in FTEC differentiation.

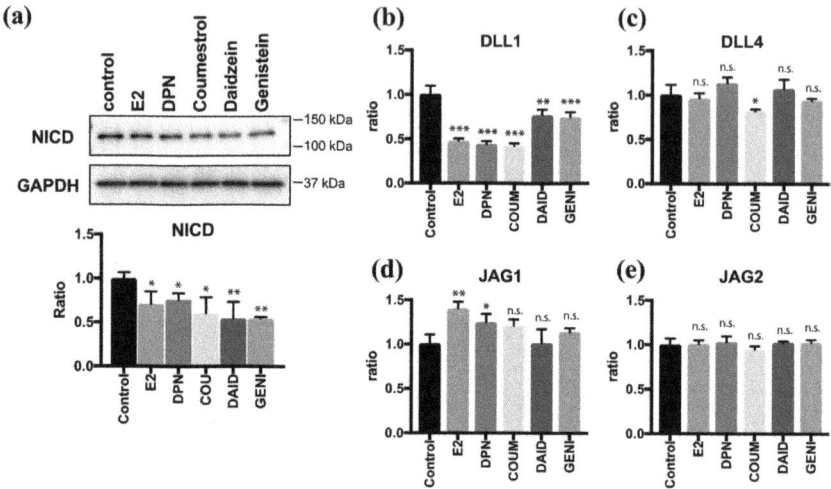

Figure 4. Phytoestrogens downregulate Notch signaling via suppression of DLL1. (**a**) Immunoblots for Notch intracellular domain (NICD) and glyceraldehyde 3-phosphate dehydrogenase (GAPDH) in lysates of cells that were treated for 24 h with E2 (2 ng/mL), DPN (100 nM), coumestrol (1 μM), daidzein (10 μM), and genistein (1 μM). The graph below the NICD blot shows the ratios of intensities of NICD to the GAPDH blots. (**b**–**e**) Quantitative RT-PCR for DLL1 (**b**), DLL4 (**c**), JAG1 (**d**), and JAG2 (**e**) expression in cells that were cultured for 24 h under each condition in (**a**) are presented. Data are presented as the mean ± SD. (n = 3 experiments). COUM, coumestrol; DAID, daidzein; GENI, genistein; GLYC, glycitin. SD, standard deviation; NICD, Notch intracellular domain; GAPDH, glyceraldehyde 3-phosphate dehydrogenase; DPN, diarylpropionitrile; RT-PCR, real-time polymerase chain reaction. Statistical significance was assigned as * $p < 0.05$, ** $p < 0.01$, and *** $p < 0.001$.

3. Discussion

This study examined the effects of phytoestrogens on the differentiation of FTECs using the ALI culture system. We used coumestrol, daidzein, genistein, and glycitin as phytoestrogens that are included in daily foodstuff. Coumestrol, daidzein, and genistein showed significant effects in promoting multi-ciliated cell differentiation, and the effects are consistent with those of the ERβ agonist DPN. Although the differentiation of secretory and basal cells was still affected, the level was not comparable to that in multi-ciliated cells. Therefore, it is suggested that some phytoestrogens, at least coumestrol, daidzein, and genistein, act as a switch to induce ciliated cell differentiation via the ERβ pathway. However, genistein slightly but significantly reduces secretory-cell differentiation and increases Ki67-positive proliferative cells. It is possible that the promotion of ciliated-cell differentiation indirectly affects the proportion of secretory cells and basal cells. Based on the higher specificity of genistein for ERβ over ERα, the strength of fate control might depend on the ERβ pathway. Future transcriptome and epigenome analyses will reveal the downstream genes regulated by each phytoestrogen. The promotion of ciliated cell differentiation is consistent with the higher binding affinity of coumestrol, genistein, and daidzein to ERβ rather than ERα [14]. Because ciliated-cell differentiation activity was suppressed by the ERβ antagonist, the responsible pathways that promote cell fate determination may be common among the phytoestrogens. Regarding the differentiation of secretory cells, other factors or pathways might be assumed instead of the ERβ pathway, because secretory cells differentiated in about 70% of cells in basal medium alone (Figure 2b,c control).

Although we used phytoestrogens at a concentration of approximately the IC$_{50}$ (half maximal inhibitory concentration) for each compound, this value (1–10 µM = 254–2542 ng/mL of daidzein and 270–2702 ng/mL of genistein) is much higher than the concentration (<100 ng/mL of daidzein and <160 ng/mL of genistein) in a UK cohort over 40 years of age [22]. However, the concentration of these compounds in a Japanese cohort was 0–2407 ng/mL and 0–4192 ng/mL for daidzein and genistein, respectively [22]. Therefore, the phytoestrogen concentration in our study was comparable to that in the Japanese cohort. Additionally, a US population did not show the presence of coumestrol in serum, although the urine was positive for coumestrol [23]. Therefore, we cannot assess the concentration of coumestrol.

Among phytoestrogens, our study showed that glycitin did not induce the multiciliogenesis. Similar to genistein and daidzein, glycitin is present in soybeans, but its structure is different from that of genistein and daidzein in terms of conjugation of glucose, and the amount of glycitin is much lower than that of other phytoestrogens [13] (Supplementary Figure S1). It has been reported that glycitin increases the ratio of Ki67-positivity in the human dermal fibroblast cells [24], although it did not induce cell proliferation in the current study. Taking the amount of glycitin in soybeans and our results into consideration, the effects of glycitin in FT epithelium would be minimal.

There are several studies that have shown different effects of genistein in different animals, such as the metabolic and secretion-stimulating action on cells, the beneficial influence on uterine homeostasis and embryonic development, and the adverse effect on implantation [24,25]. Another in vivo study in mice demonstrated that genistein reduced the efficiency of implantation [26]. Considering the very complex steps in the process of implantation, which is susceptible to various factors, it is unclear whether the adverse effect in the implantation of a mouse fertilized egg is attributable directly to genistein. Because the effect of phytoestrogens depends on the dosage and model animals that are used in each study, it is best to evaluate their effect in human cells. Although the cytoarchitecture and size of the porcine FT resembles that of humans, further elucidation of the molecular mechanism and application of phytoestrogens is required in human FTECs using primary culture system.

4. Materials and Methods

4.1. Fallopian Tube Epithelial Cell Culture

The procedures for in vitro culture and differentiation of primary porcine FTECs differentiation were described previously [20]. Briefly, porcine FT tissues were purchased from the Yamanashi Meat Logistics Center. FTECs were obtained by digesting and scraping the inside of opened porcine FTs using collagenase type IV (CLS4, Worthington, NJ, USA) and DNase I (9003-98-9, Sigma-Aldrich, St. Louis, MO, USA). To induce differentiation, cells were seeded onto a collagen type I coated 0.4-µm pore transwell (#3470, Corning, NY, USA) and basal media that included agonists or phytoestrogens were applied to the basal side in ALI culture. Reagents were as follows: β-estradiol (#E4389, Sigma-Aldrich, St. Louis, MO, USA); diarylpropionitrile (DPN) (#1428-67-7, Sigma-Aldrich, St. Louis, MO, USA); and PHTPP (#805239-56-9. Sigma-Aldrich). Phytoestrogens including genistein (#446-72-0, Wako, Osaka, Japan), daidzein (#486-66-8, Wako, Osaka, Japan), glycitin (#40246-10-4, Wako, Osaka, Japan), and coumestrol (#479-13-0, Cayman, Ann Arbor, MI, USA) were dissolved in dimethylformamide.

4.2. Immunofluorescence

The cells on the transwell were fixed using 4% paraformaldehyde (PFA) at room temperature (RT) for 10 min, permeabilized, and blocked with 0.1% Triton-X 100 and 5%

goat serum in Phosphate-buffered saline (PBS) for 30 min at RT. Cells were incubated with primary antibodies (Supplementary Table S1) at 4 °C for 24 h and with secondary antibodies at RT for 1 h. Nuclei were counterstained with DAPI (D1306, ThermoFisher Scientific, Waltham, MA, USA). Transwell membranes with cells were mounted onto glass slides using Diamond Antifade Mountant (P36961, ThermoFisher Scientific). Staining images were taken using a confocal (Olympus FV-1000, Tokyo, Japan) or fluorescent (Olympus IX71) microscopes.

4.3. Immunoblot Analysis

Cells were lysed using radioimmunoprecipitation assay (RIPA) buffer (25 mM Tris-HCl pH 7.6, 150 mM NaCl, 1% NP-40, 1% sodium deoxycholate, 0.1% SDS) with a protease inhibitor cocktail (#04693159001, Roche, Basel, Switzerland) and phosphatase inhibitor cocktail (#07575-61, Nacalai Tesque, Kyoto, Japan). Proteins in the cell lysates were separated by a 4–20% gradient polyacrylamide gel and wet-transferred to a polyvinylidene difluoride (PVDF) membrane. The membrane was blocked using Tris-buffered saline with Tween 20 containing 2% bovine serum albumin and incubated with primary antibodies (Supplementary Table S1) at 4 °C for 24 h and with secondary antibodies for 1 h at RT. Signals were developed using an enhanced chemiluminescence substrate (#02230, Nacalai Tesque, Kyoto, Japan), and blotting images were acquired using an ImageQuant LAS 4000 (GE Healthcare, Chicago, IL, USA).

4.4. Quantitative PCR

Total RNA was extracted from FTECs using the RNeasy Mini Kit (#74104, Qiagen, Germantown, MD, USA). Double-stranded cDNA was synthesized using a reverse transcription kit (#4368813, ThermoFisher Scientific, Waltham, MA, USA). Real-time quantitative polymerase chain reaction (RT-PCR) was performed by the FastStart Universal Probe Master kit (#04913957001, Roche, Basel, Switzerland) with Roche Universal Probe #2 and Probe #30 (#04684982001 and #04687639001, Roche, Basel, Switzerland) using a StepOne PCR system (Applied Biosystems, Foster, CA, USA). Relative RNA quantitation was performed using $\Delta\Delta CT$ calculations. Primer sequences are listed in Supplementary Table S2.

4.5. Statistical Analysis

Statistical analyses were performed using GraphPad Prism 7 (San Diego, CA, USA). Values were expressed as the mean ± standard deviation (SD). The Student's t-test was used to compare the variation between two samples. Analysis of variance (ANOVA) was used to compare three or more groups. Statistical significance was assigned as * $p < 0.05$, ** $p < 0.01$, and *** $p < 0.001$.

Supplementary Materials: The following are available online, Figure S1: Molecular structure of phytoestrogens that are used in this study; Figure S2: Phytoestrogens activate ERβ.; Figure S3: Phytoestrogens downregulate Notch signaling via ERβ pathway.; Table S1: List of antibodies used in this study; Table S2: List of oligonucleotides used in this study.

Author Contributions: Conceptualization, Tomohiko Iwano; Data curation, Tomohiko Iwano; Funding acquisition, Tomohiko Iwano; Investigation, Maobi Zhu and Tomohiko Iwano; Methodology, Maobi Zhu and Tomohiko Iwano; Project administration, Tomohiko Iwano; Supervision, Sen Takeda; Validation, Tomohiko Iwano; Visualization, Tomohiko Iwano; Writing—original draft, Maobi Zhu; Writing—review & editing, Sen Takeda and Tomohiko Iwano. All authors have read and agreed to the published version of the manuscript.

Funding: This research was funded by a research grant 2020 from the Kobayashi Foundation to T.I.

Institutional Review Board Statement: Not applicable.

Informed Consent Statement: Not applicable.

Data Availability Statement: The data that support the findings of this study are available from the corresponding author upon reasonable request.

Acknowledgments: We thank Kazuaki Matsumoto for helping with fallopian tube preparation. We also thank Jodi Smith, from Edanz Group (https://en-author-services.edanz.com/ac) for editing a draft of this manuscript.

Conflicts of Interest: The authors declare no conflict of interest. The funders had no role in the design of the study; in the collection, analyses, or interpretation of data; in the writing of the manuscript, or in the decision to publish the results.

Sample Availability: Samples of the compounds and cells are available from the authors.

References

1. Lyons, R.A.; Saridogan, E.; Djahanbakhch, O. The reproductive significance of human Fallopian tube cilia. *Hum. Reprod. Update* **2006**, *12*, 363–372. [CrossRef]
2. Pillai, V.V.; Weber, D.M.; Phinney, B.S.; Selvaraj, V. Profiling of proteins secreted in the bovine oviduct reveals diverse functions of this luminal microenvironment. *PLoS ONE* **2017**, *12*, 1–22. [CrossRef] [PubMed]
3. Halbert, S.A.; Tam, P.Y.; Blandau, R.J. Egg transport in the rabbit oviduct: The roles of cilia and muscle. *Science* **1976**, *191*, 1052–1053. [CrossRef] [PubMed]
4. Amso, N.N.; Crow, J.; Shaw, R.W. Endocrinology: Comparative immunohistochemical study of oestrogen and progesterone receptors in the fallopian tube and uterus at different stages of the menstrual cycle and the menopause. *Hum. Reprod.* **1994**, *9*, 1027–1037. [CrossRef]
5. Verhage, H.G.; Mavrogianis, P.A.; Boice, M.L.; Li, W.; Fazleabas, A.T. Oviductal epithelium of the baboon: Hormonal control and the immuno-gold localization of oviduct-specific glycoproteins. *Am. J. Anat.* **1990**, *187*, 81–90. [CrossRef] [PubMed]
6. Donnez, J.; Casanas-Roux, F.; Ferin, J.; Thomas, K. Changes in ciliation and cell height in human tubal epithelium in the fertile and post-fertile years. *Maturitas* **1983**, *5*, 39–45. [CrossRef]
7. Hewitt, S.C.; Korach, K.S. Estrogen receptors: New directions in the new millennium. *Endocr. Rev.* **2018**, *39*, 664–675. [CrossRef]
8. Krege, J.H.; Hodgin, J.B.; Couse, J.F.; Enmark, E.; Warner, M.; Mahler, J.F.; Sar, M.; Korach, K.S.; Gustafsson, J.A.; Smithies, O. Generation and reproductive phenotypes of mice lacking estrogen receptor β. *Proc. Natl. Acad. Sci. USA* **1998**, *95*, 15677–15682. [CrossRef]
9. Zhu, M.; Iwano, T.; Takeda, S. Estrogen and EGFR Pathways Regulate Notch Signaling in Opposing Directions for Multi-Ciliogenesis in the Fallopian Tube. *Cells* **2019**, *8*, 933. [CrossRef]
10. Domínguez-López, I.; Yago-Aragón, M.; Salas-Huetos, A.; Tresserra-Rimbau, A.; Hurtado-Barroso, S. Effects of dietary phytoestrogens on hormones throughout a human lifespan: A review. *Nutrients* **2020**, *12*, 1–25. [CrossRef]
11. Alexander, V., S. Phytoestrogens and their effects. *Eur. J. Pharmacol.* **2014**, *741*, 230–236. [CrossRef]
12. Poschner, S.; Maier-Salamon, A.; Zehl, M.; Wackerlig, J.; Dobusch, D.; Pachmann, B.; Sterlini, K.L.; Jäger, W. The Impacts of Genistein and Daidzein on Estrogen Conjugations in Human Breast Cancer Cells: A targeted metabolomics approach. *Front. Pharmacol.* **2017**, *8*, 1–11. [CrossRef] [PubMed]
13. Nakamura, Y.; Kaihara, A.; Yoshii, K.; Tsumura, Y.; Ishimitsu, S.; Tonogai, Y. Content and composition of isoflavonoids in mature or immature beans and bean sprouts consumed in Japan. *J. Heal. Sci.* **2001**, *47*, 394–406. [CrossRef]
14. Kostelac, D.; Rechkemmer, G.; Briviba, K. Phytoestrogens Modulate Binding Response of Estrogen Receptors α and β to the Estrogen Response Element. *J. Agric. Food Chem.* **2003**, *51*, 7632–7635. [CrossRef]
15. Jiang, Y.; Gong, P.; Madak-Erdogan, Z.; Martin, T.; Jeyakumar, M.; Carlson, K.; Khan, I.; Smillie, T.J.; Chittiboyina, A.G.; Rotte, S.C.K.; et al. Mechanisms enforcing the estrogen receptor β selectivity of botanical estrogens. *FASEB J.* **2013**, *27*, 4406–4418. [CrossRef]
16. Morito, K.; Hirose, T.; Kinjo, J.; Hirakawa, T.; Okawa, M.; Nohara, T.; Ogawa, S.; Inoue, S.; Muramatsu, M.; Masamune, Y. Interaction of phytoestrogens with estrogen receptors α and β. *Biol. Pharm. Bull.* **2001**, *24*, 351–356. [CrossRef]
17. Chan, K.K.L.; Siu, M.K.Y.; Jiang, Y. xin; Wang, J. jing; Leung, T.H.Y.; Ngan, H.Y.S. Estrogen receptor modulators genistein, daidzein and ERB-041 inhibit cell migration, invasion, proliferation and sphere formation via modulation of FAK and PI3K/AKT signaling in ovarian cancer. *Cancer Cell Int.* **2018**, *18*, 1–14. [CrossRef]
18. Russo, M.; Russo, G.L.; Daglia, M.; Kasi, P.D.; Ravi, S.; Nabavi, S.F.; Nabavi, S.M. Understanding genistein in cancer: The "good" and the "bad" effects: A review. *Food Chem.* **2016**, *196*, 589–600. [CrossRef]
19. Tuli, H.S.; Tuorkey, M.J.; Thakral, F.; Sak, K.; Kumar, M.; Sharma, A.K.; Sharma, U.; Jain, A.; Aggarwal, V.; Bishayee, A. Molecular mechanisms of action of genistein in cancer: Recent advances. *Front. Pharmacol.* **2019**, *10*, 1336. [CrossRef]
20. Zhu, M.; Iwano, T.; Takeda, S. Fallopian tube basal stem cells reproducing the epithelial sheets in vitro—stem cell of fallopian epithelium. *Biomolecules* **2020**, *10*, 1–15. [CrossRef]
21. Kessler, M.; Hoffmann, K.; Brinkmann, V.; Thieck, O.; Jackisch, S.; Toelle, B.; Berger, H.; Mollenkopf, H.-J.; Mangler, M.; Sehouli, J.; et al. The Notch and Wnt pathways regulate stemness and differentiation in human fallopian tube organoids. *Nat. Commun.* **2015**, *6*, 8989. [CrossRef] [PubMed]

22. Morton, M.S.; Arisaka, O.; Miyake, N.; Morgan, L.D.; Evans, B.A.J. Phytoestrogen concentrations in serum from Japanese men and women over forty years of age. *J. Nutr.* **2002**, *132*, 3168–3171. [CrossRef] [PubMed]
23. Valentín-Blasini, L.; Blount, B.C.; Caudill, S.P.; Needham, L.L. Urinary and serum concentrations of seven phytoestrogens in a human reference population subset. *J. Expo. Anal. Environ. Epidemiol.* **2003**, *13*, 276–282. [CrossRef] [PubMed]
24. Kim, Y.M.; Huh, J.S.; Lim, Y.; Cho, M. Soy isoflavone glycitin (4′-hydroxy-6-methoxyisoflavone-7-D-Glucoside) promotes human dermal fibroblast cell proliferation and migration via TGF-β signaling. *Phyther. Res.* **2015**, *29*, 757–769. [CrossRef]
25. Simintiras, C.A.; Sturmey, R.G. Genistein crosses the bioartificial oviduct and alters secretion composition. *Reprod. Toxicol.* **2017**, *71*, 63–70. [CrossRef]
26. Jefferson, W.N.; Padilla-Banks, E.; Goulding, E.H.; Lao, S.P.C.; Newbold, R.R.; Williams, C.J. Neonatal exposure to genistein disrupts ability of female mouse reproductive tract to support preimplantation embryo development and implantation. *Biol. Reprod.* **2009**, *80*, 425–431. [CrossRef]

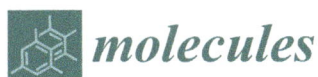

Article

Sea Buckthorn Leaf Powders: The Impact of Cultivar and Drying Mode on Antioxidant, Phytochemical, and Chromatic Profile of Valuable Resource

Lina Raudone [1,2,*], Viktorija Puzerytė [3], Gabriele Vilkickyte [2], Aurelija Niekyte [2], Juozas Lanauskas [4], Jonas Viskelis [3] and Pranas Viskelis [3]

[1] Department of Pharmacognosy, Lithuanian University of Health Sciences, Sukileliu av. 13, LT-50162 Kaunas, Lithuania
[2] Laboratory of Biopharmaceutical Research, Institute of Pharmaceutical Technologies, Lithuanian University of Health Sciences, Sukileliu av. 13, LT-50162 Kaunas, Lithuania; gabriele.vilkickyte@lsmu.lt (G.V.); aurelija.niekyte@stud.lsmu.lt (A.N.)
[3] Laboratory of Biochemistry and Technology, Institute of Horticulture, Lithuanian Research Centre for Agriculture and Forestry, Kauno Str. 30, LT-54333 Babtai, Kaunas District, Lithuania; viktorija.puzeryte@lammc.lt (V.P.); jonas.viskelis@lammc.lt (J.V.); pranas.viskelis@lammc.lt (P.V.)
[4] Department of Horticulture Technologies, Institute of Horticulture, Lithuanian Research Centre for Agriculture and Forestry, Kauno Str. 30, LT-54333 Babtai, Kaunas District, Lithuania; juozas.lanauskas@lammc.lt
* Correspondence: lina.raudone@lsmuni.lt

Citation: Raudone, L.; Puzerytė, V.; Vilkickyte, G.; Niekyte, A.; Lanauskas, J.; Viskelis, J.; Viskelis, P. Sea Buckthorn Leaf Powders: The Impact of Cultivar and Drying Mode on Antioxidant, Phytochemical, and Chromatic Profile of Valuable Resource. *Molecules* 2021, *26*, 4765. https://doi.org/10.3390/molecules26164765

Academic Editor: Toshio Morikawa

Received: 12 July 2021
Accepted: 31 July 2021
Published: 6 August 2021

Publisher's Note: MDPI stays neutral with regard to jurisdictional claims in published maps and institutional affiliations.

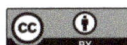

Copyright: © 2021 by the authors. Licensee MDPI, Basel, Switzerland. This article is an open access article distributed under the terms and conditions of the Creative Commons Attribution (CC BY) license (https://creativecommons.org/licenses/by/4.0/).

Abstract: Sea buckthorn (*Hippophae rhamnoides* L. (HR)) leaf powders are the underutilized, promising resource of valuable compounds. Genotype and processing methods are key factors in the preparation of homogenous, stable, and quantified ingredients. The aim of this study was to evaluate the phenolic, triterpenic, antioxidant profiles, carotenoid and chlorophyll content, and chromatic characteristics of convection-dried and freeze-dried HR leaf powders obtained from ten different female cultivars, namely 'Avgustinka', 'Botaniceskaja Liubitelskaja', 'Botaniceskaja', 'Hibrid Percika', 'Julia', 'Nivelena', 'Otradnaja', 'Podarok Sadu', 'Trofimovskaja', and 'Vorobjovskaja'. The chromatic characteristics were determined using the CIELAB scale. The phytochemical profiles were determined using HPLC-PDA (high performance liquid chromatography with photodiode array detector) analysis; spectrophotometric assays and antioxidant activities were investigated using ABTS (2,2′-Azino-bis(3-ethylbenzothiazoline-6-sulfonic acid)) and FRAP (ferric ion reducing antioxidant power) assays. The sea buckthorn leaf powders had a yellowish-green appearance. The drying mode had a significant impact on the total antioxidant activity, chlorophyll content, and chromatic characteristics of the samples; the freeze-dried samples were superior in antioxidant activity, chlorophyll, carotenoid content, and chromatic profile, compared to convection-dried leaf powder samples. The determined triterpenic and phenolic profiles strongly depend on the cultivar, and the drying technique had no impact on qualitative and quantitative composition. Catechin, epigallocatechin, procyanidin B3, ursolic acid, α-amyrin, and β-sitosterol could be used as quantitative markers in the phenolic and triterpenic profiles. The cultivars 'Avgustinka', 'Nivelena', and 'Botaniceskaja' were superior to other tested cultivars, with the phytochemical composition and antioxidant activity.

Keywords: sea buckthorn; phenolic compounds; triterpenic compounds; carotenoids; chlorophyll; freeze-drying; leaf powder ingredients

1. Introduction

In the frame of the changing climate, more attention is paid to the plants that are resistant to the environment, have ecological implications, and are important for maintaining human and animal wellness [1]. *Hippophae* L.—genus (Elaeagnaceae Juss.) consists of seven dioecious, wind-pollinated species, the most known among them is sea buckthorn, *Hippophae rhamnoides* L. (HR) [2]. The species are widely distributed in the Northern

Hemisphere and have great adaptability features to various climatic and edaphic conditions. *Hippophae* plants are native to Asia and Europe, and they can be found in North America [3,4]. The species are also cultivated in plantations as an agriculture crop using diverse genetic origin cultivars (which have possessed specific traits and suitability for different climatic zones since the 1970s) [3,5]. The HR plants can withstand a great range of temperatures and they are resistant to drought. Moreover, the HR plants can easily develop a complex root system coupled to nitrogen fixation and be used for soil erosion prevention or be suitable for planting in degraded soils [3,6]. All parts of HR plants and their extracts can be used for pharmaceutical, nutraceutical, cosmetical, food, and fodder purposes, with the most well-known materials being fruits and leaves [4,5,7,8]. The traditional medicinal systems incorporate the fruits and leaves of HR in the treatment of various ailments of digestive, hepatic, and cardiovascular systems, as well as skin diseases [3,4]. In vitro and in vivo studies have confirmed the anti-inflammatory, antitumor, hepatoprotective, immunomodulatory, anti-atherogenic, anti-stress, hepatoprotective, radioprotective, tissue repair, antibacterial, antifungal, antiviral, and antioxidant activities, which are determined by the multichemical origin compounds [4,9–13]. Fruits and leaves contain rich profiles of carotenoids, tocopherols, amino acids, triterpenic compounds, and phenolic compounds [3,5,7,8,10,14–20]. The phenolic compounds determine the pharmacological effects that are associated with the antioxidant activity [10,21,22]. Carotenoid intake is associated with a reduced risk of chronic aging-related diseases [23]. Chlorophylls can suppress radical species from mitochondria and can have antiproliferative effects on cancer cells, as well as modulate the redox status [24]. HR extracts can modulate intracellular oxidative stress, prevent mitochondrial impairment, and protect neuronal cells from damage [16]. On the other hand, the multitude of different chemical origin substances acting in different modes provide synergistic or additive effects [11,25]; therefore, the comprehensive determination of phytochemical profiles could provide information necessary for the standardization of extracts. The variable phytochemical characteristics can occur depending on the genotype, female or male plant, the climatic zone of the growing area, cultivation conditions, harvesting time, post-harvest management, and extraction methodology [3,12,20–22]. Growing promising genotypes in plantations could ensure greater homogeneity of raw materials with defined markers for standardization [26]. Due to the specific attachments of fruits, the branches are pruned during harvesting. As the leaves are also a very promising raw material, no-waste technologies could be promoted [27]. The leaves contain similar phytochemical profiles as fruits, but have significantly higher amounts of phenolic compounds, especially hydrolysable and condensed tannins, triterpenic compounds, and flavonoids [10,19–21]. Flavonol isorhamnetin, in the frame of the COVID-19 pandemic situation, gained scientific attention, due to its capabilities of in vitro inhibition on the entrance of SARS-CoV-2 spike pseudo-typed virus into cells [13]. Results suggest great potential for isorhamnetin-rich materials of HR as candidates in COVID-19 management. Literature states that the phytochemical composition and antioxidant activity of HR leaves are comparable to the green tea [9]. The drying methods also have a significant impact on the quantitative profile, as well as the color of the product [28]. Color changes can be induced by various reactions occurring in the raw materials during the drying process [29]. The elevated drying temperatures can reduce the total amounts of carotenoids and phenolic compounds [30–32]; therefore, the evaluation of the conventional drying methods and innovative techniques, such as freeze-drying, is crucial to produce high-added value products with unaltered health properties. The color characteristics have been evaluated for the HR fruit products [32], but no data were found regarding the leaves. Furthermore, the phytochemical profile data on HR cultivars' leaves is still scarce, especially on triterpenic compounds. This is the first report on the detailed triterpenic composition of leaf samples. The adaptability traits, together with rich phytochemical compositions and pharmacological potential, propose HR as a multifunctional plant for the promotion of no-waste technologies, including the better exploitation of plant material resources and growth of sustainable agriculture. The aim of this study was to evaluate the phenolic, triterpenic, antioxidant, and chromatic profiles, as well as the carotenoid and chlorophyll content of convection-dried (SD) and freeze-dried (FD) HR leaf powders obtained from ten different cultivars. To the best of our knowledge, this is the first comparative report on the processed leaf powders of ten collectional cultivars.

2. Results and Discussion

2.1. Evaluation of Chromatic Parameters in the Freeze-Dried and Convection-Dried Leaf Powders of H. rhamnoides Cultivars

The processing stage is necessary for the plant origin materials to become stable, functional ingredients or products. Thermal processing, operating in a various regimes, is applied for the preservation of materials [33]. On the other hand, it can induce the alterations in composition, as well as in color. Color is a significant quality trait for a product or ingredient linked with visual appeal, consumers' expectations and demands, intrinsic quality potential, safety, and stability [30,33,34]. The determination of color parameters can predict quality changes and aid in the standardization procedures requisite for the stable product, corresponding to purposeful quality requirements. CIELAB color parameters provide reliable, reproducible, and comparative results [34]. The applied chromatic characteristics elucidated that freeze-drying gave better color quality parameter values, with lighter, more vivid, and greener powders. Table 1 presents the data on the convection-dried and freeze-dried HR leaves, indicating the L^*, a^*, b^*, C, and h values. The significant differences between convection-dried and freeze-dried HR powders were determined for the cultivars tested. Significant correlations were established between the different drying modes for all color values (R^2 ranged 0.41–0.78 and R ranged 0.64–0.88). The L^* value represents the lightness (the closer to 100, the lighter the color). In some cases, the degradation of phytochemical compounds can be associated with the lowered values of the L^* value indicator [32,35]. The freeze-dried HR leaf powders had significantly greater ($p < 0.05$) L^* values, compared to convection-dried powders (on average, 59.88 ± 0.90 and 57.76 ± 1.62, respectively). The lightest powders were obtained from the cultivar 'Trofimovskaja' (61.76 ± 0.01 and 60.28 ± 0.03 for the FD and CD samples, respectively). The lower L^* values can be associated with the higher temperatures' regime during the drying process [31]. The a^* values represent the shift in color towards greenish (negative values) or reddish (positive values) directions. The shifts can be linked to the retention or oxidation of chlorophylls and carotenoids [31,34]. All the obtained HR sample values ranged from −8.24−−0.30. The freeze-dried HR powders were, on average, 3.5-fold more shifted toward the green scale, compared to the convection-dried HR powder samples. The powders of 'Vorobjovskaja' had the greatest a^* values ($p < 0.05$) in both drying modes. The b^* values represent the yellow and blue colors, towards positive and negative scales, respectively. Freeze-dried powders were determined with greater yellow shift (on average, b values 24.09 ± 0.86), compared to convection-dried powder samples (on average—19.71 ± 1.60).

In general, the a^* and b^* values together indicate the yellowish-green appearance of the HR powders. The chrome C value represents the chroma, or the vividness of the color [29,33,34,36]. The obtained c values were greater ($p < 0.05$) in the freeze-dried powder samples for all cultivars tested and correlated with the values of a and b (R = −0.60 and R = 98, respectively). Cultivars 'Podarok Sadu' and 'Trofimovskaja' had the greatest chroma values (>23) in convection-dried mode leaf powders, while in the freeze-dried mode cultivars, the greatest values were determined for 'Nivelena' and 'Botaniceskaja' (>26) (Table 1). The h value is a color-appearance parameter that is corresponding to the dominant wavelength and represents the degrees, herein obtained angle values from 90° (yellow) towards 180° (green) and up to 110°. The obtained values correspond to the overall trend, with the freeze-dried powder samples possessing a greater shift toward the green color. Cultivar 'Vorobjovskaja' had the greatest h values in the freeze-drying mode. The calculated ΔE values indicate the color distance between evaluated colors. Figure S4 presents the ΔE data on fresh and dried HR material. As the values of FD materials are significantly ($p < 0.05$) lower, compared to CD materials, results suggest that freeze-drying retains the color of fresh leaves greater, compared to convection-drying.

Table 1. The chromatic characteristics (L*, a*, b*, C, and h) of convection-dried (CD) and freeze-dried (FD) HR cultivars' leaf powders.

Cultivar	Drying Method	L*	a*	b*	C	h
Avgustinka	CD	58.76 ± 0.04	−1.37 ± 0.05	19.18 ± 0.15	19.23 ± 0.14	94.08 ± 0.15
Botaniceskaja Liubitelskaja	CD	55.92 ± 0.02	−0.30 ± 0.02	17.82 ± 0.07	17.82 ± 0.07	90.98 ± 0.05
Botaniceskaja	CD	57.76 ± 0.03	−1.24 ± 0.11	19.16 ± 0.08	19.20 ± 0.08	93.70 ± 0.32
Hibrid Percika	CD	59.53 ± 0.02	−2.67 ± 0.07	23.38 ± 0.13	24.66 ± 0.11	108.54 ± 0.25
Julia	CD	56.38 ± 0.03	−1.47 ± 0.14	18.56 ± 0.24	18.62 ± 0.25	94.53 ± 0.37
Nivelena	CD	57.12 ± 0.01	−0.74 ± 0.05	18.95 ± 0.07	18.96 ± 0.08	92.24 ± 0.14
Otradnaja	CD	55.79 ± 0.02	−1.37 ± 0.07	18.47 ± 0.07	18.52 ± 0.07	94.23 ± 0.05
Podarok Sadu	CD	59.84 ± 0.03	−5.03 ± 0.05	22.49 ± 0.10	23.11 ± 0.10	103.27 ± 0.14
Trofimovskaja	CD	60.28 ± 0.03	−5.22 ± 0.01	22.49 ± 0.08	23.09 ± 0.07	103.07 ± 0.07
Vorobjovskaja	CD	56.81 ± 0.02	−7.84 ± 0.09	19.93 ± 0.12	20.11 ± 0.12	97.63 ± 0.16
Avgustinka	FD	59.71 ± 0.02	−7.14 ± 0.06	24.62 ± 0.18	25.64 ± 0.19	106.18 ± 0.10
Botaniceskaja Liubitelskaja	FD	59.10 ± 0.04	−7.61 ± 0.03	24.68 ± 0.11	25.82 ± 0.11	107.14 ± 0.02
Botaniceskaja	FD	59.94 ± 0.03	−8.17 ± 0.03	25.02 ± 0.12	26.32 ± 0.10	108.09 ± 0.12
Hibrid Percika	FD	59.02 ± 0.04	−7.84 ± 0.09	23.38 ± 0.13	24.66 ± 0.11	108.54 ± 0.25
Julia	FD	59.18 ± 0.01	−7.66 ± 0.07	23.75 ± 0.13	24.95 ± 0.13	107.89 ± 0.15
Nivelena	FD	60.25 ± 0.01	−7.56 ± 0.04	25.06 ± 0.04	26.18 ± 0.04	106.79 ± 0.07
Otradnaja	FD	60.88 ± 0.02	−7.98 ± 0.04	24.35 ± 0.09	25.63 ± 0.07	108.14 ± 0.12
Podarok Sadu	FD	59.85 ± 0.04	−6.05 ± 0.10	22.40 ± 0.11	23.21 ± 0.12	105.11 ± 0.21
Trofimovskaja	FD	61.76 ± 0.01	−7.31 ± 0.08	24.35 ± 0.16	25.43 ± 0.17	106.71 ± 0.12
Vorobjovskaja	FD	58.69 ± 0.01	−8.25 ± 0.02	23.30 ± 0.17	24.71 ± 0.17	109.49 ± 0.10

2.2. Content of Chrolophyll A (Cha), Chlorophyll B (Chb), and Carotenoids in the Freeze-Dried and Convection-Dried Leaf Powders of H. rhamnoides Cultivars

The chlorophyll is an important leaf pigment, providing green color and indicating the capacity of photosynthesis [28,37,38]. The drying method influenced the content of the chlorophylls detrimentally (Figure 1). Freeze-drying, compared to convection-drying, ensured greater ($p < 0.05$) retention of chlorophyll a, chlorophyll b, and the total amount of chlorophylls, on average, 1.4-fold, 19-fold, and 1.6-fold, respectively. The greatest amounts of total chlorophyll were determined in the leaf powders of the cultivars 'Avgustinka', 'Julia', 'Otradnaja', and 'Botaniceskaja' (−3.08 ± 0.22 mg/g, 2.97 ± 0.21 mg/g, 2.97 ± 0.22 mg/g, and 2.96 ± 0.20 mg/g, respectively). The impact of the drying method on the chlorophyll content varied, depending on the cultivar. However, cultivars 'Avgustinka' and 'Julia' contained the greatest amounts of chlorophyll in both drying techniques. The amounts of chlorophylls were well-correlated with all chromatic parameters (R for L*, b*, C, and h values ranged from 0.49–0.96) (R for a* value——0.66–−0.92) and antioxidant activity (up to 0.55 and 0.61 ($p < 0.05$) with ABTS and FRAP assays, respectively). Chlorophyll b was more susceptible to drying-induced degradation, compared to chlorophyll a. Kumar et al., 2015 [38], determined that the freeze-drying method resulted in higher amounts of chlorophyll a, chlorophyll b, and the total chlorophylls, compared to thermal drying, during which auto-oxidation and various other intrinsic processes can occur. Guan et al., 2005 [30], determined that increasing the drying temperatures resulted in decreased chlorophyll content.

The amounts of total carotenoids varied significantly ($p < 0.05$) between the cultivars and drying methods (Figure 1). The greatest amounts of total carotenoids ($p < 0.05$) were determined in the freeze-dried powders of 'Avgustinka', 'Botaniceskaja', 'Otradnaja', 'Julia', and 'Nivelena' (0.41 ± 0.03 mg/g, 0.40 ± 0.03 mg/g, 0.40 ± 0.02 mg/g, 0.40 ± 0.02 mg/g, and 0.35 ± 0.02 mg/g, respectively), compared to convection-drying and other cultivars in both drying modes. No significant differences in total carotenoids, between convection-drying and freeze-drying, were determined for the other cultivars, namely 'Hibrid Percika', 'Botaniceskaja Liubitelskaja', 'Trofimovskaja', and' Vorobjovskaja'. On average, the total amount of carotenoids in the HR leaf powders was 0.34 ± 0.01 mg/g. The best preservation of phytochemical compounds, especially the lipophilic ones, is obtained using freeze-drying techniques, as the high drying temperatures in conventional modes result in compound deterioration [39]. The amounts of determined carotenoids and chlorophylls in HR leaf powders were comparable with the amounts determined in commonly used vegetables [23,30].

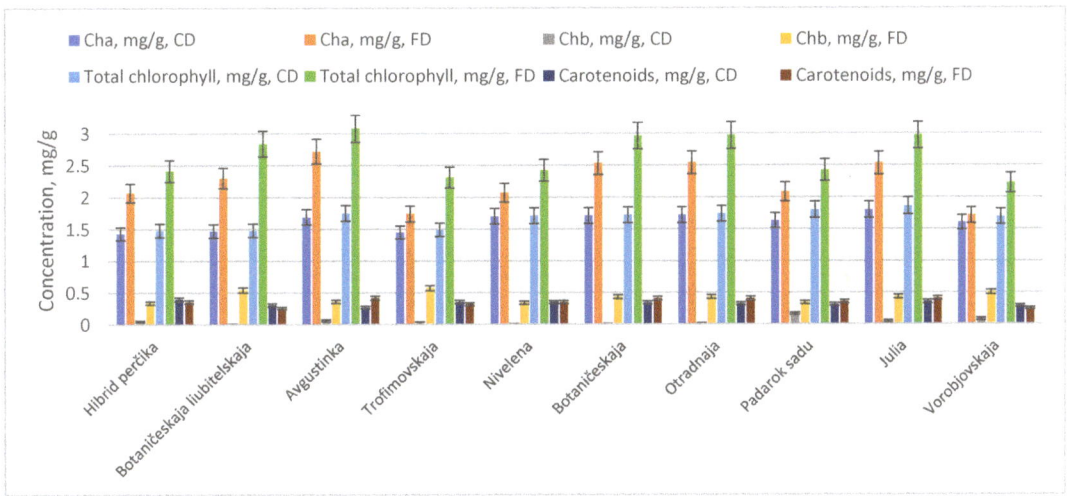

Figure 1. Total amounts (mg/g) of chrolophyll A (Cha), chlorophyll B (Chb), and carotenoids in convection-dried (CD) and freeze-dried (FD) HR cultivars' leaf powders.

2.3. Radical Scavenging and Reducing Activities of the Freeze-Dried and Convection-Dried Leaf Powders of H. rhamnoides Cultivars

The determined antioxidant activity, corresponding to the radical scavenging and reducing activities of the tested HR leaf powders, is presented in Figure 2. The drying mode had an impact on the total antioxidant activity of the samples, and the antioxidant activity of the freeze-dried samples was significantly greater than convection-dried HR leaf powder samples. The leaf powder samples of 'Avgustinka' and 'Nivelena' possessed the greatest antioxidant activities in both drying modes ($p < 0.05$). The main contributors to the antioxidant activity are phenolic origin compounds. Correlational interrelationships were determined between radical scavenging, reducing activities, and the amounts of catechin, gallic acid, ellagic acid, p-coumaric acid, rutin, kaempferol, epigallocatechin, isorhamnetin, myricetin, isoquercitrin, and procyanidin B3; additionally, with the sum of total identified phenolic compounds, the Pearson's correlation coefficients ranged from 0.44–0.74 ($p < 0.05$). Reducing activities were greater compared to radical scavenging in both drying modes and were well-correlated (R = 0.61, $p < 0.05$). Ellagic acid and flavan-3-ols, namely catechin and epigallocatechin gallate, possess greater reducing activities, compared to radical scavenging [40]. These compounds predominate the phenolic profile in all the cultivars tested and were determined to have 1.5-fold greater reduction activity, compared to radical scavenging. Our results are in agreement with Sne et al., 2013 [21], and Tzachristas et al., 2020 [41], as they determined significantly greater FRAP values, compared to DPPH in the leaves of HR [21,41]. In vitro antioxidant assays cannot be interpolated to the occurring effect in vivo; nevertheless, they elucidate the potential of antioxidant active compounds to express their effects in different modes of action. The selection of antioxidant activity methods should be based on their mechanisms of action, and due to the complexity of phytochemicals, at least two methods should be implemented [5,40]. However, other components present in the HR leaves, such as ascorbic acid, tocopherols, and carotenoids, contribute to the antioxidant activity, as well [20,22,30,41]. Gornas et al., 2014 [39], determined that lipophyllic antioxidants, such as carotenoids and tocopherols have been retained to a greater extent using freeze-drying technique, compared to conventional drying. Furthermore, raw materials of HR are void of ascorbic acid oxidase, which ensures the retention of ascorbic acid in dried products [10]. The HR leaf powders have great potential as a functional antioxidative ingredient in the vinification process [41]. HR leaf extracts, compared to green tea in cell cultures, increase glutathione levels, which causes intracellular redox homeostasis [9]. Ethanolic extracts also contain lipophyllic compounds that contribute to the total antioxidant activity significantly [39]. The multitude of lipophilic and hydrophilic chemical origin compounds present in the botanical matrix possess intrinsic and inter-relational antioxidant effects [10,39]; therefore, selection of the proper drying regime is a crucial step in the preparation of the antioxidant's active ingredients.

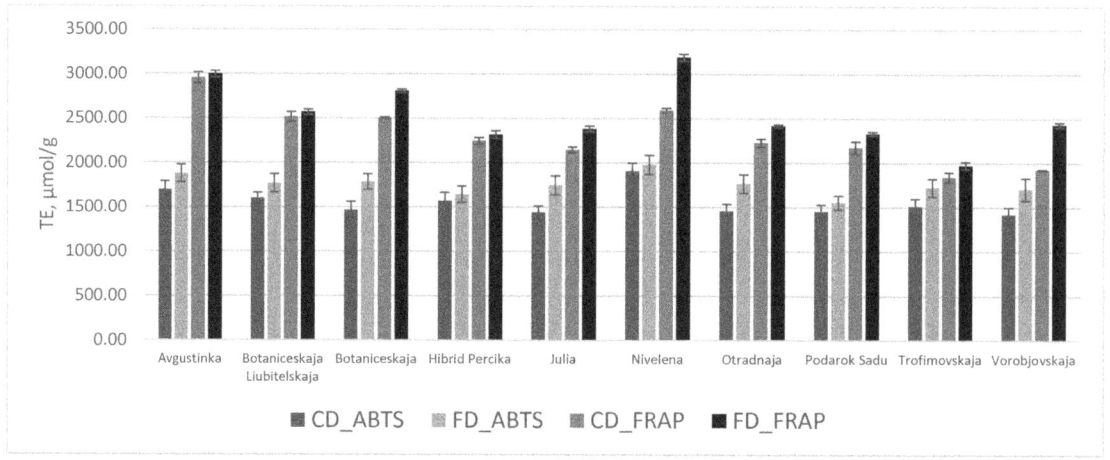

Figure 2. Trolox equivalent antioxidant activity values (TE, μmol/g) of convection-dried (CD) and freeze-dried (FD) HR cultivars' leaf powders.

2.4. Principal Component Analysis of the Freeze-Dried and Convection-Dried Leaf Powders of H. rhamnoides Cultivars

The principal component analysis was applied to distinguish the color parameters, chlorophyll content, carotenoid content, and antioxidant activity of the convection-dried and freeze-dried HR leaf powders of different cultivars. Three principal components, PC1, PC2, and PC3 were obtained, which explained 54.37%, 21.00%, and 14.41% of the total variance, respectively. The PC1 was positively correlated with L^*, b^*, C, and h values, with the correlation coefficients being 0.86, 0.93, 0.94, and 0.96, respectively; additionally, chlorophyll b (0.89) and the total chlorophylls (0.66) were negatively correlated with a value (−0.95). The PC2 highly positively correlated with the FRAP and ABTS values (0.95 and 0.71, respectively). The PC3 positively correlated with the content of total carotenoids (0.95) and chlorophyll a (0.61). The score plots (Figure 3) cultivars (with different drying modes) into groups, corresponding to the drying method and cultivar.

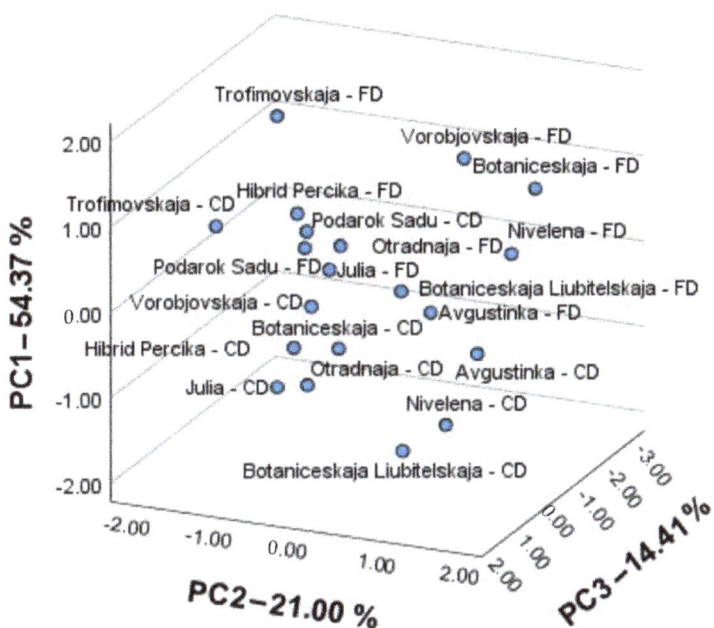

Figure 3. PCA score plots for antioxidant and chromatic characteristics of convection-dried (CD) and freeze-dried (FD) HR cultivars' leaf powders.

The first group, on the top right, consisted of the freeze-dried powders of HR cultivars, namely 'Vorobjobskaja', 'Botaniceskaja Liubitelskaja', 'Botaniceskaja', 'Avgustinka', and 'Nivelena'. They were distinguished by higher antioxidant activity and had lighter, more vivid, and closer to pure green color characteristics; additionally, they contained higher amounts of carotenoids and chlorophylls. The second group, on the bottom right, consisted of the convection-dried HR powders of three corresponding cultivars, namely 'Avgustinka', 'Nivelena', and 'Botaniceskaja Liubitelskaja'. They possessed similar antioxidant activities but were darker, shifted toward yellow color powders, and had a lower carotenoid and chlorophyll content, compared to the first group. The third group, on the bottom left, grouped convection-dried cultivars, namely 'Vorobjovskaja', 'Julia', 'Otradnaja', 'Botaniceskaja', and 'Hibrid Percika'. The fourth group, on the top left, grouped the cultivars 'Podarok Sadu' (both drying modes), 'Hibrid Percika', 'Julia', 'Otradnaja' (FD mode), and 'Trofimovskaja' (CD mode). The last two groups had significantly lower antioxidant activity, and the fourth group was characterized by its lighter, greener, and vivid colors. Cultivar 'Trofimovskaja' was distinguished by the greatest amounts of chlorophyll b and notable amounts of carotenoids. In summary, the freeze-dried powders of cultivars 'Avgustinka', 'Botaniceskaja', and 'Nivelena' were superior in antioxidant activity, carotenoid, chlorophyll content, and color characteristics. Kumar et al., 2014 [38], determined that freeze-drying retained the greatest amounts of chlorophyl, ascorbic acid, and antioxidant activity, compared to room, sun, or other thermal drying techniques [38]. Higher drying temperatures (>80 °C) induced the decay of the phenolic compounds, compared to lower drying temperatures [30]. In our study, the color parameters, radical scavenging, and reduced activities, as well as the amounts of chlorophylls and carotenoids (for certain cultivars) of the tested HR powders had greater values in the freeze-drying mode, compared to convection-thermal drying. On the other hand, the drying modes had no significant effect on the amount of identified phenolic and triterpenic compounds. This is in agreement with the results of Asofiei et al., 2019 [42], where the polyphenolic profiles were not affected by the microwave-assisted extraction. The results suggest that other compounds of the phytochemical complex with antioxidant activity can be susceptible to drying mode, such as ascorbic acid, tocopherols, carotenoids, tannins, or other unidentified compounds in the phenolic and triterpenic profiles [10].

2.5. Hierarchical Cluster Analysis of Phenolic and Triterpenic Compounds

The phytochemical profiles of individual phenolic and triterpenic compounds were determined for each HR cultivar sample for both drying modes applied. Hierarchical cluster analysis was performed to the convection-dried and freeze-dried HR leaf powder samples for the mean qualities of phenolic and triterpenic compounds (Figure 4).

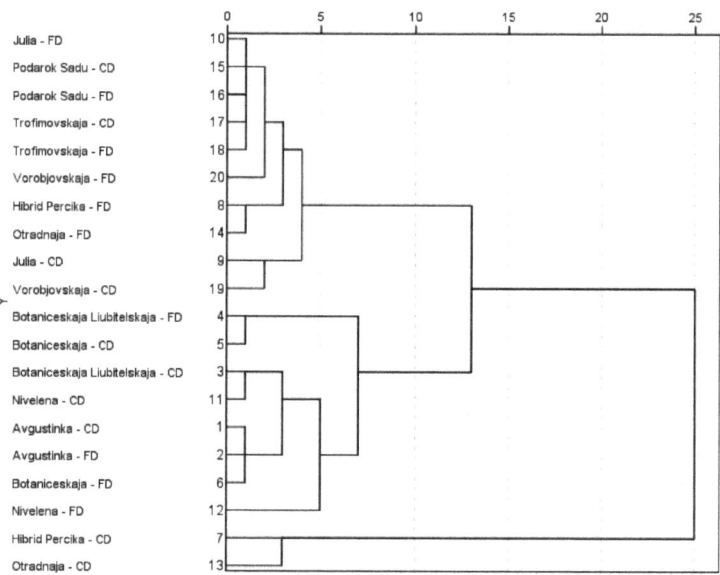

Figure 4. The dendrogram of hierarchical cluster analysis on phenolic and triterpenic compounds of convection-dried (CD) and freeze-dried (FD) HR cultivars' leaf powders. 1–cluster composed of CD and FD samples of 'Avgustinka', 'Botaniceskaja', 'Botaniceskaja Liubitelskaja', and 'Nivelena'; 2–cluster composed of CD samples of 'Hibrid Percika' and 'Otradnaja'; 3–cluster composed of CD and FD samples of 'Julia', 'Podarok Sadu', 'Trofimovskaja', 'Vorobjovskaja', and FD samples of 'Hibrid Percika' and 'Otradnaja'.

The cluster analysis grouped the samples into three clusters. The first cluster coupled all the convection-dried and freeze-dried samples from the cultivars 'Avgustinka', 'Nivelena', 'Botaniceskaja', and 'Botaniceskaja Liubitelskaja'. They can be characterized by the greatest amounts of catechin, protocatechuic acid, ellagic acid, and the total amount of triterpenic compounds. The second cluster coupled two convection-dried samples from the cultivars 'Hibrid Percika' and 'Otradnaja'. The determined amounts of the total triterpenic compounds were lower, compared to other clusters. The third cluster grouped all the convection-dried and freeze-dried samples from the cultivars, namely 'Vorobjovskaja', 'Julia', 'Trofimovskaja', and 'Podarok Sadu', as well as the freeze-dried samples from cultivars 'Hibrid Percika' and 'Otradnaja'. The clustering revealed that the triterpenic and phenolic profiles strongly depend on the cultivar, as the samples from different drying methods tended to group under the cultivar. The phenolic composition has a significant genotypic and geographic-related qualitative and quantitative variability [2,9]. The principal phenolic markers characteristic of the profiles of HR leaves are ellagic acid, gallic acid, isorhamnetin, kaempferol, and quercetin derivatives [7]. The significant differences between the amounts of determined compounds in the HR powders and the different drying methods were determined only for certain compounds, and the superiority of specific drying methods was not confirmed. Therefore, the detailed discussion on phenolic and triterpenic profiles is presented on the freeze-dried HR cultivar powder samples, as they were defined with better chlorophyll, carotenoid, and chromatic characteristics (Table 2).

2.6. Phenolic and Triterpenic Profiles of the Freeze-Dried Leaf Powders of H. rhamnoides Cultivars

The determined phenolic profiles of 10 tested cultivars of HR consisted of flavonoids, phenolic acids, and stilbene compound resveratrol. The flavonoid complex was comprised of flavan-3-ols (catechin, epigallocatechin, epicatechin gallate, and procyanidin B3) and flavonols (rutin, isorhamnetin-3-rutinoside, isorhamnetin-3-glucoside, quercetin, kaempferol, tiliroside, isorhamnetin, myricetin, quercetin 3-O-6″-acetyl-glucoside, and isoquercitrin). Flavan-3-ols were predominant compounds in the profiles of all tested cultivars, with the greatest amounts in 'Avgustinka', 'Nivelena', 'Botaniceskaja Liubitelskaja', and' Botaniceskaja' (Table 2). The total amounts of flavonol derivatives in the cultivars were in the following order: isorhamnetin derivatives > quercetin derivatives > keampferol derivatives. Their profiles were cultivar-dependent and elucidated 'Podarok Sadu', 'Trofimovskaja', and 'Vorobjovskaja' with the greatest amounts of isorhamnetin derivatives, up to 1088 µg/g of dry weight (dw). Chemophenetically isorhamnetin glycosides prevail over quercetin glycosides [19]. Recent findings on the isorhamnetin's capability to bind to human angiotensin-converting enzyme 2 and prevent the SARS-CoV-2 virus from entering the cells [13] could initiate further research on the valorization of HR leaves for the production of isorhamnetin. The leaf powders of 'Otradnaja' and 'Podarok Sadu' were determined with the greatest amounts of kaempferol derivatives. Quercetin glycosides predominated in 'Avgustinka' and 'Botaniceskaja Liubitelskaja' cultivars. Ciesarowa et al., 2020 [10], in the HR leaf profiles, determined rutin and hyperoside as the predominant quercetin derivatives, whereas in our study hyperoside was quantified only in traces (data not shown). Overall, the leaf powders of 'Avgustinka', 'Nivelena', and 'Botaniceskaja Liubitelskaja' cultivars were significantly distinguished by the greatest amounts of total identified flavonoid derivatives, on average, 111.78 mg/g dw. The qualitative profile is in agreement with the literature data, indicating rutin, epigallocatechin, and catechin as flavonoid profile markers [7,8,19,20,43,44]. The profile of specific isorhamnetin, kaempferol, and quercetin derivatives is genotype- and habitat-dependent and can be applied to chemophenetic and authenticity studies [19].

The total amounts of identified phenolic acids ranged from 4511.40 µg/g to 6150.70 µg/g in the cultivars 'Trofimovskaja' and 'Avgustinka', respectively. The profiles were predominated by the protocatechuic, ellagic, and gallic acids in all the tested cultivars (up to 3405.10 ± 117.65 µg/g, 2157.40 ± 74.43 µg/g, and 565.90 ± 19.30 µg/g, respectively), while ferulic, *p*-coumaric, and caffeic acids were the minor compounds (Table 2). Asofiei et al., 2019 [42], determined gallic acid as a predominant compound in various modes of extraction with different parameters. The greatest ($p < 0.05$) quantitative phenolic acid profiles were determined for the leaf powders of the cultivars 'Avgustinka' and 'Botaniceskaja Liubitelskaja' and corresponded to the cultivars with the greatest flavonoid profiles. On the other hand, the amounts of phenolic acids in the leaf powders of cultivar 'Julia' were comparable with the total amounts of 5421.20 µg/g. Zadernowski et al., 2005 [45], in the fruit samples of 'Nivelena', 'Otradnaja', 'Podarok Sadu', and 'Trofimovskaja' quantified 1135–1868 µg/g of phenolic acids. Fruits samples were predominated by gallic and salicylic acids. Other identified phenolic acids conform to the genotype and are in agreement with the components identified in our study. Sytarova et al., 2020 [20], in the HR leaf samples, additionally determined notable amounts of chlorogenic and neochlorogenic acids; however, leaf samples of our tested cultivars were devoid of these compounds. Studies suggest that leaves contain richer fractions of phenolic acids, and individual qualitative and quantitative profiles are genotype- and habitat-dependent [3,10,20,45].

Table 2. Phenolic and triterpenic profiles (μg/g, dw) of freeze-dried *Hippophae rhamnoides* cultivars' leaf powders.

FD	Avgustinka	Botaniceskaja	Botaniceskaja Liubitelskaja	Hibrid Percika	Julia	Nivelena	Otradnaja	Podarok Sadu	Trofimovskaja	Vorobjovskaja
Catechin	54,685.20 ± 1894.04	39,868.50 ± 1380.78	51,592.60 ± 1786.91	46,308.60 ± 1603.87	47,683.00 ± 1651.48	60,605.80 ± 2099.14	44,232.70 ± 1531.96	43,342.10 ± 1501.11	43,620.90 ± 1510.77	44,700.90 ± 1548.18
Gallic acid	462.90 ± 15.74	401.70 ± 13.62	554.1 ± 18.9	376.30 ± 12.74	460.50 ± 15.66	565.90 ± 19.30	385.80 ± 13.07	421.70 ± 14.31	404.4 ± 13.71	453.20 ± 15.40
Protocatechuic acid	3405.11 ± 117.65	2457.20 ± 84.82	2990.80 ± 103.30	2169.90 ± 74.86	3002.00 ± 103.69	1540.10 ± 53.05	2101.20 ± 72.48	2116.80 ± 73.02	2329.00 ± 80.37	2467.20 ± 85.16
Caftaric acid	243.00 ± 8.20	162.90 ± 5.36	127.90 ± 4.16	164.10 ± 5.40	130.20 ± 4.24	164.80 ± 5.43	159.10 ± 5.23	274.10 ± 9.20	244.60 ± 8.18	206.00 ± 6.85
Ellagic acid	1880.20 ± 64.83	2157.40 ± 74.43	1921.60 ± 66.26	1339.00 ± 46.08	1659.90 ± 57.20	1816.50 ± 62.64	1692.10 ± 58.31	1234.20 ± 42.80	1396.2 ± 48.06	1413.70 ± 48.67
Coumaric acid	55.20 ± 1.69	52.00 ± 1.59	50.70 ± 1.54	68.50 ± 2.13	52.70 ± 1.61	72.00 ± 2.25	45.30 ± 1.37	48.50 ± 1.47	44.5 ± 1.34	41.90 ± 1.26
Rutin	576.10 ± 19.66	343.10 ± 11.59	532.8 ± 18.16	371.40 ± 12.57	421.60 ± 14.31	386.40 ± 13.09	310.20 ± 10.45	459.20 ± 15.61	314.6 ± 10.61	360.00 ± 12.18
Isorhamnetin-3-rutinoside	585.10 ± 19.97	542.60 ± 18.50	588.30 ± 20.08	727.60 ± 24.90	640.40 ± 21.88	479.30 ± 16.31	512.30 ± 17.45	693.20 ± 23.71	671.7 ± 22.97	746.40 ± 25.56
Isorhamnetin-3-glucoside	266.40 ± 8.94	421.60 ± 14.31	287.10 ± 9.65	256.80 ± 8.61	274.30 ± 9.21	410.90 ± 13.94	301.00 ± 10.13	368.50 ± 12.47	341.5 ± 11.54	286.80 ± 9.64
Quercetin	20.40 ± 0.66	23.30 ± 0.73	22.80 ± 0.72	20.00 ± 0.66	19.70 ± 0.65	20.10 ± 0.66	19.10 ± 0.64	18.10 ± 0.62	20.00 ± 0.66	17.80 ± 0.61
Kaempferol	21.14 ± 0.68	26.74 ± 0.82	24.61 ± 0.76	20.39 ± 0.66	18.53 ± 0.63	23.82 ± 0.74	24.33 ± 0.75	20.56 ± 0.67	13.14 ± 0.55	14.24 ± 0.56
Tiliroside	540.30 ± 18.42	253.20 ± 8.48	557.5 ± 19.01	316.80 ± 10.68	321.40 ± 10.84	338.40 ± 11.43	766.00 ± 26.23	733.7 ± 25.12	308.30 ± 10.39	370.10 ± 12.53
Epigallocatechin	38,818.50 ± 1344.41	38,931.30 ± 1348.31	34,993.50 ± 1211.90	21,464.70 ± 743.25	26,194.80 ± 907.11	40,049.30 ± 1387.04	19,971.10 ± 691.51	29,104.40 ± 1007.90	24,687.20 ± 854.88	31,498.60 ± 1090.84
Isorhamnetin	25.70 ± 0.79	28.70 ± 0.87	27.40 ± 0.83	28.00 ± 0.85	26.60 ± 0.81	28.20 ± 0.85	26.80 ± 0.82	27.00 ± 0.82	25.60 ± 0.79	25.50 ± 0.78
Myricetin	45.70 ± 1.38	47.70 ± 1.45	47.30 ± 1.43	44.60 ± 1.35	45.00 ± 1.36	44.80 ± 1.35	44.50 ± 1.34	44.30 ± 1.34	45.00 ± 1.36	45.90 ± 1.39
Quercetin 3-O-(6′-acetyl-glucoside)	50.30 ± 1.53	26.60 ± 0.81	42.80 ± 1.29	47.40 ± 1.44	78.1 ± 2.46	40.80 ± 1.23	16.00 ± 0.59	12.90 ± 0.55	56.80 ± 1.74	57.00 ± 1.75
Epicatechin gallate	272.60 ± 9.15	248.00 ± 8.30	308.1 ± 10.38	372.70 ± 12.62	137.9 ± 4.5	418.20 ± 14.19	183.10 ± 6.06	212.40 ± 7.07	246.30 ± 8.24	309.00 ± 10.41
Ferulic acid	39.90 ± 1.20	37.80 ± 1.13	36.80 ± 1.10	36.95 ± 1.11	65.6 ± 2.04	59.50 ± 1.83	41.9 ± 1.26	31.70 ± 0.95	24.00 ± 0.75	25.10 ± 0.77
Caffeic acid	62.40 ± 1.93	84.00 ± 2.66	65.4 ± 2.03	65.8 ± 2.04	50.3 ± 1.53	64.2 ± 1.99	86.00 ± 2.73	80.20 ± 2.53	64.50 ± 2.00	66.9 ± 2.08
Isoquercitrin	190.62 ± 6.32	234.51 ± 7.84	197.73 ± 6.56	121.91 ± 3.95	155.44 ± 5.11	231.82 ± 7.74	107.17 ± 3.45	182.96 ± 6.06	149.43 ± 4.90	134.84 ± 4.40
Procyanidin B3	16,813.60 ± 582.13	16,120.70 ± 558.13	13,673.50 ± 473.36	8792.90 ± 304.29	9175.7 ± 317.55	16,470.40 ± 570.25	6619.20 ± 228.99	10,077.60 ± 348.79	11,734.50 ± 406.19	13,101.30 ± 453.54
Resveratrol	86.30 ± 2.74	66.90 ± 2.08	80.75 ± 2.78	75.20 ± 2.36	74.50 ± 2.34	73.4 ± 2.30	105.30 ± 3.38	106.30 ± 3.42	75.70 ± 2.38	80.80 ± 2.55
Maslinic acid	176.26 ± 5.82	71.23 ± 2.23	130.25 ± 4.24	87.77 ± 2.79	146.58 ± 4.8	189.84 ± 6.29	114.39 ± 3.69	69.21 ± 2.16	43.52 ± 1.31	147.60 ± 4.84
corosolic acid	234.20 ± 7.82	143.37 ± 4.69	184.00 ± 6.09	205.11 ± 6.82	263.05 ± 8.82	232.72 ± 7.77	84.84 ± 2.69	143.98 ± 4.71	117.73 ± 3.81	232.54 ± 7.77
Betulinic acid	12.71 ± 0.55	5.65 ± 0.54	5.16 ± 0.55	9.70 ± 0.53	4.61 ± 0.55	4.46 ± 0.55	3.60 ± 0.56	4.29 ± 0.55	8.29 ± 0.53	6.68 ± 0.54
Oleanolic acid	195.32 ± 6.48	112.16 ± 3.62	177.68 ± 5.87	148.91 ± 4.88	176.66 ± 5.84	110.53 ± 3.56	54.49 ± 1.67	95.69 ± 3.06	75.59 ± 2.37	148.49 ± 4.87
Ursolic acid	657.45 ± 22.47	396.00 ± 13.42	504.12 ± 17.17	451.51 ± 15.34	523.61 ± 17.84	397.63 ± 13.48	221.53 ± 7.39	355.07 ± 12.01	248.08 ± 8.30	467.80 ± 15.91
Betulin	212.45 ± 7.07	115.11 ± 3.72	107.06 ± 3.44	113.09 ± 3.65	116.16 ± 3.76	107.39 ± 3.46	49.58 ± 1.51	86.59 ± 2.75	57.36 ± 1.76	82.00 ± 2.59
Erythrodiol	101.86 ± 3.27	35.87 ± 1.08	32.17 ± 0.97	34.60 ± 1.04	74.52 ± 2.34	67.16 ± 2.09	47.33 ± 1.43	36.15 ± 1.08	63.34 ± 1.96	36.27 ± 1.09
Uvaol	207.73 ± 6.91	79.16 ± 2.49	31.07 ± 0.93	44.04 ± 1.33	174.34 ± 5.76	146.54 ± 4.80	66.66 ± 2.07	208.77 ± 6.95	116.72 ± 3.77	153.06 ± 5.02
Lupeol	131.37 ± 4.28	61.24 ± 1.89	58.74 ± 1.81	81.21 ± 2.56	106.98 ± 3.44	158.42 ± 5.21	68.15 ± 2.12	45.20 ± 1.37	21.21 ± 0.68	116.5 ± 3.77
β-Amyrin	145.94 ± 4.78	76.33 ± 2.4	97.88 ± 3.13	41.93 ± 1.26	54.61 ± 1.67	94.24 ± 3.01	20.1 ± 0.66	47.16 ± 1.43	22.57 ± 0.71	58.42 ± 1.80
β-Sitosterol	373.81 ± 12.65	235.34 ± 7.86	168.92 ± 5.57	256.44 ± 8.59	132.94 ± 4.33	204.77 ± 6.81	116.14 ± 3.75	277.28 ± 9.31	138.71 ± 4.53	283.84 ± 9.54
α-Amyrin	972.84 ± 33.40	498.06 ± 16.96	564.59 ± 19.26	548.5 ± 18.7	354.97 ± 12.00	690.14 ± 23.61	281.45 ± 9.46	556.35 ± 18.97	225.63 ± 7.53	727.49 ± 24.90
Friedelin	182.94 ± 6.05	144.53 ± 4.73	101.86 ± 3.27	253.44 ± 8.49	274.38 ± 9.21	180.65 ± 5.97	81.07 ± 2.56	113.29 ± 3.66	60.12 ± 1.85	139.03 ± 4.54

The greatest amounts of resveratrol (above 100 µg/g) were determined in the leaf powders of the cultivars 'Otradnaja' and 'Podarok Sadu'. Leaves of HR genotypes, cultivated in Velke Ripnany, only contained up to 7.9 µg/g of resveratrol [20]. Ghendov-Mosanu et al., 2020 [46], determined about 100 µg/g of resveratrol in the fruit extracts. The amounts of resveratrol in the leaves of HR are comparable with the amounts determined in well-known sources, such as peanuts, red wines, or itadori materials [47].

The correlational analysis revealed strong interrelationships (R = 0.38–0.66 and $p < 0.05$) between reducing activities and phenolic compounds, namely catechin, gallic acid, ellagic acid, p-coumaric acid, rutin, isorhamnetin-3-rutinoside, kaempferol, epigallocatechin, isoquercitrin, and procyanidin B3. Radical scavenging activities were correlated only to the individual amounts of isorhamnetin and myricetin, 0.53 and 0.71, respectively ($p < 0.01$). The correlations between the chromatic characteristics and individual phenolic compounds were also established. The amounts of catechin, gallic acid, ellagic acid, quercetin, kaempferol, epigallocatechin, and procyanidin B3 were positively correlated with chromatic parameters b and c (R = 0.41–0.83 and $p < 0.05$). On the other hand, the amounts of caftaric acid and isorhamnetin-3-rutinoside negatively correlated to parameters b and c (R = −0.43−−0.75 and $p < 0.05$).

The determined triterpenic profile was comprised of triterpenoid acids (maslinic, oleonolic, ursolic, corosolic, and betulinic), triterpene alcohols (erythrodiol, uvaol, lupeol, β-amyrin, and α-amyrin), neutral triterpenes (botulin and friedelin), and phytosterol—β-sitosterol (Table. 2). The predominant triterpenic compounds in the profiles occurred in the following order: α-amyrin > ursolic acid > β-sitosterol > corosolic acid. The content of α-amyrin comprised of, on average, about 24% of all identified triterpenic compounds and ranged from 225.63 ± 7.53 µg/g ('Trofimovskaja') to 972.84 ± 33.40 µg/g ('Avgustinka'). The amounts of ursolic acid ranged from 221.53 ± 7.39 µg/g ('Otradnaja') to 657.45 ± 22.47 µg/g ('Avgustinka') and constituted up to 23% of the total triterpenic compounds. The amounts of β-sitosterol in the leaf powders of HP cultivars corresponded to the quantitative pattern of ursolic acid, with the greatest amounts in 'Avgustinka' and 'Voroblevskaja' (373.81 ± 12.65 µg/g and 283.84 ± 9.54 µg/g, respectively) (Table 2). Kukin et al., 2017 [27], determined β-sitosterol as the predominant compound in the profile of triterpenoids and sterols. The leaf powders of cultivar 'Julia' were distinguished by the greatest ($p < 0.05$) amounts of corosolic acid—263.05 ± 8.82 µg/g. The greatest total amounts of identified triterpenic compounds ($p < 0.05$) were determined for the leaf powders of cultivars 'Avgustinka', 'Nivelena', and 'Vorobjevskaja' (3604.86 µg/g, 2584.47 µg/g, and 2599.71 µg/g, respectively). Individual amounts of triterpenic compounds, correlated only with reducing activity, indicated the highest coefficients for maslinic acid, α-amyrin, and β-amyrin (R= 0.70, 0.60, and 0.74, respectively). Furthermore, all triterpenic compounds (except maslinic acid, betulinic acid, erythrodiol, and uvaol) negatively correlated with the chromatic parameter L, (R = −0.35−−0.65 and $p < 0.05$) indicating their impact on the lightness of the powders. Certain triterpenic compounds were quantified in the fruit materials, with ursolic, oleanolic, and maslinic acid being the predominant compounds in different HR genotypes [48–50]. Our research proposes that HR leaves contain up to 25-fold greater amounts of triterpenes, compared to literature data on fruits. Sadowska et al., 2020 [44], reported oleanolic and ursolic acid as the predominant compounds in the leaves of HR; however, no quantitative profiles were presented. Scientific data suggests the anticancer potential of the triterpenic compounds and, particularly, ursolic acid. Grey et al., 2010 [11], determined the antiproliferative effect of ursolic acid from HR in the Caco-2 and Hep G2 cell lines by increasing apoptosis [11]. Furthermore, the synergistic effects between the triterpenic and phenolic compounds can also potentiate the anti-inflammatory and anticancer activity mechanisms [11,44,51]. Yasukawa et al., 2009 [52], determined the anti-inflammatory and antitumor activity of HR branches and identified ursolic acid and epigallocatechin as the main contributors to the activity [52]. Skalski et al., 2018 [53], determined that sea buckthorn phenolic and triterpenic fractions are promising agents for cardiovascular diseases, as they possess anticoagulant properties and inhibit plasma lipid peroxidation.

3. Materials and Methods

3.1. Plant Material and Preparation of Extracts

The leaves of sea buckthorn (*Hippophae rhamnoides* L.), from nine different female cultivars of the selection of Botanical Garden of Moscow State University, Russia, were studied: ('Avgustinka', 'Botaniceskaja Liubitelskaja', 'Botaniceskaja', 'Hibrid Percika', 'Nivelena', 'Otradnaja', 'Podarok Sadu', 'Trofimovskaja', and 'Vorobjovskaja'); 'Julia' was released in Sweden [54]. Leaf samples were collected at the Lithuanian Research Centre for Agriculture and Forestry, Institute of Horticulture (55.08911, 23.81653), in mid-August, during the phenological development stage (BBCH) 87 [55]. Leaf samples were dried using two different drying methods: convection at 60 °C and freeze-drying. Freeze-drying was performed in a Zirbus lyophilizer (Zirbus Technology GmbH, Bad Grund, Germany) at 0.01 Mbar pressure and −85 °C condenser temperature. Convection drying was performed in a UDS-150/1 hot-air laboratory dryer ("Utenos krosnys", Lithuania) at a temperature of 60 ± 1 °C and an air-flow rate of 1.5 m s^{-1}.

The dried leaves were ground in a laboratory mill Retsch ZM 200 (Retsch GmbH, Haan, Germany) using 0.2 mm ring sieve to powder and stored in tightly closed glass containers in a dark place.

For the analysis of phenolic compounds and antioxidant activity, about 0.2 g (precise weight) of HR leaf powder was weighted, and 20 mL of 70% (*v/v*) ethanol was added. For the analysis of triterpenic compounds, 1 g (precise weight) of HR leaf powder was weighted, and 10 mL of methanol was added. The extraction process continued for 15 min in an ultrasonic bath (Elmasonic P, Singen, Germany). The extracts were then centrifuged for 30 min at 3000× g in a Biofuge Stratos centrifuge and filtered through 0.22 μm pore size PVDF membrane filters (Carl Roth GmbH, Karlsruhe, Germany) to the dark glass vials. For the analysis of chlorophylls and carotenoids, about 500 mg (precise weight) of convection-dried and 200 mg (precise weight) of freeze-dried plant leaf samples were transferred to a ceramic pestle, and for the sample rehydration, 3 and 1.5 mL of ultrapure water (according to the weight of the sample) was added. The pestle was covered with aluminum foil for 2 min. The rehydrated sample was ground in a mortar and pestle with 5 g of pure quartz sand. The pigments were extracted and transferred to volumetric flask (100 mL) with an aqueous 80% solution of acetone. Homogenized sample mixture was centrifuged at 10,000 rpm for 15 min at 4 °C. The supernatant was separated and immediately subjected to analysis.

3.2. Chemicals

HPLC-grade chemicals and solvents were used for this study: acetonitrile, methanol, acetic, hydrochloric, trifluoroacetic acids, α-amyrin, β-amyrin, β-sitosterol, lupeol, erythrodiol, maslinic acid, oleanolic acid, rutin, isoquercitrin, quercetin, isorhamnetin, procyanidin B3, caffeic acid, *p*-coumaric acid, ferulic acid, gallic acid, protocatechuic acid, caftaric acid, ellagic acid, isorhamnetin-3-rutinoside, quercetin, kaempferol, tiliroside, epigallocatechin, isorhamnetin, myricetin, quercetin 3-*O*-(6''-acetyl-glucoside), epicatechin gallate, and resveratrol from Sigma-Aldrich (Steinheim, Germany); catechin, from Fluka (Buchs, Switzerland); uvaol, friedelin, betulin, betulinic acid, corosolic acid, rutin, isorhamnetin-3-*O*-glucoside, and quercitrin from Extrasynthese (Genay, France); ursolic acid from Carl Roth (Karlsruhe, Germany); ethanol 96% (*v/v*) (AB Vilniaus degtine, Vilnius, Lithuania); 2,2'-azino-bis(3-ethylbenzothiazoline-6-sulfonic acid) diammonium salt (ABTS), 2,4,6-Tri-(2-pyridyl)-S-triazine (TPTZ), ferric chloride hexahydrate (FeCl$_3 \times 6$ H$_2$O), sodium acetate (CH$_3$COONa), 3-(2-pyridyl)-5,6-bis(4-phenyl-sulfonic acid)-1,2,4-triazine (ferrozine), obtained from Sigma-Aldrich (Buchs, Switzerland); potassium persulfate (K$_2$S$_2$O$_8$), anhydrous ferrous chloride (FeCl$_2$), and 6-hydroxy-2,5,7,8-tetramethylchroman-2-carboxylic acid (Trolox), obtained from Alfa Aesar (Karlsruhe, Germany). Ultrapure water was obtained by a Milli-Q water purification system from Millipore (Bedford, MA, USA).

3.3. Evaluation of Chromatic CIELAB Parameters

The color coordinates of the samples in the uniform contrast color space, CIEL*a*b*, were measured with a MiniScan XE Plus spectrophotometer (Hunter Associates Laboratory, Inc., Reston, VA, USA), as described in [56]. The parameters evaluated during reflected-color measurements were L*, a*, and b* (brightness, red, and yellow coordinates according to the CIE L*a*b* scale, respectively), and color saturation (the chroma value) was calculated (C = $(a^{*2} + b^{*2})^{1/2}$), with a* and b* converted into hue angle (h° = arctan(b*/a*)) [57]. The values L*, a*, b*, and C* were measured in NBS units, hue angle h° was expressed in degrees from 0 to 360°. The NBS unit is a unit of the U.S. National Bureau of Standards and meets one color resolution threshold, i.e., the smallest difference in a color that can be captured by a trained human eye. Prior to each series of measurements, the spectrophotometer was calibrated with a light trap and a white standard with the following color coordinates in the XYZ color space: X = 81.3, Y = 86.2, and Z = 92.7. The value of L* indicated the ratio of white to black, the value of a* indicated the ratio of red to green, and the value of b* indicated the ratio of yellow to blue. The ΔE was calculated ($\Delta E = \sqrt{\left(L_2^* - L_1^*\right)^2 + \left(a_2^* - a_1^*\right)^2 + \left(b_2^* - b_1^*\right)^2}$). The ΔE values indicate the distance between colors of fresh and dried (in FD or CD mode) material. The ΔE values were added in Supplementary Material (Figure S4). Leaf powders of each cultivar were taken for the analysis. The color coordinates were processed by the Universal Software V.4-10.

3.4. Determination of Chlorophyll A, Chlorophyll B, and Total Carotenoid Content

The total carotenoids, chlorophyll a, and chlorophyll b content were determined spectrophotometrically, according Lichtenthaler and Buschmann [58], as described by Rubinskiene et al., 2015 [28]; the absorption was measured using a Cintra 202 spectrophotometer (GBC Scientific Equipment Pty Ltd., Australia), and the results were analyzed using the Cintral ver.2.2 program.

3.5. HPLC Analysis

Phenolics compounds were analyzed using the Waters e2695 Alliance system, (Waters, Milford, MA, USA), applying the method of Vilkickyte et al. [59]. Briefly, ACE Super C18 column (250 mm × 4.6 mm, particle size 3 µm; ACT, UK) was used with a gradient: 0.1% trifluoroacetic acid in water (A) and acetonitrile (B), 0 min, 15% B; 0–30 min, 30% B; 30–50 min, 60% B; 50–56 min, 90% B; 56–65 min, 15% B; the flow rate was 0.5 mL/min, injection volume −10 µL, and column temperature −15 °C. Detection of phenolic compounds was performed at a wavelength of 330, 280, and 360 nm for the phenolic acids, flavan-3-ols, and flavonols, respectively. The maximum absorption and the retention times were compared with standard compounds.

Triterpenic compounds were analyzed using the Waters e2695 Alliance system, (Waters, Milford, MA, USA), applying the methods of Vilkickyte et al. [60]. ACE C18 (150 × 4.6 mm, 3 µm) column (ACT, Aberdeen, UK) column was used and the injection volume was 10 µL. Maslinic, corosolic, betulinic, oleanolic, ursolic acids, betulin, erythrodiol, and uvaol were analyzed using the mobile phase of acetonitrile and water (89:11, v/v), the flow rate was 0.7 mL/min in the isocratic mode. The column temperature was set at 20 °C. Lupeol, β-amyrin, α-amyrin, friedelin, and β-sitosterol were analyzed using the mobile phase of acetonitrile and methanol (10:90, v/v). The column temperature was set at 35 °C, the flow rate was 1 mL/min. Detection of all triterpenoids was performed at a wavelength of 205 nm, corresponding to the maximum absorption and retention times, compared to standard compounds.

The obtained chromatograms have been included in the Supplementary Material.

3.6. Antioxidant Activity Assays

The ABTS assay was performed, as described by Re et al., 1999 [61], with some modifications, according to Raudone et al. [62]. The ferric reducing activity (FRAP) was determined, according to the method of Benzie and Strain (1996) [63], with some modifications, according to Raudone et al. [62]. All antioxidant activity measurements and calculations were performed using Trolox calibration curves and were expressed as μmol of the Trolox equivalent (TE) per one gram of dry weight, according to our previous research [62].

3.7. Statistical Analysis

All experiments were performed in triplicate and the results were expressed as mean ± standard deviation. Significant differences between means were evaluated using ANOVA and post-hoc Tukey's HSD multiple comparison test. Hierarchical cluster analysis was performed using squared Euclidean distances. Principal component analysis (PCA) was performed upon factors with eigenvalues higher than 1. The linear regression model was analyzed to calculate determination coefficients. Correlations were assessed using Pearson's correlation coefficients. Graphical and statistical analysis was performed using Microsoft Office Excel 2010 (Microsoft, JAV) and SPSS 20 software packages. The significance level was $p < 0.05$.

4. Conclusions

Hippophae rhamnoides leaves are still an underutilized resource of functional ingredients with notable antioxidant activity and rich phytochemical composition. The valorization of *Hippophae rhamnoides* leaves could conform to the strategy to transform agrotechnological waste into a valuables resource. Catechin, epigallocatechin, procyanidin B3, ursolic acid, α-amyrin, and β-sitosterol could be used as quantitative markers in the phenolic and triterpenic profile. The freeze-drying ensures the retainment of antioxidative active compounds, as well as notable radical scavenging and a reduction in the activities of leaf powders. The cultivars 'Avgustinka', 'Nivelena', and 'Botaniceskaja' were superior to other tested cultivars, with the greatest amounts of phenolic, triterpenic, carotenoid compounds, and content of total chlorophyll, as well as antioxidant activity. *Hippophae rhamnoides* leaf powders with defined phytochemical composition and determined antioxidant activity are perspective candidates in the production of smart and innovative pharmaceutical or functional food ingredients.

Supplementary Materials: The following are available online, Figure S1: Representative HPLC-PDA chromatogram (λ = 360 and 280nm) of Hippophae rhamnoides leaf powders, showing separation of phenolic compounds. Peak assignments: 1—gallic acid, 2—epigallocatechin, 3— protocatechuic acid acid, 4—procyanidin B3, 5—caftaric acid, 6—(+)-catechin, 7—caffeic acid, 8—rutin, 9— isoquercitrin, 10—ellagic acid, 11—isorhamnetin-3-rutinoside, 12—p-coumaric acid, 13—(-)-epicatechin gallate, 14—ferulic acid, 15—isorhamnetin-3-glucoside, 16—quercetin-3-O-(6''-acetylglucoside), 17—myricetin, 18—tiliroside, 19—resveratrol, 20—quercetin, 21—kaempferol, 22—isorhamnetin., Figure S2: Representative HPLC-PDA chromatogram (λ = 205 nm) of Hippophae rhamnoides leaf powders, showing separation of: 1—maslinic acid, 2—corosolic acid, 3—betulinic acid, 4—oleanolic acid, 5—ursolic acid, 6—betulin, 7—erythrodiol, 8—uvaol., Figure S3: Representative HPLC-PDA chromatogram (λ = 205 nm) of Hippophae rhamnoides leaf powders, showing separation of: 1—lupeol, 2—β-amyrin, 3—β-sitosterol, 4—α-amyrin, 5—friedelin., Figure S4: The difference between color of fresh Hippophae rhamnoides and dried (ΔE), using freeze-drying (FD) and convection-drying (CD).

Author Contributions: Conceptualization, L.R. and P.V.; methodology, G.V., V.P. and P.V.; formal analysis, L.R.; investigation, A.N., G.V., J.V. and V.P.; resources, J.L., J.V. and P.V.; data curation, L.R.; writing—original draft preparation, L.R.; writing—review and editing, L.R., G.V., J.L. and P.V.; supervision, L.R. and P.V.; funding acquisition, P.V. All authors have read and agreed to the published version of the manuscript.

Funding: This study was financed by the Lithuanian Research Centre for Agriculture and Forestry and attributed to the long-term research program, "Horticulture: agrobiological foundations and technologies".

Institutional Review Board Statement: Not applicable.

Informed Consent Statement: Not applicable.

Data Availability Statement: All data generated during this study are included in this article.

Conflicts of Interest: The authors declare no conflict of interest.

Sample Availability: The tested samples are available from the authors.

References

1. Parmesan, C.; Hanley, M.E. Plants and climate change: Complexities and surprises. *Ann. Bot.* **2015**, *116*, 849–864. [CrossRef] [PubMed]
2. Li, T.S.; Schroeder, W. Sea Buckthorn (*Hippophae rhamnoides* L.): A Multipurpose Plant. *HortTechnology* **1996**, *6*, 370–380. [CrossRef]
3. Pundir, S.; Garg, P.; Dviwedi, A.; Ali, A.; Kapoor, V.; Kapoor, D.; Kulshrestha, S.; Lal, U.R.; Negi, P. Ethnomedicinal uses, phytochemistry and dermatological effects of *Hippophae rhamnoides* L.: A review. *J. Ethnopharmacol.* **2021**, *266*, 113434. [CrossRef] [PubMed]
4. Suryakumar, G.; Gupta, A. Medicinal and therapeutic potential of Sea buckthorn (*Hippophae rhamnoides* L.). *J. Ethnopharmacol.* **2011**, *138*, 268–278. [CrossRef] [PubMed]
5. Kumar, M.Y.; Tirpude, R.; Maheshwari, D.; Bansal, A.; Misra, K. Antioxidant and antimicrobial properties of phenolic rich fraction of Seabuckthorn (*Hippophae rhamnoides* L.) leaves in vitro. *Food Chem.* **2013**, *141*, 3443–3450. [CrossRef] [PubMed]
6. Li, H.; Ruan, C.; Ding, J.; Li, J.; Wang, L.; Tian, X. Diversity in sea buckthorn (*Hippophae rhamnoides* L.) accessions with different origins based on morphological characteristics, oil traits, and microsatellite markers. *PLoS ONE* **2020**, *15*, e0230356. [CrossRef]
7. Ji, M.; Gong, X.; Li, X.; Wang, C.; Li, M. Advanced Research on the Antioxidant Activity and Mechanism of Polyphenols from Hippophae Species—A Review. *Molecules* **2020**, *25*, 917. [CrossRef]
8. Morgenstern, A.; Ekholm, A.; Scheewe, P.; Rumpunen, K. Changes in content of major phenolic compounds during leaf development of sea buckthorn (*Hippophae rhamnoides* L.). *Agric. Food Sci.* **2014**, *23*, 207–219. [CrossRef]
9. Cho, H.; Cho, E.; Jung, H.; Yi, H.C.; Lee, B.; Hwang, K.T. Antioxidant activities of sea buckthorn leaf tea extracts compared with green tea extracts. *Food Sci. Biotechnol.* **2014**, *23*, 1295–1303. [CrossRef]
10. Ciesarová, Z.; Murkovic, M.; Cejpek, K.; Kreps, F.; Tobolková, B.; Koplík, R.; Belajová, E.; Kukurová, K.; Daško, Ľ.; Panovská, Z.; et al. Why is sea buckthorn (*Hippophae rhamnoides* L.) so exceptional? A review. *Food Res. Int.* **2020**, *133*, 109170. [CrossRef]
11. Grey, C.; Widén, C.; Adlercreutz, P.; Rumpunen, K.; Duan, R.-D. Antiproliferative effects of sea buckthorn (*Hippophae rhamnoides* L.) extracts on human colon and liver cancer cell lines. *Food Chem.* **2010**, *120*, 1004–1010. [CrossRef]
12. Patel, C.A.; Divakar, K.; Santani, D.; Solanki, H.K.; Thakkar, J.H. Remedial Prospective of *Hippophae rhamnoides* Linn. (Sea Buckthorn). *ISRN Pharmacol.* **2012**, *2012*, 1–6. [CrossRef] [PubMed]
13. Zhan, Y.; Ta, W.; Tang, W.; Hua, R.; Wang, J.; Wang, C.; Lu, W. Potential antiviral activity of isorhamnetin against SARS-CoV-2 spike pseudotyped virus in vitro. *Drug Dev. Res.* **2021**. [CrossRef] [PubMed]
14. Zheng, W.-H.; Bai, H.-Y.; Han, S.; Bao, F.; Zhang, K.-X.; Sun, L.-L.; Du, H.; Yang, Z.-G. Analysis on the Constituents of Branches, Berries, and Leaves of *Hippophae rhamnoides* L. by UHPLC-ESI-QTOF-MS and Their Anti-Inflammatory Activities. *Nat. Prod. Commun.* **2019**, *14*. [CrossRef]
15. Raudonis, R.; Raudone, L.; Janulis, V.; Viskelis, P. Flavonoids in cultivated berries of sea buckthorn (*Hippophaë rhamnoides* L.). *Planta Med.* **2014**, *80*, LP24. [CrossRef]
16. Cho, C.H.; Jang, H.L.; Lee, M.; Kang, H.; Heo, H.J.; Kim, D.-O. Sea Buckthorn (*Hippophae rhamnoides* L.) Leaf Extracts Protect Neuronal PC-12 Cells from Oxidative Stress. *J. Microbiol. Biotechnol.* **2017**, *27*, 1257–1265. [CrossRef] [PubMed]
17. Lakušić, B.; Ristić, M.; Slavkovska, V.; Lakušić, D.; Milenković, M. Environmental and Seasonal Impacts on the Chemical Composition of Satureja horvatii Šili? (Lamiaceae) Essential Oils. *Chem. Biodivers.* **2011**, *8*, 483–493. [CrossRef]
18. Pariyani, R.; Kortesniemi, M.; Liimatainen, J.; Sinkkonen, J.; Yang, B. Untargeted metabolic fingerprinting reveals impact of growth stage and location on composition of sea buckthorn (*Hippophae rhamnoides* L.) leaves. *J. Food Sci.* **2020**, *85*, 364–373. [CrossRef]
19. Pop, R.M.; Socaciu, C.; Pintea, A.; Buzoianu, A.D.; Sanders, M.G.; Gruppen, H.; Vincken, J.-P. UHPLC/PDA-ESI/MS Analysis of the Main Berry and Leaf Flavonol Glycosides from Different Carpathian *Hippophaë rhamnoides* L. Varieties. *Phytochem. Anal.* **2013**, *24*, 484–492. [CrossRef]
20. Sytařová, I.; Orsavová, J.; Snopek, L.; Mlcek, J.; Byczyński, Ł.; Misurcova, L. Impact of phenolic compounds and vitamins C and E on antioxidant activity of sea buckthorn (*Hippophaë rhamnoides* L.) berries and leaves of diverse ripening times. *Food Chem.* **2020**, *310*, 125784. [CrossRef]

21. Šnē, E.; Seglina, D.; Galoburda, R.; Krasnova, I. Content of Phenolic Compounds in Various Sea Buckthorn Parts. *Proc. Latv. Acad. Sci. Sect. B Nat. Exact Appl. Sci.* **2013**, *67*, 411–415. [CrossRef]
22. Suvanto, J.; Tähtinen, P.; Valkamaa, S.; Engström, M.; Karonen, M.; Salminen, J.-P. Variability in Foliar Ellagitannins of *Hippophaë rhamnoides* L. and Identification of a New Ellagitannin, Hippophaenin C. *J. Agric. Food Chem.* **2018**, *66*, 613–620. [CrossRef] [PubMed]
23. Dias, M.; Borge, G.; Kljak, K.; Mandić, A.; Mapelli-Brahm, P.; Olmedilla-Alonso, B.; Pintea, A.; Ravasco, F.; Šaponjac, V.T.; Sereikaitė, J.; et al. European Database of Carotenoid Levels in Foods. Factors Affecting Carotenoid Content. *Foods* **2021**, *10*, 912. [CrossRef]
24. Vaňková, K.; Marková, I.; Jašprová, J.; Dvořák, A.; Subhanová, I.; Zelenka, J.; Novosádová, I.; Rasl, J.; Vomastek, T.; Sobotka, R.; et al. Chlorophyll-Mediated Changes in the Redox Status of Pancreatic Cancer Cells Are Associated with Its Anticancer Effects. *Oxid. Med. Cell. Longev.* **2018**, *2018*, 1–11. [CrossRef] [PubMed]
25. Stevenson, D.E.; Lowe, T. Plant-Derived Compounds as Antioxidants for Health—Are They all Really Antioxidants? *Plant Sci.* **2009**, *3*, 1–12.
26. Raudone, L.; Zymone, K.; Raudonis, R.; Vainoriene, R.; Motiekaityte, V.; Janulis, V. Phenological changes in triterpenic and phenolic composition of Thymus L. species. *Ind. Crops Prod.* **2017**, *109*, 445–451. [CrossRef]
27. Kukin, T.P.; Shcherbakov, D.N.; Gensh, K.V.; Tulysheva, E.A.; Salnikova, O.I.; Grazhdannikov, A.E.; Kolosova, E.A. Bioactive Components of Sea Buckthorn *Hippophae rhamnoides* L. Foliage. *Russ. J. Bioorgan. Chem.* **2017**, *43*, 747–751. [CrossRef]
28. Rubinskienė, M.; Viskelis, P.; Dambrauskienė, E.; Viškelis, J.; Karklelienė, R. Effect of drying methods on the chemical composition and colour of peppermint (*Mentha* × *piperita* L.) leaves. *Zemdirb. Agric.* **2015**, *102*, 223–228. [CrossRef]
29. Arabhosseini, A.; Padhye, S.; Huisman, W.; Van Boxtel, A.; Müller, J. Effect of Drying on the Color of Tarragon (*Artemisia dracunculus* L.) Leaves. *Food Bioprocess Technol.* **2011**, *4*, 1281–1287. [CrossRef]
30. Guan, T.T.Y.; Cenkowski, S.; Hydamaka, A. Effect of Drying on the Nutraceutical Quality of Sea Buckthorn (*Hippophae rhamnoides* L. ssp. sinensis) Leaves. *J. Food Sci.* **2006**, *70*, E514–E518. [CrossRef]
31. Onwude, D.I.; Hashim, N.; Janius, R.; Nawi, N.M.; Abdan, K. Color change kinetics and total carotenoid content of pumpkin as affected by drying temperature. *Ital. J. Food Sci.* **2017**, *29*, 1–18.
32. George, S.D.S.; Cenkowski, S. Influence of Harvest Time on the Quality of Oil-Based Compounds in Sea Buckthorn (*Hippophae rhamnoides* L. ssp. sinensis) Seed and Fruit. *J. Agric. Food Chem.* **2007**, *55*, 8054–8061. [CrossRef] [PubMed]
33. Krokida, M.K.; Maroulis, Z.B.; Saravacos, G.D. The effect of the method of drying on the colour of dehydrated products. *Int. J. Food Sci. Technol.* **2001**, *36*, 53–59. [CrossRef]
34. Sant'Anna, V.; Gurak, P.D.; Marczak, L.D.F.; Tessaro, I.C. Tracking bioactive compounds with colour changes in foods—A review. *Dye. Pigment.* **2013**, *98*, 601–608. [CrossRef]
35. Escuredo, O.; Rodríguez-Flores, M.S.; Rojo-Martínez, S.; Seijo, M.C. Contribution to the Chromatic Characterization of Unifloral Honeys from Galicia (NW Spain). *Foods* **2019**, *8*, 233. [CrossRef]
36. Mikulic-Petkovsek, M.; Krska, B.; Kiprovski, B.; Veberic, R. Bioactive Components and Antioxidant Capacity of Fruits from NineSorbusGenotypes. *J. Food Sci.* **2017**, *82*, 647–658. [CrossRef] [PubMed]
37. Palta, J.P. Leaf chlorophyll content. *Remote Sens. Rev.* **1990**, *5*, 207–213. [CrossRef]
38. Kumar, S.S.; Manoj, P.; Shetty, N.P.; Giridhar, P. Effect of different drying methods on chlorophyll, ascorbic acid and antioxidant compounds retention of leaves of *Hibiscus sabdariffa* L. *J. Sci. Food Agric.* **2014**, *95*, 1812–1820. [CrossRef]
39. Gornas, P.; Sne, E.; Siger, A.; Seglina, D. Sea buckthorn (*Hippophae rhamnoides* L.) leaves as valuable source oflipophilic antioxidants: The effect of harvest time, sex, drying andextraction methods. *Ind. Crops Prod* **2014**, *60*, 1–7. [CrossRef]
40. Raudonis, R.; Raudone, L.; Jakstas, V.; Janulis, V. Comparative evaluation of post-column free radical scavenging and ferric reducing antioxidant power assays for screening of antioxidants in strawberries. *J. Chromatogr. A* **2012**, *1233*, 8–15. [CrossRef]
41. Tzachristas, A.; Pasvanka, K.; Liouni, M.; Calokerinos, A.C.; Tataridis, P.; Proestos, C. Effect of *Hippophae rhamnoides* L. Leaves Treatment on the Antioxidant Capacity, Total Phenol Content and Sensory Profile of Moschofilero Wines Vinified with and without Added Sulphites. *Appl. Sci.* **2020**, *10*, 3444. [CrossRef]
42. Asofiei, I.; Calinescu, I.; Trifan, A.; Gavrila, A.I. A Semi-Continuous Process for Polyphenols Extraction From Sea Buckthorn Leaves. *Sci. Rep.* **2019**, *9*, 12044. [CrossRef] [PubMed]
43. Zu, Y.; Li, C.; Fu, I.; Zhao, C. Simultaneous determination of catechin, rutin, quercetin kaempferol and isorhamnetin in the extract of sea buckthorn (*Hippophae rhamnoides* L.) leaves by RP-HPLC with DAD. *J. Pharm. Biomed. Anal.* **2006**, *41*, 714–719. [CrossRef]
44. Sadowska, B.; Rywaniak, J.; Cichocka, A.; Cichocka, K.; Żuchowski, J.; Wójcik-Bojek, U.; Więckowska-Szakiel, M.; Różalska, B. Phenolic and Non-Polar Fractions of the Extracts from Fruits, Leaves, and Twigs of *Elaeagnus rhamnoides* (L.) A. Nelson—The Implications for Human Barrier Cells. *Molecules* **2020**, *25*, 2238. [CrossRef]
45. Zadernowski, R.; Naczk, M.; Czaplicki, S.; Rubinskienė, M.; Szałkiewicz, M. Composition of phenolic acids in sea buckthorn (*Hippophae rhamnoides* L.) berries. *J. Am. Oil Chem. Soc.* **2005**, *82*, 175–179. [CrossRef]
46. Ghendov-Mosanu, A.; Cristea, E.; Patras, A.; Sturza, R.; Padureanu, S.; Deseatnicova, O.; Turculet, N.; Boestean, O.; Niculaua, M. Potential Application of *Hippophae rhamnoides* in Wheat Bread Production. *Molecules* **2020**, *25*, 1272. [CrossRef] [PubMed]
47. Burns, J.; Yokota, T.; Ashihara, H.; Lean, M.E.J.; Crozier, A. Plant Foods and Herbal Sources of Resveratrol. *J. Agric. Food Chem.* **2002**, *50*, 3337–3340. [CrossRef] [PubMed]

48. Hu, N.; Suo, Y.; Zhang, Q.; You, J.; Ji, Z.; Wang, A.; Han, L.; Lv, H.; Ye, Y. Rapid, Selective, and Sensitive Analysis of Triterpenic Acids in *Hippophae rhamnoides* L. Using HPLC with Pre-Column Fluorescent Derivatization and Identification with Post-Column APCI-MS. *J. Liq. Chromatogr. Relat. Technol.* **2015**, *38*, 451–458. [CrossRef]
49. Michel, T.; Destandau, E.; LE Floch, G.; Lucchesi, M.E.; Elfakir, C. Antimicrobial, antioxidant and phytochemical investigations of sea buckthorn (*Hippophaë rhamnoides* L.) leaf, stem, root and seed. *Food Chem.* **2012**, *131*, 754–760. [CrossRef]
50. Sun, Y.; Feng, F.; Nie, B.; Cao, J.; Zhang, F. High throughput identification of pentacyclic triterpenes in *Hippophae rhamnoides* using multiple neutral loss markers scanning combined with substructure recognition (MNLSR). *Talanta* **2019**, *205*, 120011. [CrossRef]
51. Yang, Z.-G.; Li, H.-R.; Wang, L.-Y.; Li, Y.-H.; Lu, S.-G.; Wen, X.-F.; Wang, J.; Daikonya, A.; Kitanaka, S. Triterpenoids from *Hippophae rhamnoides* L. and Their Nitric Oxide Production-Inhibitory and DPPH Radical-Scavenging Activities. *Chem. Pharm. Bull.* **2007**, *55*, 15–18. [CrossRef] [PubMed]
52. Yasukawa, K.; Kitanaka, S.; Kawata, K.; Goto, K. Anti-tumor promoters phenolics and triterpenoid from *Hippophae rhamnoides*. *Fitoterapia* **2009**, *80*, 164–167. [CrossRef] [PubMed]
53. Skalski, B.; Kontek, B.; Olas, B.; Zuchowski, J.; Stochmal, A. Phenolic fraction and nonpolar fraction from sea buckthorn leaves and twigs: Chemical profile and biological activity. *Future Med. Chem.* **2018**, *10*, 2381–2394. [CrossRef]
54. Sriskandarajah, S.; Lundquist, P.-O. High frequency shoot organogenesis and somatic embryogenesis in juvenile and adult tissues of seabuckthorn (*Hippophae rhamnoides* L.). *Plant Cell Tissue Organ Cult. (PCTOC)* **2009**, *99*, 259–268. [CrossRef]
55. Meier, U. *Growth Stages of Mono—and Dicotyledonous Plants: BBCH Monograph*; Meier, U., Ed.; Julius Kuhn-Institut: Quedlinburg, Germany, 2018; ISBN 978-3-95547-071-5.
56. Luksiene, Z.; Paskeviciute, E. High-power pulsed light for microbial decontamination of some fruits and vegetables with different surfaces. *J. Food Agric. Environ.* **2012**, *1010*, 162–167.
57. Reporting of Objective Color Measurements. Available online: https://agris.fao.org/agris-search/search.do?recordID=US9426291 (accessed on 16 June 2021).
58. Lichtenthaler, H.K.; Buschmann, C. Chlorophylls and Carotenoids: Measurement and Characterization by UV-VIS Spectroscopy. *Curr. Protoc. Food Anal. Chem.* **2001**, *1*, F4.3.1–F4.3.8. [CrossRef]
59. Vilkickyte, G.; Raudone, L.; Petrikaite, V. Phenolic Fractions from *Vaccinium vitis-idaea* L. and Their Antioxidant and Anticancer Activities Assessment. *Antioxidants* **2020**, *9*, 1261. [CrossRef]
60. Vilkickyte, G.; Raudone, L. Optimization, Validation and Application of HPLC-PDA Methods for Quantification of Triterpenoids in *Vaccinium vitisidaea* L. *Molecules* **2021**, *26*, 1645. [CrossRef]
61. Re, R.; Pellegrini, N.; Proteggente, A.; Pannala, A.; Yang, M.; Rice-Evans, C. Antioxidant activity applying an improved ABTS radical cation decolorization assay. *Free Radic. Biol. Med.* **1999**, *26*, 1231–1237. [CrossRef]
62. Raudonė, L.; Liaudanskas, M.; Vilkickytė, G.; Kviklys, D.; Žvikas, V.; Viškelis, J.; Viškelis, P. Phenolic Profiles, Antioxidant Activity and Phenotypic Characterization of *Lonicera caerulea* L. Berries, Cultivated in Lithuania. *Antioxidants* **2021**, *10*, 115. [CrossRef] [PubMed]
63. Benzie, I.F.; Strain, J.J. The Ferric Reducing Ability of Plasma (FRAP) as a Measure of "Antioxidant Power": The FRAP Assay. *Anal. Biochem.* **1996**, *239*, 70–76. [CrossRef] [PubMed]

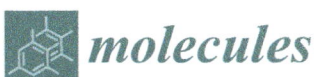

Article

Co-Treatments of Edible Curcumin from Turmeric Rhizomes and Chemotherapeutic Drugs on Cytotoxicity and FLT3 Protein Expression in Leukemic Stem Cells

Fah Chueahongthong [1,†], Singkome Tima [1,2,3,†], Sawitree Chiampanichayakul [1,2], Cory Berkland [4,*] and Songyot Anuchapreeda [1,2,3,*]

1. Division of Clinical Microscopy, Department of Medical Technology, Faculty of Associated Medical Sciences, Chiang Mai University, Chiang Mai 50200, Thailand; fahmyfah@hotmail.com (F.C.); singkome@gmail.com (S.T.); chiampanich@gmail.com (S.C.)
2. Cancer Research Unit of Associated Medical Sciences (AMS-CRU), Faculty of Associated Medical Sciences, Chiang Mai University, Chiang Mai 50200, Thailand
3. Center for Research and Development of Natural Products for Health, Chiang Mai University, Chiang Mai 50200, Thailand
4. Department of Pharmaceutical Chemistry, School of Pharmacy, University of Kansas, Lawrence, KS 66047, USA
* Correspondence: berkland@ku.edu (C.B.); sanuchapreeda@gmail.com (S.A.); Tel.: +1-785-8641-455 (C.B.); +66-539-492-37 (S.A.)
† These authors contributed equally to this work.

Abstract: This study aims to enhance efficacy and reduce toxicity of the combination treatment of a drug and curcumin (Cur) on leukemic stem cell and leukemic cell lines, including KG-1a and KG-1 (FLT3$^+$ LSCs), EoL-1 (FLT3$^+$ LCs), and U937 (FLT3$^-$ LCs). The cytotoxicity of co-treatments of doxorubicin (Dox) or idarubicin (Ida) at concentrations of the IC$_{10}$–IC$_{80}$ values and each concentration of Cur at the IC$_{20}$, IC$_{30}$, IC$_{40}$, and IC$_{50}$ values (conditions 1, 2, 3, and 4) was determined by MTT assays. Dox–Cur increased cytotoxicity in leukemic cells. Dox–Cur co-treatment showed additive and synergistic effects in several conditions. The effect of this co-treatment on FLT3 expression in KG-1a, KG-1, and EoL-1 cells was examined by Western blotting. Dox–Cur decreased FLT3 protein levels and total cell numbers in all the cell lines in a dose-dependent manner. In summary, this study exhibits a novel report of Dox–Cur co-treatment in both enhancing cytotoxicity of Dox and inhibiting cell proliferation via FLT3 protein expression in leukemia stem cells and leukemic cells. This is the option of leukemia treatment with reducing side effects of chemotherapeutic drugs to leukemia patients.

Keywords: leukemia; leukemic stem cell; FLT-3; chemotherapeutic drug; curcumin; co-treatment

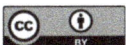

1. Introduction

Leukemia is among the top 10 cancers diagnosed globally. It is a group of cancers of early blood-forming cells, which are characterized by the uncontrolled production and accumulation of blast or immature abnormal blood cells in the peripheral blood and bone marrow. Leukemia can be divided into four major types according to the stage and cell of origin: acute myeloid leukemia (AML), acute lymphoid leukemia (ALL), chronic myeloid leukemia (CML), and chronic lymphocytic leukemia (CLL). AML is the most common type of acute leukemia in adults, with the highest incidence and death rate in both sexes. It can be distinguished by clonal expansion of abnormal myeloid blasts in bone marrow, peripheral blood, or other tissues. According to recent data, 15–25% of AML patients fail to achieve complete remission (CR) due to chemotherapy resistance and may show relapse, with the overall 5-year survival rate of approximately 40% [1,2]. Moreover, between 10 and 40% of newly diagnosed AML patients do not achieve CR with intensive induction therapy, and such patients are categorized as primary refractory or resistant [3]. Hence, AML is defined as an aggressive malignant myeloid disorder.

One theory of resistance and relapse in AML patients involves the presence of subpopulations of leukemic stem cells (LSCs) [4]. LSCs have been defined as human AML-initiating cell with a self-renewal capacity and the ability to give rise to heterogeneous lineages of cancer cells [2,5]. They can be identified by the cell surface phenotype $CD34^+$ hematopoietic stem cell and $CD38^-$ subpopulation (i.e., $CD34^+CD38^-$ cells) [6].

Traditional chemotherapeutic drugs are incapable of clearing the LSC population due to many reasons. First, these drugs have been designed to eliminate fast-dividing cells by inhibiting cell cycle progression [7]; thus, they are less effective against LSCs, which have a prolonged G_0 phase of the cell cycle [8]. Second, the expression of P-glycoprotein (MDR1), a multidrug resistance efflux pump protein in LSCs, potentially removes cytotoxic agents from cancer cells [9]. In addition, LSCs can undergo mutations and epigenetic changes, creating resistance to conventional chemotherapy toxicity [10,11]. Thus, LSCs are thought to play a fundamental role in AML pathogenesis and have become a focal point for targeted AML therapies.

Although drug resistance in AML patients is common, the traditional chemotherapy remains a popular method for leukemia treatment since these drugs can access cancer cells that have spread throughout the body. Anthracycline antibiotics such as doxorubicin (Dox (14-hydroxydaunorubicin)) and idarubicin (Ida (4-demethoxydaunorubicin)) are generally used as standard chemotherapeutic agents for AML treatment [12]. Ida is normally prepared in a 1 mg/mL solution (sterile water or normal saline). For patients with AML, the recommended intravenous dose of idarubicin for induction therapy is 12 mg/m^2 daily for 3 days by slow (10 to 15 min) infusion, while Dox is recommended to be used with a dose 50 mg/m^2 daily for 3 days [13–15]. These drugs function by inhibiting topoisomerase II activity in DNA transcription and also trigger apoptosis or autophagy in cells [16]. The combination of anthracyclines and cytarabine in the initial treatment is capable of inducing complete remission (CR) in approximately 45–70% of patients [17]; however, more than 40% of CR cases eventually experience relapse within 2 years [18]. The previous studies on AML leukemic stem cells demonstrated that anthracycline is less effective in killing LSCs ($CD34^+/CD38^-$ cells) than committed leukemic cells ($CD34^+/CD38^+$ cells) [19], and the co-treatment of cytarabine and anthracyclines is less effective against primitive AML cells than against leukemia blasts [20,21]. Furthermore, with high dose administration, anthracyclines cause side effects in patients including nausea, vomiting, hair loss, and myelosuppression [22]. Several reports expressed their concern about the presence of cardiac, renal, and liver toxicity in patients treated with Dox [23,24]. Thus, combination therapy with natural substances exhibiting chemosensitizing and chemoprotective activities may be a promising strategy to overcome LSCs and reduce the side effects of anthracyclines.

Curcumin (Cur) is a natural polyphenol constituent of turmeric (*Curcuma longa* Linn.). It exhibits a wide range of pharmacological activities, such as antioxidant, anti-cancer, anti-inflammatory, and antimicrobial effects [25–27]. Previous studies reported that Cur exhibited a potent cytotoxic effect, induced cell death in several types of leukemic cell lines [28–31], and showed inhibitory effects on WT1 and FLT3 protein expression, which are associated with cell proliferation [29,32,33]. Moreover, Cur inhibited the activity of P-glycoprotein (MDR1) [34] and exhibited cancer chemopreventive properties, especially in myocardial protection [35] by inhibiting ROS generation [36]. Consequently, it may be possible to manipulate the combination of Cur and anthracyclines for a reduction in anthracycline toxicity and to overcome drug efflux via Pgp-mediated MDR in leukemia on AML leukemic cells and LSCs. Although Dox and Cur exhibit synergistic cytotoxic effects on cancer cell models, the combination of free Dox and free Cur has shown only a modest synergistic effect in vivo [37].

The aims of this study were determined the cytotoxicity of co-treatment with anthracycline drugs and curcumin for FLT3-overexpressing leukemic stem cells (KG-1a and

KG1), FLT3-overexpressing leukemic cells (EoL-1), and non FLT3-expressing leukemic cells (U937). FLT3 protein is a member of the class III receptor tyrosine kinase (RTK) family [38]. It is overexpressed on the cell surface of AML leukemic stem cells and leukemic cells and plays an important role in cell survival and proliferation of leukemic cell blasts [39]. Cur has previously been shown to have an inhibitory effect on FLT3 protein expression in many types of FLT-3 expressing leukemic cell lines, such as EoL-1 and MV4-11 [32]. Thus, it was selected as a target protein for Dox–Cur treatment. Moreover, the effects of co-treatments on FLT3 protein expression and total cell numbers were determined.

2. Results

2.1. Determination of Cytotoxicity of Doxorubicin (Dox), Idarubicin (Ida), and Curcumin (Cur) on Leukemic Cell Viability by MTT Assay

A cell viability curve demonstrated Dox (Figure 1A) and IDa (Figure 1B) exhibited the highest cytotoxicity for EoL-1 cells, followed by U937, KG-1, and KG-1a cells. The cytotoxicity of all the treatments was assessed using an inhibitory concentration at a 50% growth (IC_{50}) value. Ida demonstrated the greatest cytotoxic effects on KG-1a, KG-1, EoL-1, and U937 cells with IC_{50} values of 19.82 ± 1.80, 5.45 ± 0.89, 2.57 ± 0.32, and 4.73 ± 2.38 ng/mL, followed by Dox with IC_{50} values of 0.69 ± 0.12, 0.21 ± 0.02, 0.02 ± 0.01, and 0.08 ± 0.02 µg/mL, respectively. The IC_{50} values of all the chemotherapeutic drugs for the leukemic cell line models are shown in Table 1.

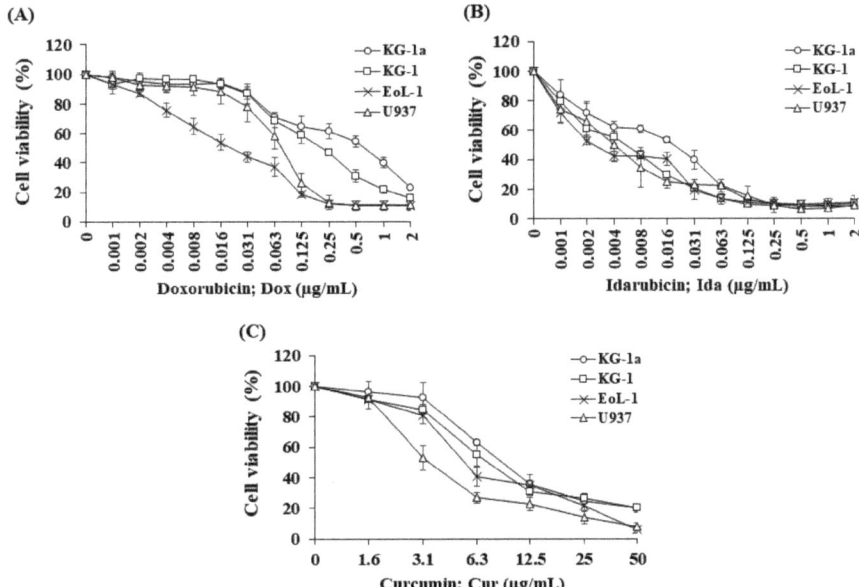

Figure 1. Cytotoxicity of (**A**) doxorubicin, (**B**) idarubicin, and (**C**) curcumin on KG-1a, KG-1, EoL-1, and U937 cells. The data are shown as mean ± SD from 3-time independent experiments.

Table 1. The IC_{50} values of chemotherapeutic drugs and curcumin on KG-1a, KG-1, EoL-1, and U937 cells.

Treatment	IC_{50} Value			
	KG-1a	KG-1	EoL-1	U937
Idarubicin (Ida) (ng/mL)	19.82 ± 1.80 [###]	5.45 ± 0.89 [***]	2.57 ± 0.32 [***]	4.72 ± 2.38 [***]
Doxorubicin (Dox) (µg/mL)	0.69 ± 0.12 [###]	0.21 ± 0.02 [***]	0.02 ± 0.01 [***,##]	0.08 ± 0.02 [***,#]
Curcumin (Cur) (µg/mL)	9.19 ± 0.49 [#]	7.31 ± 1.45 [*]	5.55 ± 0.46 [**,#]	3.55 ± 0.54 [***,##]

The significance of mean differences was assessed using one-way ANOVA. * $p < 0.05$, ** $p < 0.01$, and *** $p < 0.001$ compared with KG-1a cells. [#] $p < 0.05$, [##] $p < 0.01$, and [###] $p < 0.001$ compared with KG-1 cells.

Cur was chosen to study the combination effect in order to improve the efficacy of Dox and Ida in AML treatment. For single treatment, Cur exhibited the highest cytotoxicity for U937cells, followed by EoL-1, KG-1, and KG-1a cells (Figure 1C). The IC_{50} values of Cur for KG-1a, KG-1, EoL-1, and U937 cells were 9.19 ± 0.49, 7.31 ± 1.45, 5.55 ± 0.46, and 3.55 ± 0.54 µg/mL, respectively (Table 1).

The IC_{50} values of Dox in leukemic stem cells (KG-1a and KG-1) were found to be significantly higher than for leukemic cells, EoL-1, and U937 cells. However, KG-1 leukemic stem cells were substantially more responsive to Dox and Ida than KG-1a cells, indicating a high number of LSCs affected the chemotherapeutic treatment's sensitivity. Furthermore, the IC_{50} values of Cur in KG-1a cells were considerably higher than those in the other cells. These findings demonstrated the drug resistance in LSCs compared with LCs and suggested a possible route to improve the potency of traditional AML chemotherapeutics.

2.2. Determination of Cytotoxicity of Combined Doxorubicin–Curcumin (Dox–Cur) and Idarubicin–Curcumin (Ida–Cur) on Leukemic cell Viability by MTT Assay

Various doses of Dox and Ida (ranging from 0 to IC_{80} values) were added to Cur to investigate combination effects on the viability of AML cell lines. Dox was used to treat KG-1a (0–1.30 µg/mL), KG-1 (0–0.84 µg/mL), EoL-1 (0–0.08 µg/mL), and U937 (0–0.16 µg/mL) cells, and Ida was used to treat KG-1a (0–40.0 ng/mL), KG-1 (0–20.0 ng/mL), EoL-1 (0–8.0 ng/mL), and U937 (0–9.2 ng/mL) cells; these cells were cotreated with Cur at concentrations of the IC_{20} (condition 1), IC_{30} (condition 2), IC_{40} (condition 3), and IC_{50} (condition 4), respectively. The co-treatments of Dox–Cur and Ida–Cur exhibited higher cytotoxicity for KG-1a, KG-1, EoL-1, and U937 cells than single-drug treatments in a dose-dependent manner (see supplementary Figures S1 and S2). The IC_{50} value of each co-treatment demonstrated that curcumin enhanced the efficacy of doxorubicin and idarubicin in leukemic stem cells and non-leukemic stem cells, and also decreased the doses of drugs in co-treatment when compared with a single treatment. The IC_{50} values of Dox–Cur and Ida–Cur at different conditions in each cell line are shown in the supplementary Tables S1–S4.

2.3. Synergistic Effects of Combination Treatment

Using a combination index (CI) calculation, formulations 3 and 4 of Dox–Cur showed a synergistic effect (CI < 1) on KG-1a and EoL-1 cells and an additive effect (CI = 1) on U937 cells at the IC_{50} values, while most of the Ida–Cur treatments exhibited an antagonist effect (CI > 1) in all the leukemic cell lines (Table 2). It seemed Cur could not achieve high cytotoxicity in the Ida–Cur combination since Ida had an extremely low effective dose. Thus, most of the Ida–Cur-treated samples exhibited an antagonistic effect in AML leukemic cell lines.

2.4. Effects of Various Conditions of Combined Treatment of Dox–Cur at Concentration Value of IC_{20} on Cell Number and Cell Viability in FLT-3 Protein Expressing Leukemic Cells

Due to the synergistic and additive effect of Dox–Cur, a broader range of co-treatment conditions were chosen to investigate the effects on cell number and viability of FLT-3 protein-expressing AML leukemic cells, including KG-1a, KG-1 and EoL-1 cells. The IC_{20} values of the Dox treatments from the Section 2.2 were used to cotreat for 48 h with Cur. Dox–Cur conditions 1, 2, 3, and 4 (Dox (ng/mL) + Cur (µg/mL)) of KG-1a cells were 15.0 + 4.5, 16.0 + 5.5, 12.0 + 7.0, and 8.0 + 9.0, respectively. The conditions for KG-1 cells were 22.0 + 3.5, 10.0 + 4.5, 7.0 + 6.0, and 6.0 + 7.5, while the conditions of EoL-1 cells were 3.0 + 3.0, 0.7 + 4.0, 0.5 + 4.5, and 0.4 + 5.5, respectively. The results show that Dox concentrations at IC_{20} values and all co-treatment conditions consistently reduced the cell number of all leukemic cell lines (see supplementary Figures S3A–S5A). The total cell number of KG-1a cells (control group) was 2.59×10^5 cells/mL, and cell number gradually decreased to 1.85×10^5, 1.59×10^5, 1.42×10^5, 1.24×10^5, and 0.98×10^5 cells/mL in response to Dox and Dox–Cur treatment conditions 1, 2, 3, and 4, respectively. The total cell number of KG-1 cells decreased from 3.39×10^5 cells/mL (control group) to

2.58×10^5, 2.18×10^5, 2.00×10^5, 1.70×10^5, and 1.44×10^5 cells/mL in Dox and Dox–Cur treatment conditions 1, 2, 3, and 4, respectively. According to the cell number of EoL-1 cells after Dox and Dox–Cur conditions 1, 2, 3, and 4, the treatments reduced to 6.62×10^5, 5.77×10^5, 4.69×10^5, 4.01×10^5, and 3.27×10^5 cells/mL, respectively, compared with 12.07×10^5 cells/mL (control group). Cell viability of each sample was higher than 80% of the total cell count (see supplementary Figures S3B–S5B).

Table 2. IC_{50} values of co-treatment of Dox–Cur and Ida–Cur on KG-1a, KG-1, EoL-1, and U937 cells.

Cell Line	Dox–Cur	CI Value	Ida–Cur	CI Value
KG-1a	Dox + Cur 1 (4.5 µg/mL)	1.08	Ida + Cur 1 (4.5 µg/mL)	1.16
	Dox + Cur 2 (5.5 µg/mL)	1.12	Ida + Cur 2 (5.5 µg/mL)	1.27
	Dox + Cur 3 (7.0 µg/mL)	0.97	Ida + Cur 3 (7.0 µg/mL)	1.21
	Dox + Cur 4 (9.0 µg/mL)	1.02	Ida + Cur 4 (9.0 µg/mL)	1.09
KG-1	Dox + Cur 1 (3.5 µg/mL)	1.36	Ida + Cur 1 (3.5 µg/mL)	1.44
	Dox + Cur 2 (4.5 µg/mL)	1.07	Ida + Cur 2 (4.5 µg/mL)	1.55
	Dox + Cur 3 (6.0 µg/mL)	1.04	Ida + Cur 3 (6.0 µg/mL)	1.28
	Dox + Cur 4 (7.5 µg/mL)	1.07	Ida + Cur 4 (7.5 µg/mL)	1.11
EoL-1	Dox + Cur 1 (3.0 µg/mL)	1.23	Ida + Cur 1 (3.5 µg/mL)	1.27
	Dox + Cur 2 (4.0 µg/mL)	1.12	Ida + Cur 2 (4.0 µg/mL)	1.24
	Dox + Cur 3 (4.5 µg/mL)	0.92	Ida + Cur 3 (4.5 µg/mL)	0.85
	Dox + Cur 4 (5.5 µg/mL)	1.03	Ida + Cur 4 (5.5 µg/mL)	1.03
U937	Dox + Cur 1 (2.0 µg/mL)	1.46	Ida + Cur 1 (2.0 µg/mL)	1.35
	Dox + Cur 2 (2.5 µg/mL)	1.55	Ida + Cur 2 (2.5 µg/mL)	1.40
	Dox + Cur 3 (3.0 µg/mL)	1.42	Ida + Cur 3 (3.0 µg/mL)	1.26
	Dox + Cur 4 (3.5 µg/mL)	1.00	Ida + Cur 4 (3.5 µg/mL)	1.04

The total cell number of Cur treatments at the IC_{20}, IC_{30}, IC_{40}, and IC_{50} values were observed to gradually decrease in all the cell lines in a dose dependent manner (see supplementary Figures S3C–S5C). Moreover, these data also corresponded to the decline in the cell numbers during the Dox–Cur treatment. The cell viability for each concentration of Cur was also higher than 80% of the total cell count (see supplementary Figures S3D–S5D).

2.5. Effects of Combined Treatments of Dox–Cur at Concentration Value of IC_{20} on FLT3 Protein Expressions in FLT-3 Protein Expressing Leukemic Stem Cells and Leukemic Cells

FLT3 protein is a member of the class III receptor tyrosine kinase (RTK) family [38]. It is overexpressed on the cell surface of AML leukemic stem cells and leukemic cells and plays an important role in cell survival and proliferation of leukemic cell blasts [39]. Cur has previously been shown to have an inhibitory effect on FLT3 protein expression in many types of FLT-3 expressing leukemic cell lines, such as EoL-1 and MV4-11 [32]. Thus, it was selected as a target protein for Dox–Cur treatment.

In this study, KG-1a, KG-1, and EoL-1 cells were treated with Dox. Co-treatment was conditions at the IC_{20} value, and FLT3 protein expression levels were detected by Western blot. Dox and Dox–Cur co-treatment could decrease FLT-3 protein expression. In KG-1a cells, the FLT3 protein levels of Dox and Dox–Cur treatment conditions 1, 2, 3, and 4 were decreased by $20.4 \pm 8.8\%$, $51.6 \pm 14.5\%$, $54.6 \pm 12.2\%$, $80.2 \pm 5.7\%$, and $92.2 \pm 8.2\%$, respectively (Figure 2A,C). For KG-1 cells, FLT3 proteins were gradually decreased by $2.7 \pm 6.5\%$, $42.3 \pm 2.9\%$, $55.0 \pm 5.4\%$, $52.0 \pm 7.3\%$, and $57.9 \pm 11.5\%$ in respond to Dox and Dox–Cur conditions 1, 2, 3, and 4, respectively (Figure 3A,C). Similarly, FLT3 protein expression in EoL-1 cells was reduced to $2.7 \pm 5.6\%$, $10.7 \pm 4.2\%$, $29.9 \pm 6.8\%$, $35.2 \pm 6.4\%$, and $43.7 \pm 15.7\%$ in response to Dox and Dox–Cur conditions 1, 2, 3, and 4, respectively, compared with the control group (100% expression level; Figure 4A,C). Additionally, the ability of each concentration of Cur in the combination treatment to suppress FLT3 protein expression was evaluated. All concentrations of Cur treatments were also able to decrease the protein expression levels compared with the control group in a dose-dependent manner (Figures 2B,D, 3B,D and 4B,D).

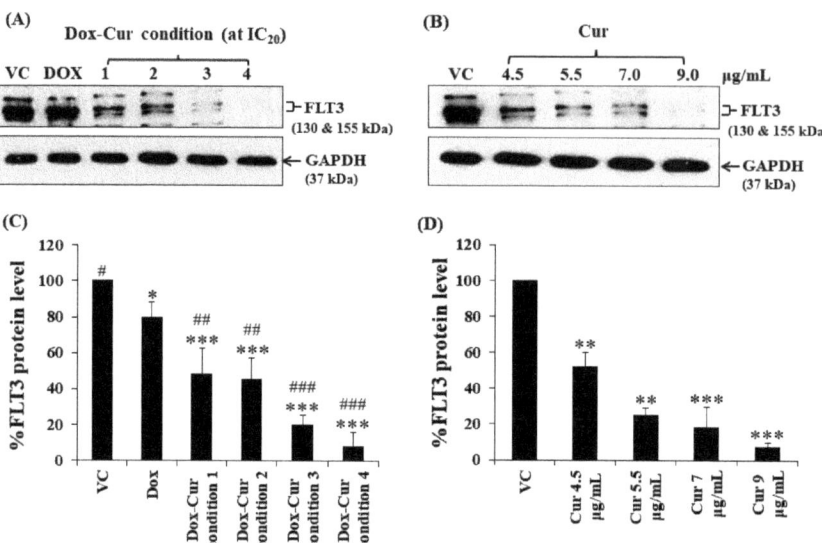

Figure 2. FLT3 protein expression of KG-1a cells after treatment with Dox and combined treatment of Dox–Cur at concentration value of IC_{20} for 48 h. Protein bands (**A**) and percentage (**C**) of FLT3 protein expression level of KG-1a cells treated with DMSO (VC), Dox at concentration of 60 ng/mL, Dox–Cur condition 1 (15 ng/mL Dox + 4.5 µg/mL Cur), Dox–Cur condition 2 (16 ng/mL Dox + 5.5 µg/mL Cur), Dox–Cur condition 3 (12 ng/mL Dox + 7 µg/mL Cur), and Dox–Cur condition 4 (8 ng/mL Dox + 9 µg/mL Cur) for 48 h. Whole protein lysates (80 µg/lane) were loaded onto SDS-PAGE. Protein bands (**B**) and percentage (**D**) of FLT3 protein expression level of KG-1a cells treated with DMSO (VC), Cur (4.5 µg/mL), Cur (5.5 µg/mL), Cur (7 µg/mL), and Cur (9 µg/mL) for 48 h. The data are shown as mean ± SD from 3 independent experiments. The significance of mean differences was assessed using one-way ANOVA. * $p < 0.05$, ** $p < 0.01$, and *** $p < 0.001$ compared with VC. # $p < 0.05$, ## $p < 0.01$, and ### $p < 0.001$ compared with single-Dox treatment.

2.6. Effects of Combination Treatments of Various Concentrations of Cur and a Fixed Concentration of Dox on Cell Number and Viability in Leukemic Stem Cells and Leukemic Cells

Thus far, Cur and Dox–Cur treatments were found to inhibit AML LSC and LC cell proliferation more effectively than Dox treatment alone. Thus, three non-toxic concentrations within the range of Cur IC_{20} value and a fixed concentration of Dox from Dox–Cur condition 1 were tested using KG-1a, KG-1, and EoL-1 cells for 48 h. Co-treatments of Dox–Cur significantly decreased the cell number of both cell lines in a dose-dependent manner when compared with a single-Dox treatment and control (Figure 5). The cell number of KG-1a cells in the control group was 3.44×10^5 cells/mL, and decreased to 2.96×10^5, 2.21×10^5, 1.91×10^5, and 1.46×10^5 cells/mL in response to Dox, Dox + Cur at 4 µg/mL, Dox + Cur at 4.5 µg/mL, and Dox + Cur at 5 µg/mL, respectively (Figure 5A). In addition, the cell number of KG-1 cells decreased from 4.18×10^5 cells/mL in the control group to 3.48×10^5, 2.93×10^5, 2.47×10^5, and 2.22×10^5 cells/mL in response to Dox, Dox + Cur at 3 µg/mL, Dox + Cur at 3.5 µg/mL, and Dox + Cur at 4 µg/mL, respectively (Figure 5C). Moreover, the number of EoL-1 cells also decreased from 10.43×10^5 cells/mL in the control group to 8.99×10^5, 6.82×10^5, 6.08×10^5, and 4.94×10^5 cells/mL in response to the treatments of Dox, Dox + Cur at 2.5 µg/mL, Dox + Cur at 3 µg/mL, and Dox + Cur at 3.5 µg/mL, respectively (Figure 5E). All samples exhibited viable cells higher than 80% of the total cell count (Figure 5B,D,F).

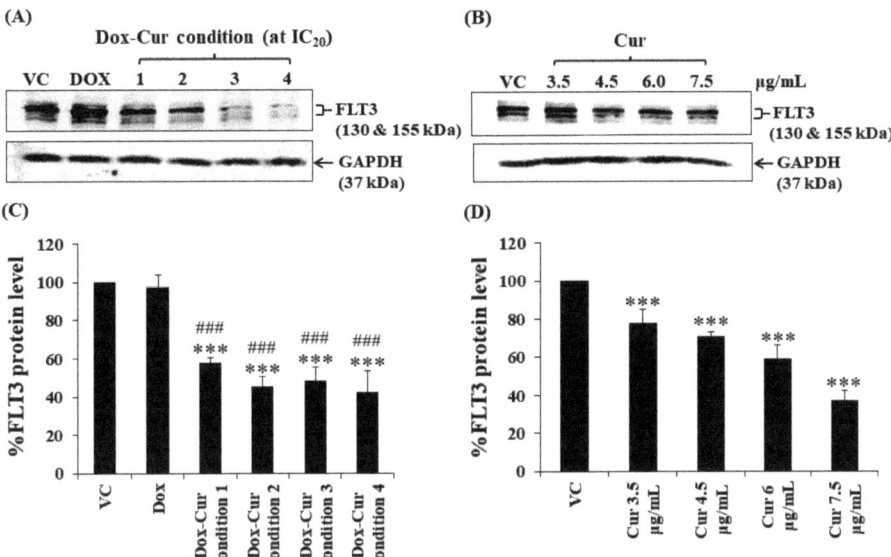

Figure 3. FLT3 protein levels of KG-1 cells after treatment with Dox and Dox–Cur at concentration value of IC$_{20}$ for 48 h. Protein bands (**A**) and percentage (**C**) of FLT3 protein levels of KG-1 cells were from DMSO (VC), Dox (58 ng/mL), Dox–Cur condition 1 (22 ng/mL Dox + 3.5 μg/mL Cur), condition 2 (10 ng/mL Dox + 4.5 μg/mL Cur), condition 3 (7 ng/mL Dox + 6 μg/mL Cur), and condition 4 (6 ng/mL Dox + 7.5 μg/mL Cur). Protein bands (**B**) and percentage (**D**) of FLT3 protein level of KG-1 cells were from DMSO (VC), Cur (3.5 μg/mL), Cur (4.5 μg/mL), Cur (6 μg/mL), and Cur (7.5 μg/mL) for 48 h. Whole protein lysates (80 μg/lane) were loaded onto SDS-PAGE. The data are shown as mean ± SD from 3 independent experiments. The significance of mean differences was assessed using one-way ANOVA. *** $p < 0.001$ compared with VC. ### $p < 0.001$ compared with single-Dox treatment.

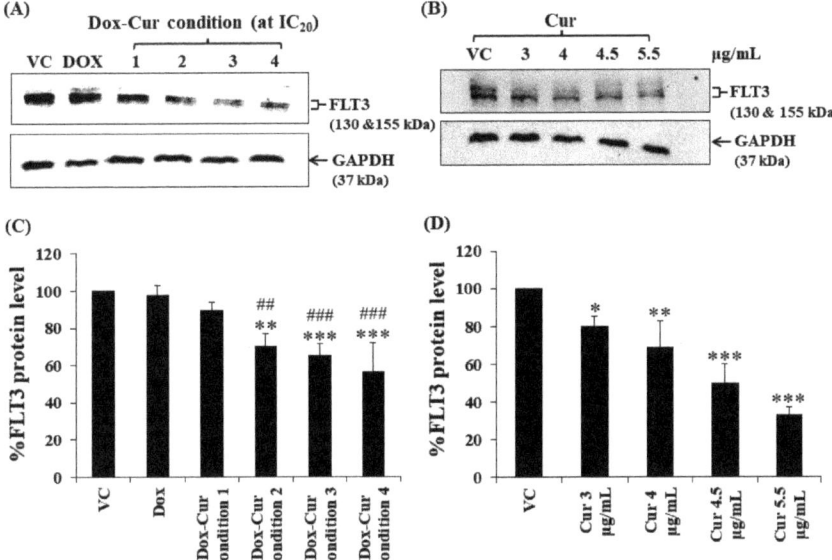

Figure 4. FLT3 protein expression of EoL-1 cells after treatment with Dox and combined treatment of Dox–Cur at concentration value of IC$_{20}$ for 48 h. Protein bands (**A**) and percentage (**C**) of FLT3 protein expression level of EoL-1 cells treated with DMSO (VC), Dox at concentration of 6 ng/mL, Dox–Cur condition 1 (3 ng/mL Dox + 3 μg/mL Cur), Dox–Cur condition 2

(0.7 ng/mL Dox + 4 µg/mL Cur), Dox–Cur condition 3 (0.5 ng/mL Dox + 4.5 µg/mL Cur), and Dox–Cur condition 4 (0.4 ng/mL Dox + 5.5 µg/mL Cur) for 48 h. Whole protein lysates (80 µg/lane) were loaded onto SDS-PAGE. Protein bands (**B**) and percentage (**D**) of FLT3 protein expression level of EoL-1 cells treated with DMSO (VC), Cur (3 µg/mL), Cur (4 µg/mL), Cur (4.5 µg/mL), and Cur (5.5 µg/mL) for 48 h. The data are shown as Mean ± SD from 3 independent experiments. The significance of mean differences was assessed using one-way ANOVA. * $p < 0.05$, ** $p < 0.01$, and *** $p < 0.001$ compared with VC. ## $p < 0.01$ and ### $p < 0.001$ compared with single-Dox treatment.

2.7. Effects of Combination Treatments of Various Concentrations of Cur and a Fixed Concentration of Dox on FLT3 Protein Expressions in Leukemic Stem Cells

Cur and Dox–Cur co-treatments were more effective in suppressing FLT3 protein expression in all AML leukemic cell lines than single-Dox treatment. Moreover, the percentages of FLT3 protein in all conditions of co-treatments were also similar to those of Cur treatment alone. To confirm the effect of Cur in increasing the inhibitory effect of Dox on FLT3 expression, co-treatment of Dox–Cur condition 1 was used. Western blot clearly showed all the non-toxic concentrations of Cur remarkably increased FLT3 protein expression in all three AML cell lines when combined with Dox. The FLT3 expression level of KG-1a cells after treatment with Dox (15 ng/mL), Dox + Cur (4 µg/mL), Dox + Cur (4.5 µg/mL), and Dox + Cur (5 µg/mL) were decreased by 14.1 ± 5.2%, 35.8 ± 8.5%, 38.2 ± 3.3%, and 37.8 ± 7.0%, respectively, compared with the vehicle control (100% FLT3 protein expression level) (Figure 6A,B). For KG-1 cells, the FLT3 protein levels were decreased by 17.9 ± 7.6%, 38.2 ± 13.0%, 39.7 ± 11.4%, and 47.2 ± 5.4% in response to Dox (22 ng/mL), Dox + Cur (3 µg/mL), Dox + Cur (3.5 µg/mL), and Dox + Cur (4 µg/mL), respectively (Figure 6C,D). Finally, while the FLT3 protein expression levels in EoL-1 cells were reduced to 3.5 ± 8.9%, 10.2 ± 8.1%, 15.6 ± 7.1%, and 34.6 ± 8.9% in response to the treatments of Dox (2.8 ng/mL), Dox + Cur (2.5 µg/mL), Dox + Cur (3 µg/mL), and Dox + Cur (3.5 µg/mL), respectively, from 100% protein expression level of the vehicle control (Figure 6E,F).

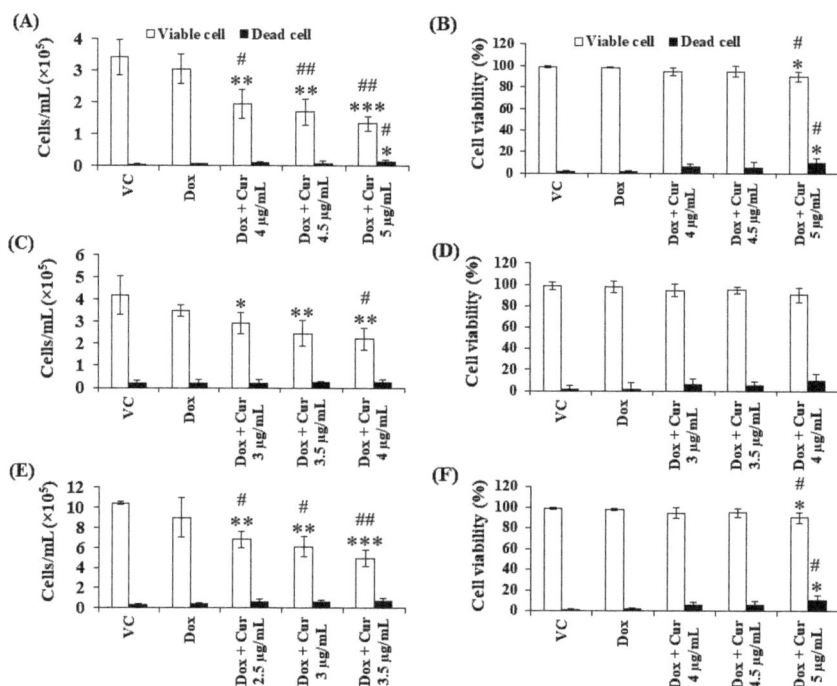

Figure 5. Total cell number and cell viability of KG-1a, KG-1, and EoL-1 cells after treatment with Dox and combination of

fixed concentration of Dox and various non-toxic concentration of Cur for 48 h. Total cell number (**A**) and cell viability (**B**) of KG-1a cells were treated with DMSO (VC), Dox (15 ng/mL), Dox + Cur (4 μg/mL), Dox + Cur (4.5 μg/mL), and Dox + Cur (5 μg/mL) for 48 h. Total cell number (**C**) and cell viability (**D**) of KG-1 cells were treated with DMSO (VC), Dox (22 ng/mL), Dox and Cur (3 μg/mL), Dox and Cur (3.5 μg/mL), and Dox and Cur (4 μg/mL) for 48 h. Total cell number (**E**) and cell viability (**F**) of EoL-1 cells were treated with DMSO (VC), Dox (2.8 ng/mL), Dox and Cur (2.5 μg/mL), Dox and Cur (3 μg/mL), and Dox and Cur (3.5 μg/mL) for 48 h. The data are shown as mean ± SD from 3 independent experiments. The significance of mean differences was assessed using one-way ANOVA. * $p < 0.05$, ** $p < 0.01$, and *** $p < 0.001$ compared with VC. # $p < 0.05$ and ## $p < 0.01$ compared with single-Dox treatment.

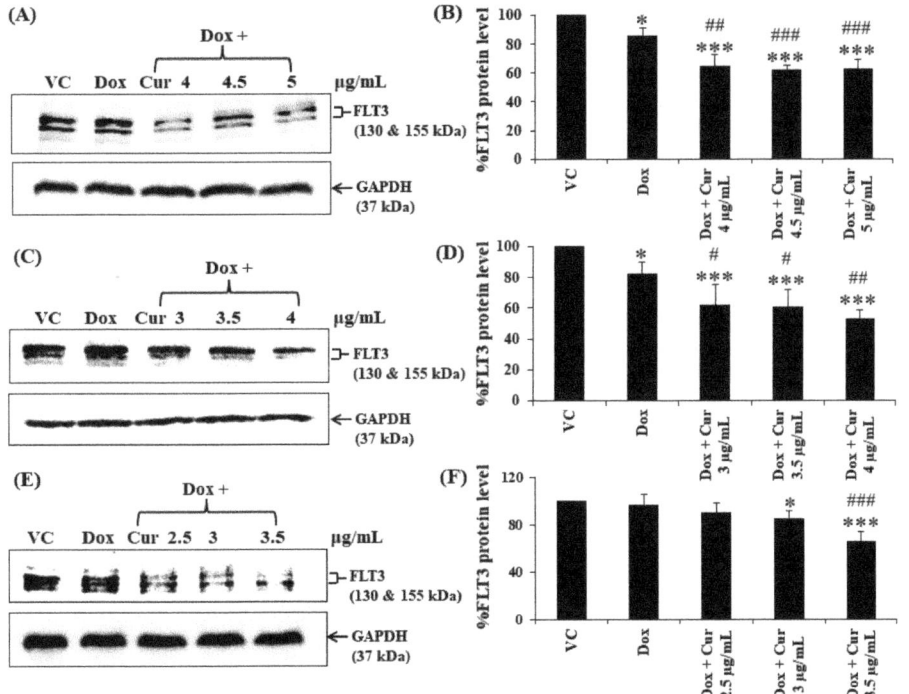

Figure 6. FLT3 protein expression of KG-1a, KG-1, and EoL-1 cells following treatment with Dox and combination of fixed concentration of Dox and various non-toxic concentrations of Cur for 48 h. Protein bands (**A**) and percentage (**B**) of KG-1a cells treated with DMSO (VC), Dox (15 ng/mL), Dox + Cur (4 μg/mL), Dox + Cur (4.5 μg/mL), and Dox + Cur (5 μg/mL), for 48 h. Protein band (**C**) and percentage (**D**) of KG-1 cells treated with DMSO (VC), Dox (22 ng/mL), Dox + Cur (3 μg/mL), Dox + Cur (3.5 μg/mL), and Dox + Cur (4 μg/mL) for 48 h. Protein band (**E**) and percentage (**F**) of EoL-1 cells were treated with DMSO (VC), Dox (2.8 ng/mL), Dox + Cur (2.5 μg/mL), Dox + Cur (3 μg/mL), and Dox + Cur (3.5 μg/mL) for 48 h. Whole protein lysates (80 μg/lane) were loaded onto SDS-PAGE. The data are shown as mean ± SD from 3 independent experiments. The significance of mean differences was assessed using one-way ANOVA. * $p < 0.05$ and *** $p < 0.001$ compared with VC. # $p < 0.05$, ## $p < 0.01$, and ### $p < 0.001$ compared with single-Dox treatment.

3. Discussion

Doxorubicin (Dox) and idarubicin (Ida) are the standard chemotherapy treatments for AML patients. These compounds can destroy leukemic cells by binding to DNA and inhibiting topoisomerase II activity in DNA transcription, thereby triggering apoptosis or autophagy [16,40,41]. The cytotoxic activity of these anthracyclines was determined in each leukemic cell line by MTT assays. Both drugs showed the greatest cytotoxicity for EoL-1 cells, followed by U937, KG-1, and KG-1a cells. The inhibitory concentrations at cell growth values of 50 (IC$_{50}$) for Ida on KG-1a and KG-1 cells were 19.82 ± 1.80 and

5.45 ± 0.89 ng/mL, respectively. In contrast, Dox showed lower cytotoxicity than Ida with IC_{50} values of 0.65 ± 0.13 and 0.21 ± 0.02 µg/mL, respectively. Ida and Dox doses in a previous report in vitro were 1–100 ng/mL and 0.1–1.5 µg/mL, respectively, in normal and leukemic human bone marrow progenitors [42]. Drug doses were within the range of our studies. However, doses used in this study presented activity at low levels when compared with the previous report. Looking at intravenous injections of Ida and Dox in a rat model, the maximum tolerated doses of both drugs were 3 mg/kg and 0.75 mg/kg per injection. Moreover, the cardiac toxicity of Ida remained significantly lower than that of Dox [43].

Next, studies were conducted to determine the effect of combining the natural product curcumin with these AML chemotherapeutics. Cur tended to increase the cytotoxicity of Dox and Ida on all leukemic cell lines; however, several conditions of Dox + Cur co-treatment showed additive and synergistic manners, whereas most conditions of Ida + Cur co-treatment suggested that Cur was antagonistic. Ida appears to have a mechanism similar to Dox in that it can intercalate DNA and block topoisomerase II activity [44], thus differences may be due to the chemical structures of Ida and Dox. The absence of the methoxyl group at position 4 of idarubicin's structure increased the lipophilicity and rate of cellular uptake, leading to greater toxicity than that of daunorubicin or doxorubicin [45]. Furthermore, Ida is relatively more potent than doxorubicin in suppressing the growth of low or nonproliferating progenitor cells [42]. Thus, it is likely that the concentrations of Cur used in the combination treatment were too low to achieve a synergistic effect when combined with Ida. As a result, increasing the concentration of Cur combined with Ida may be explored in future research.

In addition, the cytotoxicity of curcumin (Cur), a natural substance with chemosensitizing and chemoprotective activities [26], was also examined with four leukemic cell lines by MTT assay. Cur demonstrated the highest cytotoxic effect on U937 cells, followed by EoL-1, KG-1, and KG-1a cells. Thus, Cur was selected as a supplementary substance for enhancing the efficiency and decreasing the toxicity of anthracycline drugs in this study.

Appropriate concentrations of Dox, Ida, and Cur were chosen for the combination effect, based on the results of the preliminary screening study. The co-treatments of Ida and Dox at concentrations in the range of IC_{10} to IC_{50} values and low concentrations of Cur at 1, 2, and 3 µg/mL did not show a different effect on cell viability of KG-1a and KG-1 cells, when compared with a single treatment (data not shown). Thus, KG-1a, KG1-a, EoL-1, and U937 cells were treated with Dox and Ida at the concentration values of IC_{10}–IC_{80} combined with Cur at concentrations of IC_{20}, IC_{30}, IC_{40}, and IC_{50} values, respectively. To investigate the combination effect, the percentage of cell viability of each treatment was calculated and compared with that for the single drug and vehicle control, and the inhibitory concentrations at 20% (IC_{20}) and 50% (IC_{50}) were determined.

Co-treatment of Dox–Cur and Ida–Cur tended to increase the cytotoxicity for KG-1a, KG-1, EoL-1, and U937 cells in dose-dependent manners as compared with single-drug treatment. Moreover, Cur also enhanced the cytotoxic efficacy for both chemotherapeutic drugs in dose dependent manners, based on the lower IC_{50} values of anthracyclines used in co-treatment in each cell line.

Dox and Ida are usually ineffective due to an increase in LSCs, drug resistance, and relapse in AML patients. In this study, the natural substance Cur was found to improve the cytotoxicity of Dox and Ida in all the cell lines due to its anti-leukemic (apoptotic induction) [46] and chemosensitizing (decreasing MDR-1 gene expression) [34] activities. For these reasons, Cur improved both chemotherapies by lowering IC_{50} values for Dox and Ida in co-treatments when compared with single drug treatments.

It is notable that effective doses of the co-treatments used to treat KG-1a cells were higher than those for KG-1, EoL-1, and U937 cells. KG-1a and KG-1 cells are leukemic stem cell lines with a high percentage of leukemic stem cells (~95% and ~55%, respectively). These cells are well-known for their chemotherapy resistance, which includes a prolonged stage G_0 of the cell cycle and high expression of the drug efflux pump. Since the EoL-1 and U937 cells lack these stem cell features, they were more vulnerable to the co-treatments.

The combination treatment of Dox–Cur showed synergistic and additive cytotoxic effects on both AML leukemic stem cell lines (KG-1a and KG-1 cells) and AML leukemic cell lines (EoL-1 and U937 cells). Even though only Dox–Cur condition 3 showed synergism on KG-1a and EoL-1 cells, Cur was able to lower chemotherapeutic agent doses. The combination treatment also reduced the concentration at the IC_{50} value of Dox in each cell line which could be a useful formulation to decrease the cytotoxicity of Dox on normal cells. However, the poor solubility and short biological half-life of Cur, as well as the non-specific activity of Dox, may result in low absorption and cytotoxicity of these drugs in tumor cells [16,27].

FLT3 is a key driver of AML, and its mutations are associated with the development of high risk of relapse in patients. Previous studies demonstrated that Cur has an inhibitory effect on FLT3 protein expression in leukemic cells [32]. Thus, the combination of Dox and Cur for AML treatment may lead to FLT3 protein expression reduction, which in turn could denote reduced proliferation of leukemic cells.

In this study, non-toxic doses at IC_{20} of the four conditions of Dox–Cur co-treatments decreased the cell number and showed a higher inhibitory effect on FLT3 protein expression than single Dox in both stem cell and leukemic cell lines. However, when compared with Cur alone, none of the co-treatments showed any differences. To confirm, Dox–Cur condition 1 was selected for the inhibitory effect of various concentrations of Cur with a fixed concentration of Dox on cell number and FLT3 protein expression. Dox–Cur-treated samples exhibited a lower cell number and FLT3 protein level than treatment with Dox alone in all cell lines. It is possible that Cur was the main compound in co-treatment that could suppress the FLT3 protein expression in a dose-dependent manner, leading to a decrease in cell proliferation, while the main functions of Dox, in order to eradicate tumor cells, involved inhibiting cell cycle progression, producing oxidation, and inducing apoptosis, which is unrelated to the inhibition of FLT3 protein expression [16]. In addition, these functions of Dox could affect cell proliferation, resulting in the decrease in cell number in single-Dox-treated samples. The co-treatment had an inhibitory effect on FLT3 protein expression. Notably, the IC_{20} values of Dox in Dox–Cur condition 1 (Dox 15 ng/mL + Cur 4.5 µg/mL) and 2 (Dox 16 ng/mL + Cur 5.5 µg/mL) in KG-1a cells were not reduced in a dose-dependent response to the Cur increase. This might be because the chosen Cur concentration was too low, making the lowering of the Dox concentration in the reaction impractical, as shown by the cell number and FLT3 protein expression level.

Co-treatment likely assists in enhancing the cytotoxic effects of Dox by inhibiting the cell proliferation activity of AML leukemic stem cells and leukemic cells as a result of the decrease in the cell proliferation rate of each co-treatment condition compared with the single treatment and vehicle control. These findings are consistent with a previous study in which the combination of Dox with SU11657, a FLT3 inhibitor, increased the survival rate of APL mice and overcame resistance to traditional chemotherapies in AML [47].

4. Materials and Methods

4.1. Reagents and Chemicals

Curcumin (Cur) was purchased from Thai-China Flavours and Fragrances Industry Co., LTD (Nonthaburi, Thailand). MTT dye (3-[4,5-dimethylthiazol-2-yl]-2,5-diphenyl-tetrazolium bromide), trypan blue, and DMSO were purchased from Sigma-Aldrich (St. Louis, MO, USA). IMDM, RPMI-1640, penicillin-streptomycin, L-glutamine, and fetal calf serum were purchased from Invitrogen™ Life (Carlsbad, CA, USA). Rabbit polyclonal anti-GAPDH was purchased from Santa Cruz Bitechnology (Santa Cruz, CA, USA). HRP-conjugated goat anti-rabbit IgG was purchased from Promega (Madison, WI, USA). Rabbit polyclonal anti-FLT3 and Luminata™ Forte Western HRP Substrate were purchased from Merck Millipore Corporation (Billerica, MA, USA).

4.2. Cell Culture

KG-1a (acute myeloblastic leukemic cell line; ATCC® CCL-246.1™), KG-1 (acute myeloblastic leukemic cell line; ATCC® CCL-246™), and EoL-1 (acute myeloblastic leukemic cell line) were used as human leukemic cell line models in this study. KG-1a and KG-1 cells were cultured in IMDM medium (Invitrogen™, CA, USA) supplemented with 20% fetal bovine serum, 2 mM L-glutamine, 100 units/mL penicillin, and 100 µg/mL streptomycin. EoL-1 (Eosinophilic leukemic cell line), a model of FLT3 overexpressing leukemic cells, was purchased from RIKEN BRC Cell Bank (Ibaraki, Japan). U937 (monoblastic leukemic cell line) was purchased from ATCC®. These were cultured in RPMI-1640 medium containing 10% fetal calf serum, 1 mM L-glutamine, 100 units/mL penicillin, and 100 µg/mL streptomycin. All the leukemic cell lines were cultured at 37 °C in a humidified incubator with 5% CO_2.

4.3. Cytotoxicity of Single Doxorubicin, Idarubicin, and Curcumin (Curcuminoid Mixture) on Leukemic Stem Cell and Leukemic Cell Viability by MTT Assay

KG-1a and KG-1 cell lines were adjusted to 1.5×10^4 cells, while EoL-1 and U937 cells were adjusted to 3.0×10^4 and 1.0×10^4 cells in 100 µL of complete medium, and then seeded into flat-bottom 96-well plate and incubated at 37 °C under 5% CO_2 atmosphere for 24 h. Following that, doxorubicin (Dox), idarubicin (Ida), and curcumin (Cur) were diluted in 100 µL of medium with the 2-fold dilution technique and applied to the cells to obtain the final concentrations from 0.001 to 2 µg/mL for Dox and Ida and 1.56 to 50 µg/mL for Cur for 48 h. Complete medium and DMSO were used as cell control and vehicle control, respectively. Afterwards, 100 µL of medium was removed, and 15 µL of MTT dye solution was added and further incubated for 4 h. After removing the supernatant, 200 µL of DMSO were added to dissolve the formazan crystals (cell viability indication). The optical density was measured using an ELISA plate reader at 578 nm with the reference wavelength at 630 nm. The percentage of cell survival was calculated from the absorbance of test and control wells using the equation below, and the inhibitory concentration at 20% (IC_{20}) and 50% (IC_{50}) growth of Dox, Ida, and Cur were determined.

$$\% \text{ Cell viability} = \frac{\text{Absorbance of test}}{\text{Absorbance of vehicle control}} \times 100$$

4.4. Assessing Cytotoxic Effects of Combination of the Chemotherapeutic Drug and Curcumin on Leukemic Stem Cell and Leukemic Cell Viability by MTT Assay

KG-1a, KG-1, EoL-1, and U937 cells were seeded into flat-bottom 96-well plate and incubated at 37 °C under 5% CO_2 atmosphere for 24 h. Then, various concentrations of Dox and Ida in the range of IC_{10}–IC_{80} (from the cytotoxic effects of single treatment) were mixed with each concentration of Cur at IC_{20}, IC_{30}, IC_{40}, and IC_{50} values, as well as DMSO, to prepare the combination and single drug treatments, respectively. All the treatments were added to the cells and incubated for 48 h. The cell viability in each treatment was determined by the MTT assay, as described in Section 4.3.

4.5. Synergistic Effects of Combination Treatment

The combination index (CI) is used to quantitatively define the synergistic (CI < 1), additive (CI = 1), and antagonist effect (CI > 1) of a drug–drug interaction [48]. It can be calculated by using the following equation:

$$CI = \frac{\text{Dose of drug in combination at ICx}}{\text{Dose of single drug at ICx}} \times \frac{\text{Dose of Cur in combination at ICx}}{\text{Dose of single Cur at ICx}}$$

ICx = The concentrations required to produce the given effect, such as IC_{50}.

4.6. Cell Number and Cell Viability of FLT3-Exprssing Cells Determined by the Trypan Blue Exclusion Method

KG-1a, KG-1, and EoL-1 cells were adjusted to 1.5×10^5 and 3.0×10^5 cells/mL, respectively, and incubated with non-toxic concentrations (IC_{20}) of Dox, Cur, and combination treatment at 37 °C under 5% CO_2 atmosphere for 48 h. Then, the treated cells were collected, and their cell number and percent of cell viability were estimated using the trypan blue exclusion method by mixing the cells and the 0.4% trypan blue solution in a ratio of 1:1; following this, the cells were counted in a hemacytometer under a light microscope.

4.7. Western Blotting

KG-1a, KG-1, and EoL-1 cells were prepared and treated with Dox, Cur, and the co-treatment as discussed in Section 4.6. After that, the cells were harvested after 48 h of incubation, and the whole proteins were extracted using RIPA buffer. The protein concentration was measured with the Folin-Lowry method. The protein lysates were separated through 7.5% SDS-PAGE and then transferred to PVDF membranes. For the antibody–protein reaction step, the membrane was cut to separate FLT3 (target protein) and GAPDH (internal control protein), and then blocked in 5% skim milk. The part of the membrane containing FLT3 protein was probed with rabbit polyclonal anti-FLT3 at a dilution 1:1000, whereas the part containing GAPDH was probed with rabbit polyclonal anti-GAPDH antibody at a dilution of 1:1000. After that, the reaction was followed by a 1:15,000 dilution of HRP-conjugated goat anti-rabbit IgG. The proteins were visualized using Luminata™ Forte Western HRP substrate. Finally, the protein band signal (chemiluminescence) was detected by X-ray film or Fluorchem E Western blot and gel imager (ProteinSimple, San Jose, CA, USA) and quantified using a scan densitometer (Bio-Rad, Hercules, CA, USA) or Fluorchem Q program (ProteinSimple, CA, USA).

4.8. Statistical Analysis

The average of triplicate experiments and standard derivation (SD) were used for quantification. The levels of target protein expressions were compared with those of the vehicle control in each experiment. The results are shown as mean ± SD. The differences between the means of each sample were analyzed by one-way analysis of variance (one-way ANOVA). Statistical significance was considered at $p < 0.05$, $p < 0.01$, and $p < 0.001$.

5. Conclusions

Overall, anthracyclines (Dox and Ida) and Cur, a natural phenolic compound with antitumor activity, were shown to be effective AML chemotherapeutic agents. The combination of Dox and Cur had a synergistic effect and could improve Dox anti-tumor activity in AML cells, particularly leukemic stem cells, by inhibiting cell proliferation through FLT-3 protein suppression. This study demonstrated the benefit of co-treatment combining the natural product curcumin and chemotherapeutic drugs (Dox and Ida) in leukemia therapy as a potential approach to decrease chemotherapy dose and thereby reduce associated side effects. Adding nontoxic doses of edible Cur to chemotherapeutic drugs enhanced the cytotoxicity of Dox and suppressed leukemic stem cell proliferation. This finding presents an alternative choice that may be useful in the development of a promising regimen for the treatment of AML relapse in the future.

Supplementary Materials: The following are available online, Figure S1: Cytotoxic effects of co-treatment of doxorubicin and curcumin (Dox–Cur) on KG-1a, KG-1, EoL-1, and U937 cell lines, Figure S2: Cytotoxic effects of co-treatment of Idarubicin and curcumin (Ida–Cur) on KG-1a, KG-1, EoL-1, and U937 cell lines, Figure S3: Cell number and cell viability of KG-1a cells after treatment with Dox, Cur, and combined treatment of Dox–Cur for 48 h, Figure S4: Cell number and cell viability of KG-1 cells after treatment with Dox, Cur, and combined treatment of Dox–Cur for 48 h, Figure S5: Cell number and cell viability of EoL-1 cells after treatment with Dox, Cur, and combined treatment of Dox–Cur for 48 h, Table S1: IC_{50} values of single and co-treatment of Dox or Ida and Cur on KG-1a cells, Table S2: IC$_{50}$ values of single and co-treatment of Dox or Ida and Cur on KG-1 cells, Table S3: IC$_{50}$ values of single and co-treatment of Dox or Ida and Cur on EoL-1 cells, Table S4: IC$_{50}$ values of single and co-treatment of Dox or Ida and Cur on U937 cells.

Author Contributions: Conceptualization, S.A. and C.B.; methodology, F.C.; validation, F.C. and S.T.; investigation, F.C. and S.T.; writing—original draft preparation, F.C. and S.A.; writing—review and editing, S.A., C.B., S.T. and S.C.; supervision, S.A. and C.B.; project administration, S.A.; funding acquisition, S.A., S.T. and C.B. All authors have read and agreed to the published version of the manuscript.

Funding: This research was funded by the Thailand Research Fund (TRF), grant number RSA6280034, MRG6180124, and the TRF through the Royal Golden Jubilee Ph.D. Program of Thailand (Grant No. PHD/0086/2559).

Institutional Review Board Statement: Not applicable.

Informed Consent Statement: Not applicable.

Data Availability Statement: Not applicable.

Acknowledgments: This research was partially supported by Chiang Mai University, the Center for Research and Development of Natural Products for Health (Chiang Mai University) and Department of Medical Technology, Faculty of AMS (Chiang Mai University). The authors are grateful to Department of Pharmaceutical Sciences, School of Pharmacy (The University of Kansas), and Vaccine Analytics and Formulation Center (The University of Kansas) for supporting research space and laboratory instruments.

Conflicts of Interest: The authors declare no conflict of interest.

Sample Availability: Not available.

References

1. Juliusson, G.; Antunovic, P.; Derolf, A.; Lehmann, S.; Mollgard, L.; Stockelberg, D.; Tidefelt, U.; Wahlin, A.; Hoglund, M. Age and acute myeloid leukemia: Real world data on decision to treat and outcomes from the Swedish Acute Leukemia Registry. *Blood* **2009**, *113*, 4179–4187. [CrossRef] [PubMed]
2. Roboz, G.J.; Guzman, M. Acute myeloid leukemia stem cells: Seek and destroy. *Expert Rev. Hematol.* **2009**, *2*, 663–672. [CrossRef] [PubMed]
3. Dohner, H.; Estey, E.H.; Amadori, S.; Appelbaum, F.R.; Buchner, T.; Burnett, A.K.; Dombret, H.; Fenaux, P.; Grimwade, D.; Larson, R.A.; et al. Diagnosis and management of acute myeloid leukemia in adults: Recommendations from an international expert panel, on behalf of the European LeukemiaNet. *Blood* **2010**, *115*, 453–474. [CrossRef]
4. Sperr, W.R.; Hauswirth, A.W.; Florian, S.; Ohler, L.; Geissler, K.; Valent, P. Human leukaemic stem cells: A novel target of therapy. *Eur. J. Clin. Investig.* **2004**, *34* (Suppl. S2), 31–40. [CrossRef] [PubMed]
5. Dick, J.E. Acute myeloid leukemia stem cells. *Ann. N. Y. Acad. Sci.* **2005**, *1044*, 1–5. [CrossRef] [PubMed]
6. Bonnet, D.; Dick, J.E. Human acute myeloid leukemia is organized as a hierarchy that originates from a primitive hematopoietic cell. *Nat. Med.* **1997**, *3*, 730–737. [CrossRef] [PubMed]
7. Tallman, M.S.; Gilliland, D.G.; Rowe, J.M. Drug therapy for acute myeloid leukemia. *Blood* **2005**, *106*, 1154–1163. [CrossRef] [PubMed]
8. Guan, Y.; Gerhard, B.; Hogge, D.E. Detection, isolation, and stimulation of quiescent primitive leukemic progenitor cells from patients with acute myeloid leukemia (AML). *Blood* **2003**, *101*, 3142–3149. [CrossRef] [PubMed]
9. Dean, M.; Fojo, T.; Bates, S. Tumour stem cells and drug resistance. *Nat. Rev. Cancer* **2005**, *5*, 275–284. [CrossRef]
10. Zhou, S.; Schuetz, J.D.; Bunting, K.D.; Colapietro, A.M.; Sampath, J.; Morris, J.J.; Lagutina, I.; Grosveld, G.C.; Osawa, M.; Nakauchi, H.; et al. The ABC transporter Bcrp1/ABCG2 is expressed in a wide variety of stem cells and is a molecular determinant of the side-population phenotype. *Nat. Med.* **2001**, *7*, 1028–1034. [CrossRef]
11. Ravandi, F.; Estrov, Z. Eradication of leukemia stem cells as a new goal of therapy in leukemia. *Clin. Cancer Res.* **2006**, *12*, 340–344. [CrossRef]
12. Blasiak, J.; Gloc, E.; Wozniak, K.; Mlynarski, W.; Stolarska, M.; Skorski, T.; Majsterek, I. Genotoxicity of idarubicin and its modulation by vitamins C and E and amifostine. *Chem. Biol. Interact.* **2002**, *140*, 1–18. [CrossRef]
13. Gerson, S.L.; Caimi, P.F.; William, B.M.; Creger, R.J. Pharmacology and molecular mechanisms of antineoplastic agents for hematologic malignancies. In *Hematology*; Elsevier: Amsterdam, The Netherlands, 2018; pp. 849–912.
14. Ohtake, S.; Miyawaki, S.; Fujita, H.; Kiyoi, H.; Shinagawa, K.; Usui, N.; Okumura, H.; Miyamura, K.; Nakaseko, C.; Miyazaki, Y. Randomized study of induction therapy comparing standard-dose idarubicin with high-dose daunorubicin in adult patients with previously untreated acute myeloid leukemia: The JALSG AML201 Study. *Blood J. Am. Soc. Hematol.* **2011**, *117*, 2358–2365. [CrossRef] [PubMed]

15. Bittencourt, R.; Bortolheiro, T.C.; Chauffaille, M.d.L.L.F.; Fagundes, E.M.; Pagnano, K.B.B.; Rego, E.M.; Bernardo, W.M. Guidelines on the treatment of acute myeloid leukemia: Associação Brasileira de Hematologia, Hemoterapia e Terapia Celular. *Rev. Bras. Hematol. Hemoter.* **2016**, *38*, 58–74. [CrossRef] [PubMed]
16. Tacar, O.; Sriamornsak, P.; Dass, C.R. Doxorubicin: An update on anticancer molecular action, toxicity and novel drug delivery systems. *J. Pharm. Pharmacol.* **2013**, *65*, 157–170. [CrossRef] [PubMed]
17. Szakacs, G.; Paterson, J.K.; Ludwig, J.A.; Booth-Genthe, C.; Gottesman, M.M. Targeting multidrug resistance in cancer. *Nat. Rev. Drug Discov.* **2006**, *5*, 219–234. [CrossRef] [PubMed]
18. Yagi, T.; Morimoto, A.; Eguchi, M.; Hibi, S.; Sako, M.; Ishii, E.; Mizutani, S.; Imashuku, S.; Ohki, M.; Ichikawa, H. Identification of a gene expression signature associated with pediatric AML prognosis. *Blood* **2003**, *102*, 1849–1856. [CrossRef] [PubMed]
19. Costello, R.T.; Mallet, F.; Gaugler, B.; Sainty, D.; Arnoulet, C.; Gastaut, J.A.; Olive, D. Human acute myeloid leukemia $CD34^+/CD38^-$ progenitor cells have decreased sensitivity to chemotherapy and Fas-induced apoptosis, reduced immunogenicity, and impaired dendritic cell transformation capacities. *Cancer Res.* **2000**, *60*, 4403–4411.
20. Ayton, P.M.; Cleary, M.L. Molecular mechanisms of leukemogenesis mediated by MLL fusion proteins. *Oncogene* **2001**, *20*, 5695–5707. [CrossRef]
21. Armstrong, S.A.; Kung, A.L.; Mabon, M.E.; Silverman, L.B.; Stam, R.W.; Den Boer, M.L.; Pieters, R.; Kersey, J.H.; Sallan, S.E.; Fletcher, J.A.; et al. Inhibition of FLT3 in MLL. Validation of a therapeutic target identified by gene expression based classification. *Cancer Cell* **2003**, *3*, 173–183. [CrossRef]
22. Carvalho, C.; Santos, R.X.; Cardoso, S.; Correia, S.; Oliveira, P.J.; Santos, M.S.; Moreira, P.I. Doxorubicin: The good, the bad and the ugly effect. *Curr. Med. Chem.* **2009**, *16*, 3267–3285. [CrossRef]
23. Vergely, C.; Delemasure, S.; Cottin, Y.; Rochette, L. Preventing the cardiotoxic effects of anthracyclines: From basic concepts to clinical data. *Heart Metab.* **2007**, *35*, 1–7.
24. Mohan, M.; Kamble, S.; Gadhi, P.; Kasture, S. Protective effect of Solanum torvum on doxorubicin-induced nephrotoxicity in rats. *Food Chem. Toxicol.* **2010**, *48*, 436–440. [CrossRef]
25. Jobin, C.; Bradham, C.A.; Russo, M.P.; Juma, B.; Narula, A.S.; Brenner, D.A.; Sartor, R.B. Curcumin blocks cytokine-mediated NF-kappa B activation and proinflammatory gene expression by inhibiting inhibitory factor I-kappa B kinase activity. *J. Immunol.* **1999**, *163*, 3474–3483.
26. Qian, H.; Yang, Y.; Wang, X. Curcumin enhanced adriamycin-induced human liver-derived Hepatoma G2 cell death through activation of mitochondria-mediated apoptosis and autophagy. *Eur. J. Pharm. Sci.* **2011**, *43*, 125–131. [CrossRef]
27. Anand, P.; Sundaram, C.; Jhurani, S.; Kunnumakkara, A.B.; Aggarwal, B.B. Curcumin and cancer: An "old-age" disease with an "age-old" solution. *Cancer Lett.* **2008**, *267*, 133–164. [CrossRef] [PubMed]
28. Anuchapreeda, S.; Tima, S.; Duangrat, C.; Limtrakul, P. Effect of pure curcumin, demethoxycurcumin, and bisdemethoxycurcumin on WT1 gene expression in leukemic cell lines. *Cancer Chemother. Pharmacol.* **2008**, *62*, 585–594. [CrossRef] [PubMed]
29. Tima, S.; Anuchapreeda, S.; Ampasavate, C.; Berkland, C.; Okonogi, S. Stable curcumin-loaded polymeric micellar formulation for enhancing cellular uptake and cytotoxicity to FLT3 overexpressing EoL-1 leukemic cells. *Eur. J. Pharm. Biopharm.* **2017**, *114*, 57–68. [CrossRef] [PubMed]
30. Kong, Y.; Ma, W.; Liu, X.; Zu, Y.; Fu, Y.; Wu, N.; Liang, L.; Yao, L.; Efferth, T. Cytotoxic Activity of Curcumin towards CCRF-CEM Leukemia Cells and Its Effect on DNA Damage. *Molecules* **2009**, *14*, 5328–5338. [CrossRef] [PubMed]
31. Seghetti, F.; Di Martino, R.M.C.; Catanzaro, E.; Bisi, A.; Gobbi, S.; Rampa, A.; Canonico, B.; Montanari, M.; Krysko, D.V.; Papa, S.; et al. Curcumin-1,2,3-Triazole Conjugation for Targeting the Cancer Apoptosis Machinery. *Molecules* **2020**, *25*, 3066. [CrossRef]
32. Tima, S.; Okonogi, S.; Ampasavate, C.; Pickens, C.; Berkland, C.; Anuchapreeda, S. Development and Characterization of FLT3-Specific Curcumin-Loaded Polymeric Micelles as a Drug Delivery System for Treating FLT3-Overexpressing Leukemic Cells. *J. Pharm. Sci.* **2016**, *105*, 3645–3657. [CrossRef]
33. Gao, S.-m.; Yang, J.-j.; Chen, C.-q.; Chen, J.-j.; Ye, L.-p.; Wang, L.-y.; Wu, J.-b.; Xing, C.-y.; Yu, K. Pure curcumin decreases the expression of WT1 by upregulation of miR-15a and miR-16-1 in leukemic cells. *J. Exp. Clin. Cancer Res.* **2012**, *31*, 1–9. [CrossRef] [PubMed]
34. Shukla, S.; Zaher, H.; Hartz, A.; Bauer, B.; Ware, J.A.; Ambudkar, S.V. Curcumin inhibits the activity of ABCG2/BCRP1, a multidrug resistance-linked ABC drug transporter in mice. *Pharm. Res.* **2009**, *26*, 480–487. [CrossRef]
35. Chen, T.H.; Yang, Y.C.; Wang, J.C.; Wang, J.J. Curcumin treatment protects against renal ischemia and reperfusion injury-induced cardiac dysfunction and myocardial injury. *Transplant. Proc.* **2013**, *45*, 3546–3549. [CrossRef] [PubMed]
36. Cohly, H.H.; Taylor, A.; Angel, M.F.; Salahudeen, A.K. Effect of turmeric, turmerin and curcumin on H_2O_2-induced renal epithelial (LLC-PK1) cell injury. *Free Radic. Biol. Med.* **1998**, *24*, 49–54. [CrossRef]
37. Wang, J.; Ma, W.; Tu, P. Synergistically Improved Anti-tumor Efficacy by Co-delivery Doxorubicin and Curcumin Polymeric Micelles. *Macromol. Biosci.* **2015**, *15*, 1252–1261. [CrossRef] [PubMed]
38. Matthews, W.; Jordan, C.T.; Wiegand, G.W.; Pardoll, D.; Lemischka, I.R. A receptor tyrosine kinase specific to hematopoietic stem and progenitor cell-enriched populations. *Cell* **1991**, *65*, 1143–1152. [CrossRef]
39. Zheng, R.; Levis, M.; Piloto, O.; Brown, P.; Baldwin, B.R.; Gorin, N.C.; Beran, M.; Zhu, Z.; Ludwig, D.; Hicklin, D.; et al. FLT3 ligand causes autocrine signaling in acute myeloid leukemia cells. *Blood* **2004**, *103*, 267–274. [CrossRef]
40. Hope, K.J.; Jin, L.; Dick, J.E. Human acute myeloid leukemia stem cells. *Arch. Med. Res.* **2003**, *34*, 507–514. [CrossRef] [PubMed]
41. Luo, L.; Han, Z.C. Leukemia stem cells. *Int. J. Hematol.* **2006**, *84*, 123–127. [CrossRef]

42. Minderman, H.; Linssen, P.; Van der Lely, N.; Wessels, J.; Boezeman, J.; De Witte, T.; Haanen, C. Toxicity of idarubicin and doxorubicin towards normal and leukemic human bone marrow progenitors in relation to their proliferative state. *Leukemia* **1994**, *8*, 382–387. [PubMed]
43. Platel, D.; Pouna, P.; Bonoron-Adèle, S.; Robert, J. Comparative cardiotoxicity of idarubicin and doxorubicin using the isolated perfused rat heart model. *Anti-Cancer Drugs* **1999**, *10*, 671–676. [CrossRef]
44. Taymaz-Nikerel, H.; Karabekmez, M.E.; Eraslan, S.; Kırdar, B. Doxorubicin induces an extensive transcriptional and metabolic rewiring in yeast cells. *Sci. Rep.* **2018**, *8*, 13672. [CrossRef]
45. Hollingshead, L.M.; Faulds, D. Idarubicin. A review of its pharmacodynamic and pharmacokinetic properties, and therapeutic potential in the chemotherapy of cancer. *Drugs* **1991**, *42*, 690–719. [CrossRef]
46. Reuter, S.; Eifes, S.; Dicato, M.; Aggarwal, B.B.; Diederich, M. Modulation of anti-apoptotic and survival pathways by curcumin as a strategy to induce apoptosis in cancer cells. *Biochem. Pharmacol.* **2008**, *76*, 1340–1351. [CrossRef] [PubMed]
47. Lee, B.D.; Sevcikova, S.; Kogan, S.C. Dual treatment with FLT3 inhibitor SU11657 and doxorubicin increases survival of leukemic mice. *Leuk. Res.* **2007**, *31*, 1131–1134. [CrossRef] [PubMed]
48. Chou, T.-C. Drug combination studies and their synergy quantification using the Chou-Talalay method. *Cancer Res.* **2010**, *70*, 440–446. [CrossRef] [PubMed]

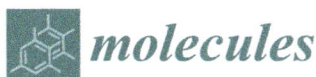 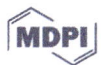

Article

Lycoperoside H, a Tomato Seed Saponin, Improves Epidermal Dehydration by Increasing Ceramide in the Stratum Corneum and Steroidal Anti-Inflammatory Effect

Shogo Takeda [1], Kenchi Miyasaka [1], Sarita Shrestha [2], Yoshiaki Manse [2], Toshio Morikawa [2] and Hiroshi Shimoda [1,*]

1. Research and Development Division, Oryza Oil and Fat Chemical Co., Ltd., 1 Numata, Kitagata-cho, Ichinomiya 493-8001, Aichi, Japan; kgohedasato2@gmail.com (S.T.); kgohedasato3@gmail.com (K.M.)
2. Pharmaceutical Research and Technology Institute, Kindai University, 3-4-1 Kowakae, Higashi-osaka 577-8502, Osaka, Japan; japan.sarita@gmail.com (S.S.); manse@phar.kindai.ac.jp (Y.M.); morikawa@kindai.ac.jp (T.M.)
* Correspondence: kaihatsu@mri.biglobe.ne.jp; Tel.: +81-586-86-5141

Abstract: Tomatoes are widely consumed, however, studies on tomato seeds are limited. In this study, we isolated 11 compounds including saponins and flavonol glycosides from tomato seeds and evaluated their effects on epidermal hydration. Among the isolated compounds, tomato seed saponins (10 µM) significantly increased the mRNA expression of proteins related to epidermal hydration, including filaggrin, involucrin, and enzymes for ceramide synthesis, by 1.32- to 1.91-fold compared with the control in HaCaT cells. Tomato seed saponins (10 µM) also decreased transepidermal water loss by 7 to 13 g/m^2·h in the reconstructed human epidermal keratinization (RHEK) models. Quantitative analysis of the ceramide content in the stratum corneum (SC) revealed that lycoperoside H (1–10 µM) is a promising candidate to stimulate ceramide synthesis via the upregulation of ceramide synthase-3, glucosylceramide synthase, and β-glucocerebrosidase, which led to an increase in the total SC ceramides (approximately 1.5-fold) in concert with ceramide (NP) (approximately 2-fold) in the RHEK models. Evaluation of the anti-inflammatory and anti-allergic effects of lycoperoside H demonstrated that lycoperoside H is suggested to act as a partial agonist of the glucocorticoid receptor and exhibits anti-inflammatory effects (10 mg/kg in animal test). These findings indicate that lycoperoside H can improve epidermal dehydration and suppress inflammation by increasing SC ceramide and steroidal anti-inflammatory activity.

Keywords: tomato seed; lycoperoside; steroidal saponin; ceramide; transepidermal water loss; anti-inflammation

Citation: Takeda, S.; Miyasaka, K.; Shrestha, S.; Manse, Y.; Morikawa, T.; Shimoda, H. Lycoperoside H, a Tomato Seed Saponin, Improves Epidermal Dehydration by Increasing Ceramide in the Stratum Corneum and Steroidal Anti-Inflammatory Effect. *Molecules* **2021**, *26*, 5860. https://doi.org/10.3390/molecules26195860

Academic Editors: Karel Šmejkal and Juraj Majtan

Received: 31 August 2021
Accepted: 22 September 2021
Published: 27 September 2021

Publisher's Note: MDPI stays neutral with regard to jurisdictional claims in published maps and institutional affiliations.

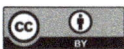

Copyright: © 2021 by the authors. Licensee MDPI, Basel, Switzerland. This article is an open access article distributed under the terms and conditions of the Creative Commons Attribution (CC BY) license (https://creativecommons.org/licenses/by/4.0/).

1. Introduction

Tomato (*Solanum lycopersicum*) is a popular food consumed around the world. It contains various nutritional phytochemicals, including vitamins, carotenoids, saponins, and flavonoids [1]. Among these, previous works regarding tomato saponins are limited. The spirosolane types of steroidal saponins have been isolated as lycoperosides [2,3] and escleosides [4–7] from tomato. Regarding the biological activities of these steroidal saponins, Fujiwara et al. have reported that the oral administration of esculeoside A reduced serum cholesterol and low-density lipoprotein-cholesterol in apolipoprotein E-deficient mice [8]. On the other hand, Zhou et al. have reported that orally administered esculeoside B isolated from tomato juice improved 2,4-dinitrochlorobenzene-induced type IV allergic dermatitis in mice [9]. However, research specific to the seeds is limited.

We had an opportunity to obtain dried tomato seeds, and hence we performed a chemical study on low molecular components in the tomato seeds and found that they contain several types of saponins and flavonol glycosides (Figure 1). Among them, we have recently demonstrated that oral administration of lycoperoside H, a steroidal saponin isolated from tomato seeds, ameliolated atopic dermatitis (AD)-like skin inflammation and transepidermal water loss (TEWL), in concert with a decrease in accumulation of mast cells, eosinophils in dermis, the secretion of serum total IgE, and the Th2/Th1 cytokine ratio in IL-33 transgenic mice [10]. However, the mechanism of lycoperoside H in this study was not evaluated in detail and the anti-inflammtory and/or epidermal hydrating effect of isolated compounds other than lycoperoside H remain unknown.

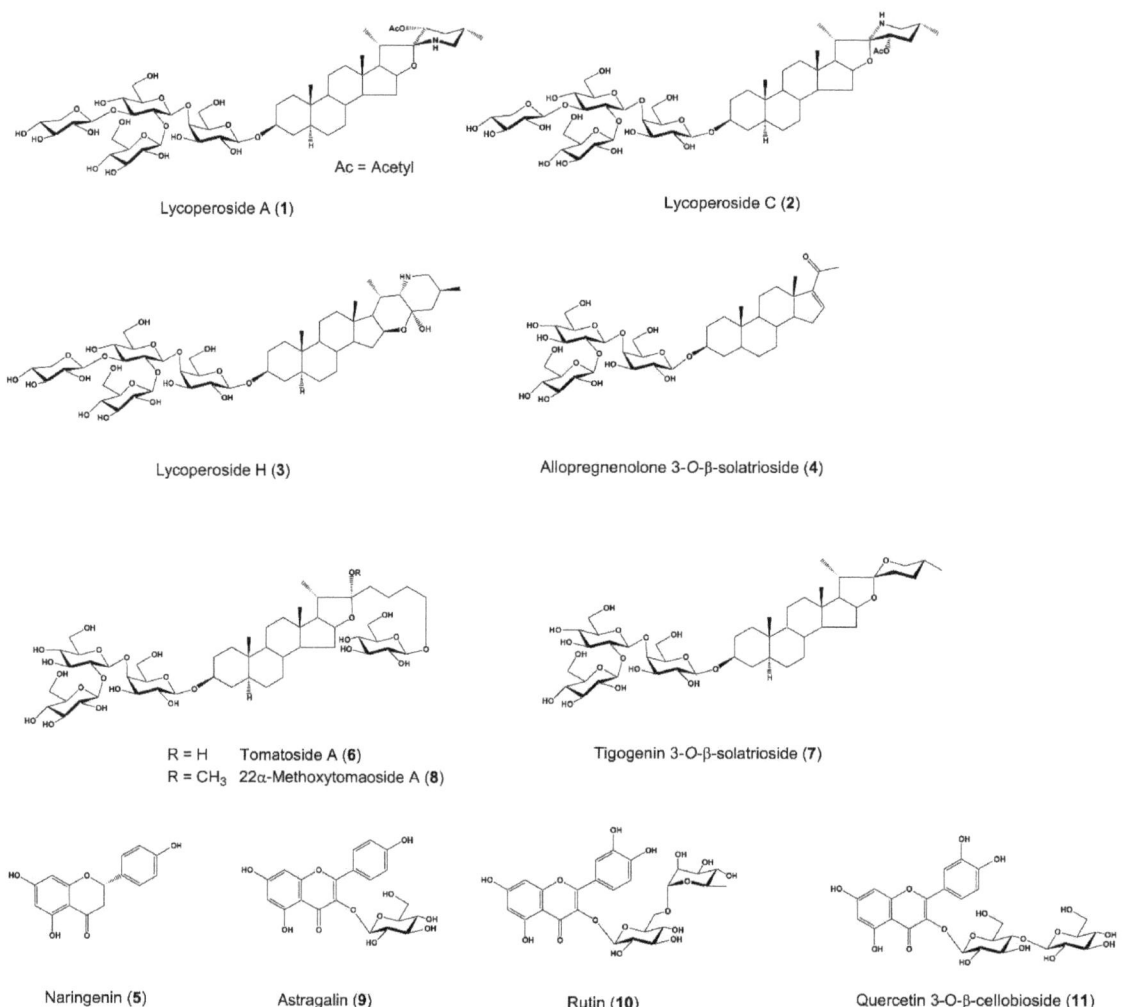

Figure 1. Chemical structures of the isolated compounds (1–11) from tomato seeds.

Generally, saponins exhibit a variety of biological activities. Among them, the anti-inflammatory effects [11] and wound healing effects [12] of saponins on human skin have been recognized as beneficial effects for decades. For example, Korean ginseng is well-known for containing specific saponins, ginsenosides. Lee et al. have reported that the oral administration of Korean ginseng extract containing ginsenosides improved TEWL in AD mice, meaning an increase in anti-inflammatory effects and skin hydration [13]. Especially, ginsenoside Rg1, a principal ginsenoside, ameliorated the increase in TEWL in hairless mouse skin damaged by UV rays [14]. In addition to the anti-inflammatory effects, ginsenoside Rc enhances filaggrin expression in HaCaT cells, a keratinocyte cell line, which contributes to the retention of epidermal moisture [15]. On the other hand, gracillin, a spirostan-type saponin, isolated from *Dioscorea quinqueloba*, improved TEWL in an AD mouse model [16], and centella saponins in the leaves and stems of *Centella (C.) asiatica* are famous for their wound healing effect by promoting collagen production [17]. Centella saponins also reduce epidermal dehydration. Madecassoside, a major pentacyclic triterpene saponin in *C. asiatica*, reduces TEWL and enhances several moisturizing molecules, including aquaporin-3, loricrin, and involucrin [17]. Moreover, topical application of a cosmetic formulation containing *C. asiatica* extract has been used for skin moisturizing and anti-inflammation [18].

In consideration of the above references, we built the hypothesis that tomato seed extract (TSE) and tomato seed saponins affect epidermal hydration by improving TEWL or increasing moisturizing factors. Since several factors, including ceramide, a dominant lipid in the stratum corneum (SC), filaggrin, and involucrin, contribute to epidermal hydration, we conducted a study on the epidermal hydrating effect of tomato seed saponins including lycoperoside H and flavonoids through epidermal molecule expressions contributing toward hydration and TEWL suppression.

2. Results

2.1. Effect of TSE and Isolated Compounds (1–11) on the mRNA Expression of Proteins Related to Epidermal Hydration in HaCaT Cells

We evaluated the effect of isolated compounds from tomato seeds on the mRNA expression of filaggrin, involucrin, serine palmitoyltransferase-2 (SPT2), ceramide synthase-3 (CerS3), and glucosylceramide synthase (GCS), which play crucial roles in epidermal hydration. As shown in Table 1, TSE significantly upregulated the mRNA expression of involucrin, SPT2, CerS3, and GCS, and tended to increase that of filaggrin. Similar to TSE, lycoperoside C (**2**) significantly increased the mRNA expression of all the proteins examined. Lycoperoside H (**3**) significantly enhanced the mRNA expression of proteins, except filaggrin and SPT2. On the other hand, lycoperoside A (**1**) did not affect any mRNA expression of proteins. As for allopregnenolone 3-*O*-β-solatrioside (**4**), only significant upregulation of involucrin was observed.

Table 1. Effects of TSE and isolated compounds (**1–11**) on the mRNA expression of proteins related to epidermal hydration in HaCaT cells.

	Relative mRNA Expression				
	Filaggrin	Involucrin	SPT2	CerS3	GCS
Control	1.00 ± 0.03	1.00 ± 0.01	1.00 ± 0.02	1.00 ± 0.02	1.00 ± 0.01
TSE	1.42 ± 0.06	1.56 ± 0.12 **	1.49 ± 0.07 *	1.78 ± 0.04 **	1.62 ± 0.13 **
Lycoperoside A (**1**)	1.47 ± 0.16	0.91 ± 0.04	0.98 ± 0.05	1.26 ± 0.04	1.00 ± 0.04
Lycoperoside C (**2**)	1.91 ± 0.26 **	1.59 ± 0.14 **	1.70 ± 0.21 **	1.72 ± 0.07 **	1.32 ± 0.01 *
Lycoperoside H (**3**)	1.56 ± 0.15	1.67 ± 0.07 **	1.45 ± 0.05	1.50 ± 0.17 **	1.47 ± 0.11 **
Allopregnenolone 3-*O*-β-solatrioside (**4**)	1.57 ± 0.14	1.40 ± 0.06 *	1.01 ± 0.17	1.20 ± 0.06	1.01 ± 0.03
Tomatoside A (**6**)	1.31 ± 0.11	0.96 ± 0.04	1.35 ± 0.09	1.33 ± 0.07 *	1.66 ± 0.15 **
Tigogenin 3-*O*-β-solatrioside (**7**)	1.30 ± 0.13	1.03 ± 0.12	1.59 ± 0.28 *	1.18 ± 0.05	1.58 ± 0.04 **
22α-Methoxytomatoside A (**8**)	1.50 ± 0.09 **	1.21 ± 0.08	1.37 ± 0.09	1.32 ± 0.08 *	1.28 ± 0.08
Naringenin (**5**)	1.30 ± 0.11	1.14 ± 0.12	1.84 ± 0.09 *	1.09 ± 0.08	0.83 ± 0.07
Astragalin (**9**)	1.07 ± 0.09	1.16 ± 0.02	1.82 ± 0.09 **	1.18 ± 0.09	0.81 ± 0.03
Rutin (**10**)	0.80 ± 0.11	1.01 ± 0.13	1.03 ± 0.03	0.66 ± 0.09 **	0.81 ± 0.05 *
Quercetin 3-*O*-β-cellobioside (**11**)	0.72 ± 0.01 *	0.82 ± 0.12	0.79 ± 0.02 *	0.56 ± 0.03 **	0.62 ± 0.03 **

HaCaT cells were treated with TSE (10 μg/mL) or isolated compounds (**1–11**, 10 μM) for 6 h. Extraction of total RNA and real-time RT-PCR analysis were performed as described in the Materials and Methods section. Data are expressed as mean ± SE ($n = 3$). * $p < 0.05$, ** $p < 0.01$ vs. control. Each value was corrected by the mRNA expression level of β-actin and shown as the value relative to the control.

Tomatoside A (**6**) significantly increased CerS3 and GCS expression, and tigogenin 3-*O*-β-solatrioside (**7**) enhanced SPT2 and GCS expression. In contrast to the effects of tigogenin 3-*O*-β-solatrioside (**7**), 22α-methoxytomatoside A (**8**) significantly increased the mRNA expression of filaggrin and CerS3. In terms of the flavonoids, only naringenin (**5**) and astragalin (**9**) exhibited significant upregulation of SPT2, whereas rutin (**10**) significantly downregulated the mRNA expression of CerS3 and GCS, and quercetin 3-O-β-cellobioside (**11**) significantly decreased the expression of filaggrin, SPT2, CerS3, and GCS and tended to diminish involucrin expression.

2.2. Effects of TSE and Saponins (1–4,6–8) on TEWL in RHEK Models

As a result of the screening for active compounds for skin hydration using HaCaT cells, tomato seed saponins (**1–4,6–8**) were selected as the candidates which upregulate the mRNA expression of factors related to epidermal hydration. As a next step, we evaluated the effect of TSE and tomato seed saponins (**1–4,6–8**) on TEWL in RHEK models and whether they have hydrating activity. TSE (10 μg/mL) significantly decreased TEWL on days 5 and 7 (Figure 2A). As for the tomato seed saponins, 10 μM of **1**, **3**, and **7** significantly suppressed TEWL on days 5 and 7 (Figure 2A,B). Compound **8** significantly decreased TEWL on day 5 and **2** and **6** reduced TEWL on day 7 (Figure 2B). On the other hand, **4** had no effect on TEWL.

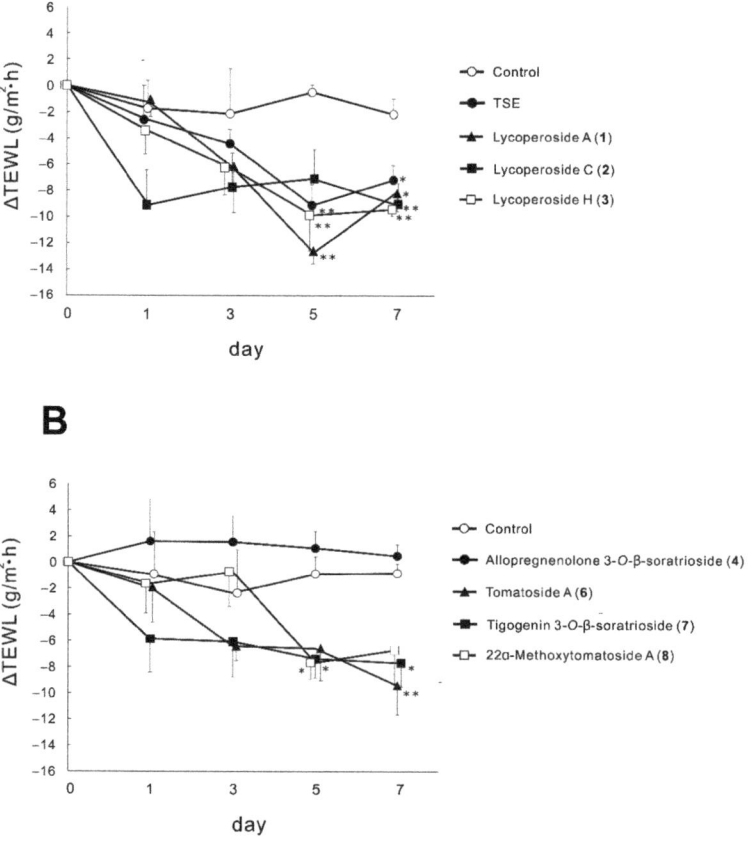

Figure 2. Effects of TSE and tomato seed saponins (**1–4,6–8**) on TEWL in RHEK models. RHEK models were treated with each sample ((**A**) TSE: 10 μg/mL, **1–3**: 10 μM, (**B**) **4–8**: 10 μM) for 7 days. TEWL measurements were performed on days 0, 1, 3, 5, and 7 using Tewitro TW24. Data are expressed as mean ± SE (n = 4). * $p < 0.05$, ** $p < 0.01$ vs. control.

2.3. Effects of Tomato Seed Saponins (1–4,6–8) on the Ceramide Contents in SC of RHEK Models

Figure 3A shows the effects of tomato seed saponins (**1–4,6–8**) on SC ceramide contents in RHEK models. Among tomato seed saponins, only lycoperoside H (**3**) significantly increased the total ceramide contents, and tigogenin 3-O-β-solatrioside (**7**) slightly increased the total ceramide contents but the difference was not significant. In terms of the ceramide species, ceramide (NP) was significantly increased by lycoperoside H (**3**) and tended to increase with treatment of tigogenin 3-O-β-solatrioside (**7**) and 22α-methoxytomatoside A (**8**). Although similar trends were observed in the contents of ceramide (NS, NDS), (EOH), (AS), and (AP), significant differences were not confirmed. Other tomato seed saponins did not affect the SC ceramide contents.

As described above, only lycoperoside H (**3**) significantly increased the SC ceramide contents at 10 μM among the tomato seed saponins (**1–4,6–8**). Thus, we next evaluated the concentration dependency of lycoperoside H (**3**). The effect of 1 and 10 μM of lycoperoside H (**3**) on the SC ceramide contents in RHEK models is shown in Figure 3B. Lycoperoside H (**3**) increased the total ceramide contents dose-dependently, and a significant difference was observed at 10 μM. In addition, lycoperoside H (**3**) significantly increased the ceramide (NP) contents at 1 and 10 μM with dose dependency. As for the ceramide (NS, NDS), (EOS), (EOH), (AS), and (AP), lycoperoside H (**3**) tended to increase their contents.

2.4. Effects of Lycoperoside H (3) on the mRNA Expression of Enzymes Related to Ceramide Synthesis in RHEK Models

Lycoperoside H (**3**) significantly increased the SC ceramide contents in RHEK models, as described above. Therefore, we evaluated the effects of lycoperoside H (**3**) on the expression of enzymes involved in SC ceramide synthesis. Figure 4 shows the effects of lycoperoside H (**3**) on the mRNA expression of enzymes related to SC ceramide synthesis, SPT2, CerS3, GCS, β-glucocerebrosidase (GBA), sphingomyelin synthase-2 (SMS2), and acid sphingomyelinase (ASM) in RHEK models. Lycoperoside H (**3**) significantly upregulated the mRNA expression of CerS3, GCS, and GBA at 1, 3, and 10 μM, 3 and 10 μM, and 10 μM, respectively. On the other hand, the mRNA expression of SPT2 and SMS2 were significantly downregulated by the treatment of lycoperoside H (**3**) at 1, 3, and 10 μM. No significant change was observed in the mRNA expression of ASM.

2.5. Anti-Inflammatory and Anti-Allergic Effects of Lycoperoside H (3)

The anti-inflammatory and anti-allergic effects of lycoperoside H (**3**) were evaluated to clarify the mechanism that contributes to the suppression of skin barrier deterioration, other than ceramide production enhancement. TSE and lycoperoside H (**3**) did not affect the compound 48/80-induced and histamine-induced scratching behavior in mice (Figure 5A). On the other hand, significant suppression of the IgE-mediated passive cutaneous anaphylaxis (PCA) reaction in mice was observed with a high dose of TSE administration, but not with lycoperoside H (**3**) (Figure 5B). Figure 5C shows the effects of TSE, lycoperoside H (**3**), and tigogenin 3-O-β-solatrioside (**7**) on the acetic acid-induced writhing (upper) and vascular permeability (lower) in mice. TSE and lycoperoside H (**3**) significantly suppressed writhing and vascular permeability, while tigogenin 3-O-β-solatrioside (**7**) did not show any effects. As a result of the glucocorticoid receptor competitive assay, lycoperoside H (**3**) exhibited partial glucocorticoid receptor binding ability (Figure 5D). Figure 5E shows the effects of TSE and lycoperoside H (**3**) on histamine-induced guinea pig tracheal muscle contraction. TSE and lycoperoside H (**3**) did not show an antihistaminic effect in tracheal muscle contraction.

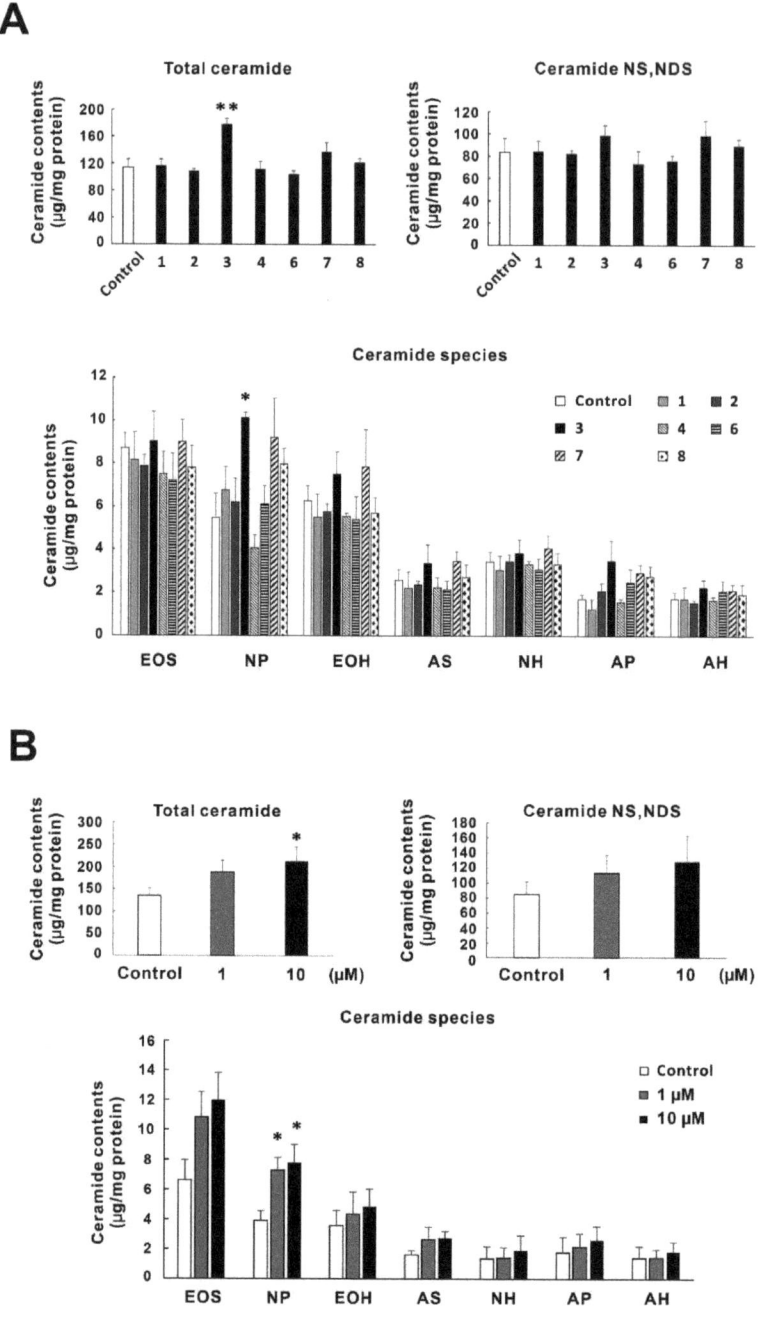

Figure 3. Effects of TSE and tomato seed saponins (**1–4,6–8**) on TEWL in RHEK models. RHEK models were treated for 5 days in culture with 10 μM of tomato seed saponins (**A**) or 1 and 10 μM of lycoperoside H (**B**). The extraction of lipids from the SC of the RHEK model and high-performance thin-layer chromatography (HPTLC) analysis were performed as described in the Materials and Methods section. Data are expressed as mean ± SE ($n = 4$). * $p < 0.05$, ** $p < 0.01$ vs. control.

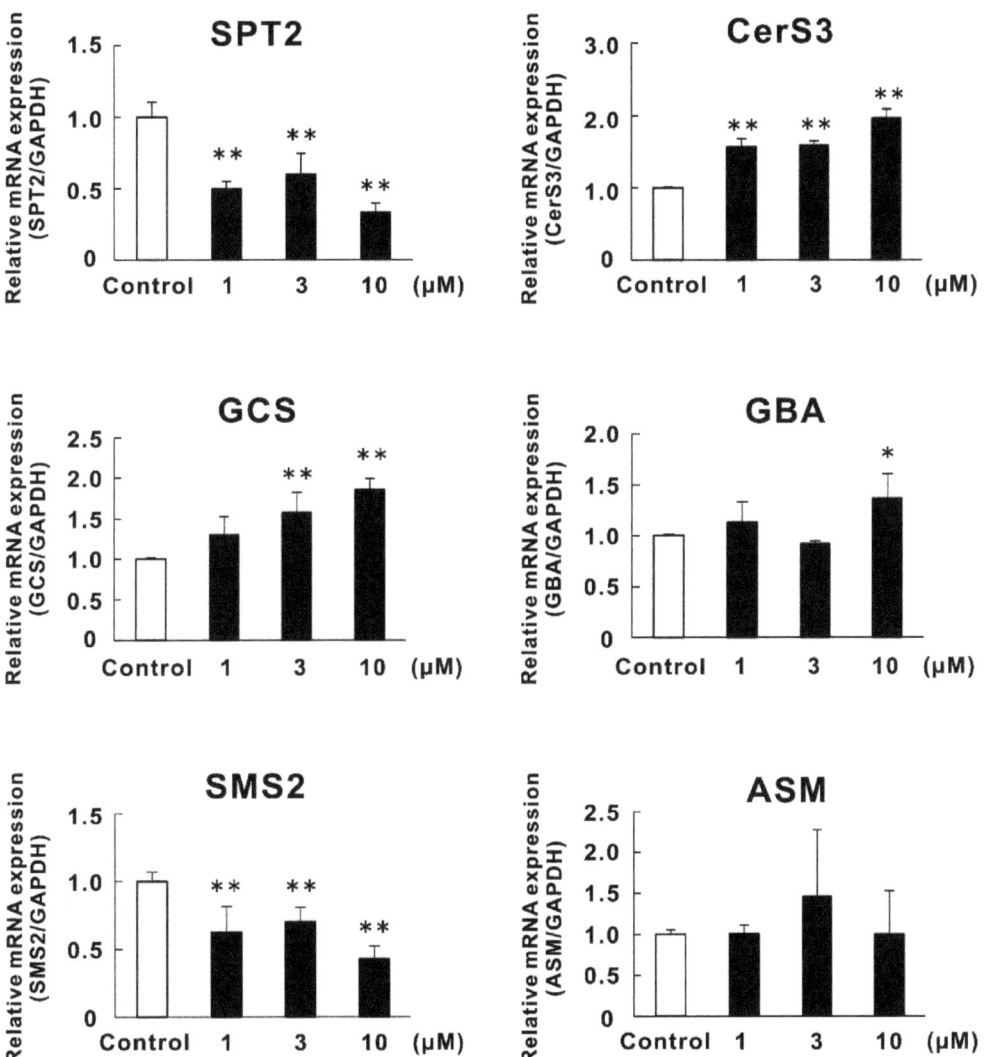

Figure 4. Effects of lycoperoside H (**3**) on the mRNA expression of enzymes related to SC ceramide synthesis. RHEK models were treated for 4 days in culture with 1, 3, and 10 µM of lycoperoside H (**3**). Extraction of total RNA and real-time RT-PCR analysis was performed as described in the Materials and Methods section. Data are expressed as mean ± SE (n = 3). * $p < 0.05$, ** $p < 0.01$ vs. control.

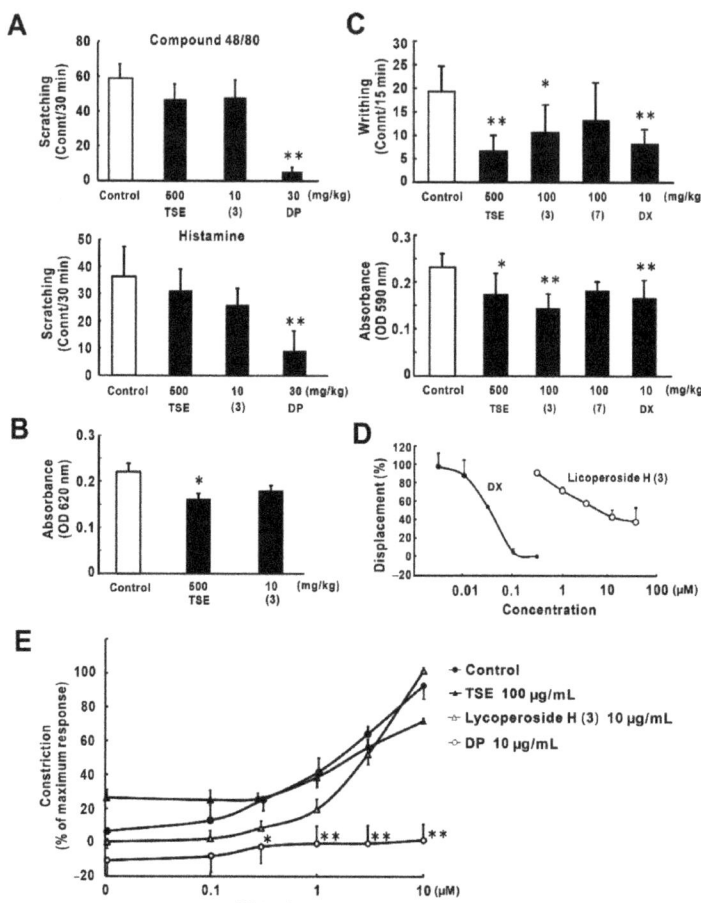

Figure 5. Anti-inflammatory and anti-allergic effects of lycoperoside H (3) and its relations to glucocorticoid and histamine. (**A**) Effect on compound 48/80- and histamine-induced scratching behaviors in mice (n = 5–7). Pruritus was induced by the subcutaneous administration of compound 48/80 or histamine dihydrochloride. Diphenhydramide hydrochloride (DP) was used as a positive control. (**B**) Effect on the PCA reaction in mice (n = 10–14). Both the right and left mouse auricles were sensitized by anti-2,4-dinitrophenyl (DNP). After test sample administration, intravenous administration of 2,4-dinitrophenylated bovine serum albumin (DNP-BSA) and Evans blue was performed, and the pigment that leaked into the auricles was measured. (**C**) Effect on acetic acid-induced writhing behavior and vascular permeability in mice (n = 5–7). Two percent pontamine sky blue was intravenously administered to mice after test sample administration. One percent acetic acid was injected intraperitoneally and writhing behavior and leaked pigment into the peritoneal cavity were measured. Dexamethasone (DX) was used as a positive control. (**D**) Glucocorticoid receptor binding ability (n = 4). Glucocorticoid receptor competitive assay was performed using a PolarScreen™ Glucocorticoid Receptor Competitor Assay Kit, Red. (**E**) Effect on histamine-induced guinea pig tracheal muscle contraction (n = 3–4). An excised tracheal strip was fixed to a Magnus apparatus. Changes in contraction induced by histamine were assessed after test sample addition. DP was used as a positive control. All data are expressed as mean ± SE, * $p < 0.05$, ** $p < 0.01$ vs. control.

3. Discussion

In previous studies on tomato saponins, steroidal saponins, such as lycoperosides (**1–3**), had been isolated from whole fruits [2,19–21]. Furthermore, flavonoids including naringenin (**5**), astragalin (**9**), and rutin (**10**) had been reported to exist in the fruits [22]. On the other hand, as for the constituent study of tomato seeds, these compounds had not been isolated, while hydrophobic compounds, such as β-sitosterol, stigmasterol, and γ-tocopherol, have been found [23]. In the present study, we isolated 7 saponins and 4 flavonoids from tomato seeds. Thus, our findings may be the first report that tomato seeds contain steroidal saponins and flavonoids as secondary metabolites.

Aiming to find the candidate compounds for skin hydration, the effects of 11 isolated compounds on the mRNA expression of proteins related to epidermal hydration, filaggrin, involucrin, SPT2, CerS3, and GCS were evaluated. Filaggrin provides natural moisturizing amino acids by its self-decomposition in SC [24] and acts as a filament-aggregating protein [25]. Involucrin is one of the essential proteins for the formation of the cornified envelope which contributes to the barrier function of the skin [26,27]. SPT2, CerS3, and GCS are involved in the synthesis of SC ceramides, which exist as dominant lipids in the SC of human skin and play important roles in the moisturization and barrier function [28]. SPT and CerS are involved in the de novo synthesis of ceramides [29,30] and GCS acts as a glucosyltransferase enzyme to synthesize glucosylceramides, which are precursors of SC ceramides [31]. In the present study, tomato seed saponins (**1–4,6–8**), especially lycoperoside C (**2**), significantly upregulated the mRNA expression of these enzymes in HaCaT cells. On the other hand, tomato seed flavonoids (**5,9–11**) exhibited a trend to downregulate the expression of enzymes for ceramide synthesis. These results suggest that tomato seed saponins appeared to be leading candidates that contribute to epidermal hydration. Regarding previous reports of saponins on skin health, Oh et al. reported that ginsenoside Rc isolated from *Panax ginseng* protects the epidermis from UVB-induced photooxidative damage with the upregulation of filaggrin expression in HaCaT cells [15]. Likewise, madecassoside, an ursane-type saponin from *C. asiatica*, has been reported to increase the mRNA and protein expressions of involucrin in HaCaT cells [17]. These findings may support our present findings of the hydrating effects of tomato seed saponins observed in HaCaT cells. In terms of the flavonols (**9–11**), we have demonstrated that tiliroside, a flavonol glycoside isolated from strawberry seeds, upregulated the expression of GCS and increased SC ceramide [32]. Regarding this finding, which is contrary to the present result, the presence of coumaroyl moiety in the structure of tiliroside is suggested to be involved in these effects. Li et al. demonstrated that tiliroside exhibits much greater antioxidant and cytoprotective activities compared to astragalin (**9**), which has the same structure, other than the coumaroyl moiety [33]. Thus, it is considered that the difference between tomato seed flavonoids and tiliroside in the effect on GCS expression is also due to the presence or absence of the coumaroyl moiety.

TEWL is the most frequently used parameter for the evaluation of the epidermal barrier function [34]. Significant elevation of TEWL is commonly observed in dry skin diseases such as AD [35], xerosis, and psoriasis [36]. To measure TEWL in vitro and in vivo, several TEWL devices have been developed. Recently, Tewitro TW24, a device which can directly and simultaneously measure the TEWL of RHEK models on a 24-well plate, has been developed [37,38]. However, there are no reports that evaluated the effect of natural compounds on TEWL using this device. Thus, we used this device to assess the effects of tomato seed saponins on changes in TEWL in RHEK models in this study. As a result of the measurements, all tomato seed saponins (**1–3,6–8**) except **4** significantly decreased TEWL during the 7 days of treatment. Considering the difference in the effect between **4** and the other saponins, it is suggested that the difference in aglycon structure might be involved. Allopregnenolone 3-*O*-β-solatrioside (**4**) has a pregnane steroid structure which consists of only steroidal A- to D-rings. On the other hand, saponins (**1–3,6–8**) which affected the TEWL have a furostanol, a spirosolanol, or a spirostanol steroid structure which consist of not only steroidal A- to D-rings but also an E-ring or E- to F-rings [39]. Similarly, it has been reported that topical application of gracillin, a spirostanol-type steroidal saponin isolated from *Dioscorea quinqueloba*, prevented TEWL elevation on 2,4-dinitrochlorobenzen-induced AD-like skin in mice [16]. Gracillin also has steroidal A- to F-rings. Therefore, it is suggested that the TEWL-lowering effect of saponins requires at least an E-ring in the structure.

Ceramides are a family of sphingolipids consisting of a sphingoid base and a fatty acid. Ceramides dominantly exist in the SC and play pivotal roles as a water reservoir and a barrier [28]. In the profiling study of ceramide species, 12 major classes of ceramides have been found in the human SC [40]. SC ceramide significantly decreased in patients with AD [41] or xerosis [42], and decreasing ceramide correlates to epidermal water evaporation [43]. Among the tomato seed saponins, only lycoperoside H (**3**) significantly increased the total SC ceramide contents in the RHEK models in concert with a significant increase of ceramide (NP). Lycoperoside H (**3**) is the most abundant saponin in TSE, and its concentration-dependent effect (1 and 10 μM) was observed in ceramide production. Our previous studies demonstrated that tiliroside isolated from strawberry seeds increases the ceramide (NS, NDS) contents [32], and β-sitosterol 3-*O*-glucoside isolated from rice bran increased ceramide (EOS) [44]. On the other hand, the present study demonstrated that lycoperoside H (**3**) increased ceramide (NP), which was not observed in tiliroside and β-sitosterol 3-*O*-glucoside. Therefore, the mechanism of increasing SC ceramide may be different to tiliroside and β-sitosterol 3-*O*-glucoside.

Since a positive effect of lycoperoside H (**3**) on the SC ceramide contents was observed, we evaluated the effects of lycoperoside H (**3**) on the mRNA expression of enzymes related to SC ceramide synthesis in the RHEK models. In addition to SPT2, CerS3, and GCS, as mentioned above, GBA, SMS2, and ASM are involved in SC ceramide synthesis. GBA hydrolyzes glucosylceramide, which is synthesized by GCS to SC ceramide [45]. SMS catalyzes the synthesis of sphingomyelin [46] and ASM synthesizes the SC ceramide from sphingomyelin [47]. Lycoperoside H (**3**) significantly upregulated the mRNA expression of CerS3, GCS, and GBA. On the other hand, significant downregulation of the mRNA expression of SPT2 and SMS2 was also observed. The ceramide synthesis pathway in the epidermis was regulated by two distinct streams, which involve glucosylceramide or sphingomyelin as intermediate products, and a major part of SC ceramide species are synthesized from glucosylceramides [31]. Thus, it is considered that the upregulation of GCS and GBA by lycoperoisde H (**3**) mainly led to an increase in SC ceramide. However, the effect of downregulation of SPT2, which is the most upstream enzyme of the pathway, remains unclear in this study. Taken together, these results suggest that lycoperoside H (**3**) is a promising compound to increase the level of SC ceramide by the upregulation of CerS3, GCS, and GBA expression, in turn leading to TEWL improvement.

Although lycoperoside H (**3**) significantly increased the SC ceramide contents, we thought that only the decrease in TEWL was not sufficient to ameliorate severe AD inflammation, as previously reported [9,11]. Therapy with steroidal medicines improves TEWL due to anti-inflammatory and anti-allergic effects [48,49]. Therefore, we evaluated whether lycoperoside H (**3**) has anti-inflammation and/or anti-allergic effects. As a result, lycoperoside H (**3**) did not exhibit suppressive effects on compound 48/80-induced pruritus and IgE-mediated PCA reaction in mice. From these results, lycoperoside H (**3**) is not considered to be effective against type-I allergy involving histamine as a mediator. Actually, lycoperoside H (**3**) did not affect histamine-induced scratching behavior in mice and histamine-induced guinea pig tracheal muscle contraction. These results suggest that lycoperoside H (**3**) is not an antihistaminic agent. On the other hand, lycoperoside H (**3**) significantly suppressed acetic acid-induced writhing behavior and vascular permeability in mice, while tigogenin 3-*O*-β-solatrioside (**7**) did not exhibit any effect. Similarly, escins, the oleanane-type saponins isolated from the seeds of *Aesculus hippocastanum* L., have been reported to show a suppressive effect on acetic acid-induced vascular permeability in mice [50]. Shehu et al. also reported that the saponin-rich fraction of *Laggera aurita* suppressed the acetic acid-induced writhing [51]. Thus, the mechanism of lycoperoside

H (**3**) in this experiment is considered similar to that of these saponins. Finally, as a result of the glucocorticoid receptor competitive assay, the partial glucocorticoid receptor binding ability of lycoperoside H (**3**) was observed. A previous report demonstrated that ginsenoside Rg1, a steroidal saponin derived from *Panax ginseng*, was shown to fully bind to the human glucocorticoid receptor in the glucocorticoid receptor competitive assay, and docking simulation revealed that the ginsenoside molecule marginally fits into the hydrophobic cavity around the ligand-binding domain of the glucocorticoid receptor, in spite of the sugar moiety causing steric bumps [52]. Ginsenoside Rg1 has steroidal A- to D-rings with 2 sugar moieties which bind to A- and B-rings, respectively. Similarly, lycoperoside H also has steroidal A- to D-rings with 4 sugars which bind to the A-ring. Thus, it is reasonable to understand that both compounds could exhibit steroidal activity through the glucocorticoid receptor, and lycoperoside H has less and partial ability to bind to the glucocorticoid receptor because of disrupted binding by 4 sugars on the A-ring. In the other study, the glucocorticoid receptor binding assay using FTO2B rat hepatoma cells demonstrated that ginsenoside Rg1 binds to the glucocorticoid receptor with 1/10 to 1/100 ability of Dx [53]. Therefore, these findings suggest that lycoperoside H (**3**) is a partial agonist of the glucocorticoid receptor and acts as a natural steroidal agent to exhibit anti-inflammatory effects. Taken together, it is suggested that lycoperoside H (**3**) improved TEWL by acting as a partial glucocorticoid receptor agonist with suppression of the acute inflammatory effect. This activity is also considered to be the mechanism of our previous results, which demonstrated that oral administration of lycoperoside H suppressed AD-like skin inflammation in IL-33 transgenic mice [10].

In conclusion, we identified 11 compounds from tomato seeds, and among them, lycoperoside H (**3**) has the potential to improve TEWL by the SC ceramide increasing effect, in concert with significantly increased ceramide (NP) contents and by anti-inflammatory effects via acting as a partial glucocorticoid receptor agonist. Therefore, lycoperoside H (**3**) is a promising skin hydrating and anti-inflammatory compound that can be expected to have excellent effects on epidermal hydration.

4. Materials and Methods

4.1. Preparation of Tomato Seed Extract and Its Compounds

To isolate lycoperoside A (**1**), lycoperoside C (**2**), lycoperoside H (**3**), allopregnanolone 3-O-β-solatrioside (**4**), and naringenin (**5**), tomato seeds (2 kg) obtained from JiuQuan Jiuzhou Seed Co., Ltd. (Gansu, China) were defatted with hexane. The defatted seeds were ground and MeOH (10 L) was used for extraction at 70 °C for 3 h, and then the solvent was evaporated to yield the tomato seed extract (TSE, 44 g, yield 2.2%). The TSE was suspended in water (500 mL) and extraction was performed with EtOAc (500 mL, twice) and *n*-BuOH (500 mL, twice). These solvents were evaporated to obtain the EtOAc layer (0.63 g, yield 0.03%), *n*-BuOH layer (2.41 g, yield 0.12%), and H$_2$O layer (5.05 g, yield 0.26%). The *n*-BuOH layer underwent silica-gel column chromatography [CHCl$_3$:MeOH (9:1→7:3)→CHCl$_3$:MeOH:water (6:4:1)→MeOH] to obtain fraction (Fr.) 1 (183.4 mg), Fr.2 (623.5 mg), Fr.3 (1.12 g), and Fr.4 (246.4 mg). Fr.3 was purified by reversed-phase HPLC (Inertsil Ph-3, 20 φ × 250 mm; GL Science Inc., Tokyo, Japan) with 70% MeOH to obtain lycoperoside A (**1**, 9.4 mg, yield 0.0005%), lycoperoside C (**2**, 1.9 mg, yield 0.00001%), lycoperoside H (**3**, 12.2 mg, yield 0.0006%), and allopregnenolone 3-O-β-solatrioside (**4**, 11.2 mg, yield 0.0006%). The EtOAc layer was purified by reversed-phase HPLC (Inertsil ODS-SP, 20 φ × 250 mm; GL Science Inc. Tokyo, Japan) with 80% MeOH to obtain naringenin (**5**, 3.3 mg, yield 0.0002%).

To isolate tomatoside A (**6**), tigogenin 3-O-β-solatrioside (**7**), 22α-methoxytomatoside A (**8**), astragalin (**9**), rutin (**10**), and quercetin 3-O-β-cellobioside (**11**), the H$_2$O layer (60.0 g) after EtOAc extraction underwent Diaion® HP-20 column chromatography (water→MeOH) to obtain the MeOH-eluted Fr. (22.94 g, yield 2.15%) and the water-eluted Fr. (33.18 g, yield 3.11%). The MeOH-eluted Fr. was fractionated by ODS column chromatography (40% MeOH→60% MeOH→90% MeOH→MeOH) to obtain Fr.1 (1.47 g), Fr.2 (0.82 g),

Fr.3 (1.59 g), Fr.4 (0.77 g), Fr.5 (10.37 g), Fr.6 (5.49 g), Fr.7 (2.06 g), and Fr.8 (0.84 g). Fr. 8 was purified by reversed-phase HPLC (Cosmosil $5C_{18}$-MS-II, 20 φ × 250 mm; Nacalai Tesque Inc., Kyoto, Japan) with 90% MeOH–1% acetic acid to obtain tomatoside A (**6**, 12.0 mg, yield 0.0034%) and tigogenin 3-O-β-solatrioside (**7**, 19.5 mg, yield 0.0055%). Fr. 5 was purified by reversed-phase HPLC (Cosmosil $5C_{18}$-MS-II, 20 φ × 250 mm) with 50% MeOH–1% acetic acid to obtain 22α-methoxytomatoside A (**7**, 289.9 mg, yield 0.939%). Fr. 3 was purified by reversed-phase HPLC (Cosmosil $5C_{18}$-MS-II, 20 φ × 250 mm) with 50% MeOH–1% acetic acid to obtain astragalin (**9**, 31.0 mg, 0.0247%), rutin (**10**, 10.0 mg, 0.0080%), and quercetin 3-O-β-cellobioside (**11**, 14.6 mg, 0.0112%). The chemical structures of the isolated compounds were identified by a comparison of the ^{1}H- and ^{13}C- NMR spectra with References [2,19,20,54–60]. The chemical structures of the isolated compounds (**1–11**) are shown in Figure 1.

4.2. Reagents

Dulbecco's modified Eagle medium (DMEM), 0.25 w/v% trypsin 1 mmol/L/EDTA 4Na solution with phenol red (trypsin/EDTA aqueous solution), phosphate-buffered saline (PBS), skim milk, DP, DX, histamine dihydrochloride, gum Arabic, Evans blue, and pontamine sky blue were obtained from FUJIFILM Wako Pure Chemical Co. Ltd. (Osaka, Japan). The RNeasy® Mini Kit was purchased from QIAGEN (Hilden, Germany). PrimeScript™ Reverse Transcriptase and TB Green® Premix Dimer Eraser™ were purchased from Takara Bio Inc. (Kusatsu, Japan). The dNTP mixture, random primer, and PolarScreen™ Glucocorticoid Receptor Competitor Assay Kit, Red, were purchased from Invitrogen (Waltham, MA, USA). HPTLC plate and DNP-BSA were purchased from Merck Millipore (Darmstadt, Germany). Fetal bovine serum (FBS) was purchased from Biosera (Boussens, France). The ceramide standards of ceramide (NS, NDS) and (AS) were purchased from Matreya LLC. (Philadelphia, PA, USA). Anti-DNP IgE was obtained from Seikagaku Industry (Tokyo, Japan).

4.3. Cells and Animals

Immortalized human keratinocytes, HaCaT cells, were kindly supplied by Kindai University (Osaka, Japan). RHEK models (LabCyte EPI-MODEL) obtained from Japan Tissue Engineering Co., Ltd. (Gamagori, Japan) were used for the measurement of TEWL, quantification of ceramide, and enzymes related to ceramide synthesis expression. LabCyte EPI-MODEL was used for the measurement of TEWL, and LabCyte EPI-MODEL 6D, which was cultured under pre-keratinization conditions before the formation of the SC layer, was used for the other experiments.

Different animal sources were selected according to the experimental method. Male ddY mice aged 5 and 8 weeks old and male Hartley guinea pigs aged 5 weeks old were purchased from Japan SLC Inc. (Hamamatsu, Japan). The mice and guinea pigs were acclimated for 7 days under 22 ± 2 °C and 50% ± 5% RH before the experiments and were fed a standard CE-2 non-purified diet (Clea Japan Inc., Shizuoka, Japan) and LRC4 (Oriental Yeast Co. Ltd., Tokyo, Japan), respectively. The animal experiments were performed in accordance with the Guidelines for Animal Experimentation (Japan Association for Laboratory Animal Science, 1987). All the animal experiments were approved by the ethics committee of Oryza Oil and Fat Chemical Co., Ltd. (Aichi, Japan).

4.4. Culture of HaCaT Cells for the Screening of Candidate Compounds with Hydration Activity

HaCaT cells (1.0 × 10^5 cells/well) were seeded onto a 24-well culture plate and maintained in DMEM with 10% FBS at 37 °C, 5% CO_2 atmosphere. After incubation for 1 night, the medium was changed to DMEM without FBS and incubated for 24 h, and the cells were treated with TSE (10 μg/mL) or isolated compounds (10 μM) which were dissolved in dimethyl sulfoxide (DMSO) for 6 h. The final concentration of DMSO was adjusted to 0.1%. The total RNA was extracted using a RNeasy® Mini Kit and automated

RNA purification system (QIAcube; QIAGEN, Hilden, Germany), which includes the procedure of RNase inhibition and DNase treatment.

4.5. Culture of the RHEK Models for the Evaluation of Hydration Factors

Each cup of the RHEK models was placed onto a 24-well culture plate and assay medium was added under the cup. After incubating the plate at 37 °C, 5% CO_2 atmosphere for 1 day, the RHEK models were treated with a solution of TSE or isolated compounds (final DMSO concentration: 0.1%). Depending on each experiment, the culture time was selected. Namely, RHEK models were cultured for 7 days for TEWL measurement, for 4 days for real-time RT-PCR, and for 5 days for ceramide analysis. The medium containing the test samples was replaced every day.

4.6. Measurement of TEWL in RHEK Models

TEWL measurement was performed before treatment and at 1, 3, 5, and 7 days after treatment by Tewitro TW24 (Courage+Khazaka, Cologne, Germany), which can simultaneously measure TEWL in 24-well RHEK models [36,37]. The RHEK model was placed on a thermal insulation mat (HIENAI Mat; Cosmo Bio Co., Ltd., Tokyo, Japan) which keeps the entire bottom surface at 32 °C without a lid for 5 min before measurement. TEWL was measured for 30 min maintaining the bottom surface at 32 °C, and the mean value for the last 10 min was used for the analysis. The measurements were performed under sterile conditions.

4.7. Real-Time RT-PCR

The mRNA expression of enzymes related to ceramide synthesis in HaCaT cells and RHEK models were measured by quantitative real-time RT-PCR. After the extraction, 0.1 µg of total RNA was reverse transcribed using PrimeScript™ Reverse Transcriptase to obtain cDNA. Real-time RT-PCR reaction was conducted using TB Green® Premix Dimer Eraser™ and Thermal Cycler Dice® Real-Time System Single (TM 800, Takara Bio Inc.). The specific primers were used as follows: SPT2, 5′-AGCCGCCAAAGTCCTTGAG-3′ as forward and 5′-CTTGTCCAGGTTTCCAATTTCC-3′ as reverse; CerS3, 5′-CCAGGCTGAAGAAATTCCAG-3′ as forward and 5′-AACGCAATTCCAGCAACAGT-3′ as reverse; GCS, 5′-ATGTGTCATT-GCCTGGCATG-3′ as forward and 5′-CCAGGCGACTGCATAATCAAG-3′ as reverse; GBA, 5′-TGGCATTGCTGTACATTGG-3′ as forward and 5′-CGTTCTTCTGACTGGCAACC-3′ as reverse; SMS2, 5′-AAGTGTATAACATCAGCTGTGAA-3′ as forward and 5′-CAGTACCAG-TTGTGCTAGACTAC-3′ as reverse; ASM, 5′-TGGCTCTATGAAGCGATGG-3′ as forward and 5′-AGGCCGATGTAGGTAGTTGC-3′ as reverse; β-actin, 5′-CATGTACGTTGCTATCC-AGGC-3′ as forward and 5′-CTCCTTAATGTCACGCACGAT-3′ as reverse; GAPDH, 5′-AAGGTGAAGGTCGGAGTCAAC-3′ as forward and 5′-GGGGTCATTGATGGCAACAATA-3′ as reverse. The mRNA expression level of each enzyme was determined by the 2-ΔΔCt method and corrected by the expression level of β-actin or GAPDH.

4.8. Lipid Extraction and Ceramide Determination

The whole tissue of the RHEK models was carefully peeled from the membrane. The separation of SC was initially carried out by incubation (37 °C, 5% CO_2 atmosphere) of the tissue in trypsin (2.5 mg/mL)/EDTA (0.25 mg/mL) aqueous solution (1 mL) for 15 min. Then, 10% FBS diluted in PBS (1 mL) was added to stop the trypsin activity and SC separation was carried out under a microscope. The separated SC samples were washed with PBS and stored at −80 °C until the determination of ceramides. The extraction method described in previous studies [32,44] was used for lipid extraction. Namely, the SC samples were homogenized with an ultrasonic homogenizer (AGC Techno Glass Co., Ltd. Shizuoka, Japan) in a 4 mL mixture of chloroform, methanol, and PBS (1:2:0.8). The mixture was centrifuged (3000 rpm, 15 min) at room temperature and the supernatants were collected in test tubes. Chloroform (1 mL) and PBS (1 mL) were added to each supernatant and mixed using a shaker for 20 min. After mixing, the mixture was centrifuged (3000 rpm, 15 min) and the bottom layer was collected using a 1 mL glass syringe with a 22G needle. The collected bottom layer was dried at 30 °C by N_2 gas blowing. The remaining precipitates were used for the quantification of total protein contents to correct the ceramide contents. The precipitates obtained after lipid extraction were dissolved in a mixture (300 µL) of 10% sodium lauryl sulfate (SDS) and 1 N NaOH (1:9) at 60 °C for 2 h. Then, the mixture was neutralized with 2N HCl (30 µL) and the total protein amounts were determined by the bicinchoninic acid (BCA) method.

The ceramide contents in SC were measured by HPTLC. The quantification method as described by previous studies [32,44] was carried out for TLC analysis. The dried lipid samples were dissolved in a mixture of chloroform and methanol (2:1) and were developed on a TLC plate (10 × 10 cm). The lipid samples were developed twice. Namely, a mixture of chloroform, methanol, and acetic acid (190:9:1) was used for the first development and a mixture of chloroform, methanol, and acetic acid (197:2:1) was used for the second development. After the development, the spots were visualized by 10% copper sulfate in 8% phosphoric acid aqueous solution, followed by heating at 180 °C for 7 min. The spots for the ceramides were scanned and analyzed using an imaging system (ImageQuant LAS500; GE Health Care, CT, USA). The spot areas of ceramides were corrected by the spot areas of ceramide standard.

4.9. Compound 48/80- and Histamine-Induced Mice Pruritus (In Vivo Anti-Inflammation Models)

Male ddY mice aged 5 weeks old were fasted for 18–20 h prior to the experiment. Gum Arabic (5%) in water was administrated orally to the control group. TSE (500 mg/kg), lycoperoside H (10 mg/kg), and DP (30 mg/kg) suspended with 5% gum Arabic in water were orally administered to each group. One hour after administration of the test samples, 3% compound 48/80 solution dissolved in saline was subcutaneously administered (50 µL) to the back of the neck, and the number of scratching behaviors were counted for 30 min [61].

Male ddY mice aged 5 weeks old were fasted for 18–20 h prior to the experiment. The test samples were orally administered to each group. One hour after administration of the test samples, histamine dihydrochloride solution (2 µM) dissolved in saline (50 µL) was subcutaneously administered to the back of the neck, and the number of scratching behaviors were counted for 30 min [62].

4.10. PCA Reaction in Mice (In Vivo Anti-Allergy Model)

Anti-DNP IgE diluted with saline (×2000) was intradermaly administered (20 µL) to both the right and left auricles in male ddY mice aged 8 weeks old. One day after the sensitization, the mice were fasted for 18–20 h. Gum Arabic (5%) in water was administrated orally to the control group. TSE (500 mg/kg) and lycoperoside H (10 mg/kg) suspended with 5% gum Arabic in water were orally administered to each group. Two hours after administration of the test samples, saline containing DNP-BSA (1 mg/mL) and Evans blue (5 mg/mL) was injected (10 mL/kg) into the tail vein. The mice were sacrificed 30 min later, and the auricles were excised. The removed auricles were suspended into 1N KOH (1 mL) and incubated with slow shaking (37 °C, overnight). After incubation, 2 mL of the mixture of 2.5N phosphoric acid and acetone (3:17) was added and centrifuged (2000 rpm, 10 min) to obtain a clean supernatant. The absorbance (620 nm) of the supernatants (200 µL) was measured using a microplate reader (Sunrise RAINBOW, Tecan Group Ltd., Manne Dorf, Switzerland) [63].

4.11. Acetic Acid-Induced Writhing and Vascular Permeability in Mice (In Vivo Anti-Inflammation Model)

Male ddY mice aged 5 weeks old were fasted for 15 h. Gum Arabic (5%) in water was administrated orally to the control group. TSE (500 mg/kg), lycoperoside H (10 mg/kg), tigogenin 3-O-β-soratrioside (10 mg/kg), or DX (10 mg/kg) suspended with 5% gum Arabic in water were orally administered to each group. Two percent pontamine sky blue dissolved in saline was injected (10 mL/kg) into the tail vein 55 min after the test samples were administered orally. Five minutes later, 1% acetic acid in saline was injected (10 mL/kg) intraperitoneally and the number of writhings were counted for 15 min. The mice were sacrificed, and the abdomen was immediately opened. After washing of the peritoneal cavity with approximately 8 mL of saline, the washed solution was collected in a glass tube and 0.1 mL of 1N NaOH was added. The solution was topped-up to 10 mL with saline, and the absorbance (590 nm) was measured using a microplate reader to assess the vascular permeability [50].

4.12. Glucocorticoid Receptor Competitive Assay (In Vitro Assay for Glucocorticoid Receptor Ligand)

A PolarScreen™ Glucocorticoid Receptor Competitor Assay Kit, Red, was used according to the manufacturer's protocols. Briefly, lycoperoside H diluted with GR screening buffer to adjust the final concentrations to 0.3, 1, 3, 10, and 30 μM was added to a 96-well black plate. Similarly, DX diluted to adjust the final concentrations to 3, 10, 30, 100, and 300 nM was added. Then, 25 μL of 4× Fluormone™ GS Red solution was added and mixed by shaking on a plate shaker. After shaking, 4× glucocorticoid receptor was added and shaken on a plate shaker. The mixed solutions were incubated in the dark at room temperature for 2 h, and then the fluorescence polarization values were measured at 535 nm (excitation) and 590 nm (emission) using a fluorescence microplate reader (Infinit® 200 PRO, Tecan Group Ltd.).

4.13. Histamine-Induced Guinea Pig Tracheal Muscle Contraction (In Vitro Anti-Histaminic Model)

Male Hartley guinea pigs were anesthetized and sacrificed. The tracheal muscle was harvested and cut horizontally into 5 or 6 strips. One muscle strip was opened and fixed to a Magnus apparatus and placed in Krebs-Henselite solution (NaCl: 117 mM, KCl: 4.7 mM, $CaCl_2$: 2.5 mM, $MgSO_4$: 1.2 mM, KH_2PO_4: 1.2 mM, $NaHCO_3$: 24.8 mM, glucose: 11 mM) gently bubbled with 5% CO_2 and 95% O_2.

The organ bath was kept at 37 °C and the specimen was set under a tension of 1 g. Changes in contraction were assessed with an isotonic transducer (Powerlab, AD Instruments, Dunedin, New Zealand) and contractions were recorded (Lab chart 6, AD Instruments). After the tension became stable (30 min), histamine dihydrochloride (final concentration 10 μM) was added to the organ bath to confirm muscle contraction. After washing 5 times with Krebs-Henselite solution, the specimen was allowed to stabilize again. Then, the TSE (final concentration 100 μg/mL) and lycoperoside H (3, final concentration 10 μg/mL) diluted in DMSO were added to the bath and the response was assessed for 10 min. Histamine dihydrochloride diluted in buffer (final concentration: 0.1–10 μM) was added cumulatively and the responses were recorded. DP was used as a positive control [63].

4.14. Statistics

All the results are expressed as means ± standard error (SE). The significance of the differences was examined by one-way analysis of variance (ANOVA) followed by Dunnett's test. Bartlett's test was performed before Dunnett's test to confirm that all data were parametric. Values of $p < 0.05$ or $p < 0.01$ were considered significant.

Author Contributions: Conceptualization, S.T.; Data curation, S.T., K.M., S.S., Y.M., T.M. and H.S.; Formal analysis, S.T., K.M., S.S. and Y.M.; Funding acquisition, S.T. and H.S.; Investigation, S.T., T.M. and H.S.; Resources, S.T.; Methodology, S.T. and H.S.; Project administration, H.S.; Supervision, T.M. and H.S.; Visualization, S.T. and H.S.; Writing—original draft, S.T. and H.S.; Writing—review and editing, T.M. and H.S. All authors have read and agreed to the published version of the manuscript.

Funding: This work was supported by the New Aichi Creative Research and Development Subsidy (grant numbers: 118–20, 2019) and Oryza Oil and Fat Chemical Co., Ltd.

Institutional Review Board Statement: All animal experiments were approved by the ethics committee of Oryza Oil and Fat Chemical Co., Ltd.

Informed Consent Statement: Not applicable.

Data Availability Statement: The data that support the findings of this study are available from the corresponding author upon reasonable request.

Conflicts of Interest: The authors declare no conflict of interest. The funders had no role in the design of the study; in the collection, analyses, or interpretation of data; in the writing of the manuscript or in the decision to publish the results.

Sample Availability: Samples of the compounds are available from the authors.

Abbreviations

The following abbreviations are used in this manuscript.

TSE	tomato seed extract
TEWL	transepidermal water loss
AD	atopic dermatitis
DP	diphenhydramine hydrochloride
C	Centella
DMEM	Dulbecco's modified Eagle medium
PBS	phosphate-buffered saline
DX	dexamethasone
HPTLC	high-performance thin-layer chromatography
DNP-BSA	2,4-dinitrophenylated bovine serum albumin
FBS	fetal bovine serum
RHEK	reconstructed human epidermal keratinization
SC	stratum corneum
DMSO	dimethyl sulfoxide
SDS	sodium lauryl sulfate
BCA	bicinchoninic acid
PCA	passive cutaneous anaphylaxis
SPT	serine palmitoyltransferase
CerS	ceramide synthase
GCS	glucosylceramide synthase
GBA	β-glucocerebrosidase
SMS	sphingomyelin synthase
ASM	acid sphingomyelinase

References

1. Chaudhary, P.; Sharma, A.; Singh, B.; Nagpal, A.K. Bioactivities of phytochemicals present in tomato. *J. Food Sci. Technol.* **2018**, *55*, 2833–2849. [CrossRef]
2. Yahara, S.; Uda, N.; Nohara, T. Lycoperosides A–C, three stereoisomeric 23-acetoxyspirosolan-3β-ol β-lycotetraosides from *Lycopersicon esculentum*. *Phytochemistry* **1996**, *42*, 169–172. [CrossRef]
3. Yoshizaki, M.; Matsushita, S.; Fujiwara, Y.; Ikeda, T.; Ono, M.; Nohara, T. Tomato new sapogenols, isoesculeogenin A and esculeogenin B. *Chem. Pharm. Bull.* **2005**, *53*, 839–840. [CrossRef] [PubMed]
4. Fujiwara, Y.; Takaki, A.; Uehara, Y.; Ikeda, T.; Okawa, M.; Yamauchi, K.; Ono, M.; Yoshimitsu, H.; Nohara, T. Tomato steroidal alkaloid glycosides, esculeosides A and B, from ripe fruits. *Tetrahedron* **2004**, *60*, 4915–4920. [CrossRef]
5. Fujiwara, Y.; Yahara, S.; Ikeda, T.; Ono, M.; Nohara, T. Cytotoxic major saponin from tomato fruits. *Chem. Pharm. Bull.* **2003**, *51*, 234–235. [CrossRef]
6. Nohara, T.; Fujiwara, Y.; Zhou, J.R.; Urata, J.; Ikeda, T.; Murakami, K.; El-Aasr, M.; Ono, M. Saponins, esculeosides B-1 and B-2, in tomato juice and sapogenol, esculeogenin B1. *Chem. Pharm. Bull.* **2015**, *63*, 848–850. [CrossRef]
7. Ono, M.; Takara, Y.; Egami, M.; Uranaka, K.; Yoshimitsu, H.; Matsushita, S.; Fujiwara, Y.; Ikeda, T.; Nohara, T. Steroidal alkaloid glycosides, esculeosides C and D, from the ripe fruit of cherry tomato. *Chem. Pharm. Bull.* **2006**, *54*, 237–239. [CrossRef]
8. Fujiwara, Y.; Kiyota, N.; Hori, M.; Matsushita, S.; Iijima, Y.; Aoki, K.; Shibata, D.; Takeya, M.; Ikeda, T.; Nohara, T.; et al. Esculeogenin A, a new tomato sapogenol, ameliorates hyperlipidemia and atherosclerosis in ApoE-deficient mice by inhibiting ACAT. *Arterioscler. Thromb. Vasc. Biol.* **2007**, *27*, 2400–2406. [CrossRef]
9. Zhou, J.R.; Urata, J.; Shiraishi, T.; Tanaka, C.; Nohara, T.; Yokomizo, K. Tomato juice saponin, esculeoside B ameliorates mice experimental dermatitis. *FFHD* **2018**, *8*, 228–241. [CrossRef]

10. Takeda, S.; Miyasaka, K.; Shimoda, H. Lycoperoside H, a steroidal alkaloid saponin in tomato seeds, ameliorates atopic dermatitis-like symptoms in IL-33 transgenic mice. *J. Food Biochem.* **2021**, *45*, e13877. [CrossRef]
11. Im, D.S. Pro-resolving effect of ginsenosides as an anti-inflammatory mechanism of Panax ginseng. *Biomolecules* **2020**, *10*, 444. [CrossRef]
12. Agra, L.C.; Ferro, J.N.; Barbosa, F.T.; Barreto, E. Triterpenes with healing activity: A systematic review. *J. Dermatolog. Treat.* **2015**, *26*, 465–470. [CrossRef]
13. Lee, H.J.; Cho, S.H. Therapeutic effects of Korean red ginseng extract in a murine model of atopic dermatitis: Anti-pruritic and anti-inflammatory mechanism. *J. Korean Med. Sci.* **2017**, *32*, 679–687. [CrossRef]
14. Jimbo, N.; Kawada, C.; Nomura, Y. Herb extracts and collagen hydrolysate improve skin damage resulting from ultraviolet-induced aging in hairless mice. *Biosci. Biotechnol. Biochem.* **2015**, *79*, 1624–1628. [CrossRef]
15. Oh, Y.; Lim, H.W.; Park, K.H.; Huang, Y.H.; Yoon, J.Y.; Kim, K.; Lim, C.J. Ginsenoside Rc protects against UVB-induced photooxidative damage in epidermal keratinocytes. *Mol. Med. Rep.* **2017**, *16*, 2907–2914. [CrossRef]
16. Jegal, J.; Park, N.J.; Jo, B.G.; Bong, S.K.; Jegal, H.; Yang, M.H.; Kim, S.N. Anti-atopic properties of gracillin isolated from *Dioscorea quinqueloba* on 2,4-dinitrochlorobenzene-induced skin lesions in mice. *Nutrients* **2018**, *10*, 1205. [CrossRef]
17. Shen, X.; Guo, M.; Yu, H.; Liu, D.; Lu, Z.; Lu, Y. *Propionibacterium acnes* related anti-inflammation and skin hydration activities of madecassoside, a pentacyclic triterpene saponin from *Centella asiatica*. *Biosci. Biotechnol. Biochem.* **2019**, *83*, 561–568. [CrossRef] [PubMed]
18. Ratz-Lyko, A.; Arct, J.; Pytkowska, K. Moisturizing and antiinflammatory properties of cosmetic formulations containing *Centella asiatica* extract. *Indian J. Pharm. Sci.* **2016**, *78*, 27–33. [CrossRef] [PubMed]
19. Yahara, S.; Uda, N.; Yoshio, E.; Yae, E. Steroidal alkaloid glycosides from tomato (*Lycopersicon esculentum*). *J. Nat. Prod.* **2004**, *67*, 500–502. [CrossRef]
20. Yamanaka, T.; Vincken, J.P.; de Waard, P.; Sanders, M.; Takada, N.; Gruppen, H. Isolation, characterization, and surfactant properties of the major triterpenoid glycosides from unripe tomato fruits. *J. Agric. Food Chem.* **2008**, *56*, 11432–11440. [CrossRef] [PubMed]
21. Dall'Asta, C.; Falavigna, C.; Galaverna, G.; Sforza, S.; Dossena, A.; Marchelli, R. A multiresidual method for the simultaneous determination of the main glycoalkaloids and flavonoids in fresh and processed tomato (*Solanum lycopersicum* L.) by LC-DAD-MS/MS. *J. Sep. Sci.* **2009**, *32*, 3664–3671. [CrossRef] [PubMed]
22. Slimestad, R.; Verheul, M. Review of flavonoids and other phenolics from fruits of different tomato (*Lycopersicon esculentum* Mill.) cultivars. *J. Sci. Food Agric.* **2009**, *89*, 1255–1270. [CrossRef]
23. Kaunda, J.S.; Zhang, Y.J. The genus Solanum: An ethnopharmacological, phytochemical and biological properties review. *Nat. Prod. Bioprospect.* **2019**, *9*, 77–137. [CrossRef] [PubMed]
24. McLean, W.H. Filaggrin failure-from ichthyosis vulgaris to atopic eczema and beyond. *Br. J. Dermatol.* **2016**, *175*, 4–7. [CrossRef]
25. Kezic, S.; Jakasa, I. Filaggrin and skin barrier function. *Curr. Probl. Dermatol.* **2016**, *49*, 1–7.
26. Eckert, R.L.; Yaffe, M.B.; Crish, J.F.; Murthy, S.; Rorke, E.A.; Welter, J.F. Involucrin-structure and role in envelope assembly. *J. Investig. Dermatol.* **1993**, *100*, 613–617. [CrossRef] [PubMed]
27. Nishifuji, K.; Yoon, J.S. The stratum corneum: The rampart of the mammalian body. *Vet. Dermatol.* **2013**, *24*, 60–72. [CrossRef]
28. Huang, H.C.; Chang, T.M. Ceramide 1 and ceramide 3 act synergistically on skin hydration and the transepidermal water loss of sodium lauryl sulfate-irritated skin. *Int. J. Dermatol.* **2008**, *47*, 812–819. [CrossRef]
29. Hanada, K. Serine palmitoyltransferase, a key enzyme of sphingolipid metabolism. *Biochim. Biophysi. Acta* **2003**, *1632*, 16–30. [CrossRef]
30. Levy, M.; Futerman, A.H. Mammalian ceramide synthases. *IUBMB Life* **2010**, *62*, 347–356. [CrossRef]
31. Hamanaka, S.; Hara, M.; Nishio, H.; Otsuka, F.; Suzuki, A.; Uchida, Y. Human epidermal glucosylceramides are major precursors of stratum corneum ceramides. *J. Invest. Dermatol.* **2002**, *119*, 416–423. [CrossRef]
32. Takeda, S.; Shimoda, H.; Takarada, T.; Imokawa, G. Strawberry seed extract and its major component, tiliroside, promote ceramide synthesis in the stratum corneum of human epidermal equivalents. *PLoS ONE* **2018**, *13*, e0205061. [CrossRef] [PubMed]
33. Li, X.; Tian, Y.; Wang, T.; Lin, Q.; Feng, X.; Jiang, Q.; Liu, Y.; Chen, D. Role of the p-coumaroyl moiety in the antioxidant and cytoprotective effects of flavonoid glycosides: Comparison of astragalin and tiliroside. *Molecules* **2017**, *22*, 1165. [CrossRef]
34. Fluhr, J.W.; Feingold, K.R.; Elias, P.M. Transepidermal water loss reflects permeability barrier status: Validation in human and rodent in vivo and ex vivo models. *Exp. Dermatol.* **2006**, *15*, 483–492. [CrossRef] [PubMed]
35. Seidenari, S.; Giusti, G. Objective assessment of the skin of children affected by atopic dermatitis: A study of pH, capacitance and TEWL in eczematous and clinically uninvolved skin. *Acta Derm. Venereol.* **1995**, *75*, 429–433.
36. Tezuka, T.; Fang, K.T.; Yamaura, T.; Masaki, H.; Sakon, K.; Suzuki, K. Changes of TEWL value at various skin diseases. *Ski. Res.* **1989**, *31*, 153–156.
37. Alexander, H.; Brown, S.; Danby, S.; Flohr, C. Research techniques made simple: Transepidermal water loss measurement as a research tool. *J. Investig. Dermatol.* **2018**, *138*, 2295–2300. [CrossRef] [PubMed]
38. Joly-Tonetti, N.; Ondet, T.; Monshouwer, M.; Stamatas, G.N. EGFR inhibitors switch keratinocytes from a proliferative to a differentiative phenotype affecting epidermal development and barrier function. *BMC Cancer* **2021**, *21*, 1–10. [CrossRef] [PubMed]
39. Upadhyay, S.; Jeena, G.S.; Shukla, R.K. Recent advances in steroidal saponins biosynthesis and in vitro production. *Planta* **2018**, *248*, 519–544. [CrossRef]

40. Masukawa, Y.; Narita, H.; Shimizu, E.; Kondo, N.; Sugai, Y.; Oba, T.; Homma, R.; Ishikawa, J.; Takagi, Y.; Kitahara, T.; et al. Characterization of overall ceramide species in human stratum corneum. *J. Lipid Res.* **2008**, *49*, 1466–1476. [CrossRef]
41. Imokawa, G.; Abe, A.; Jin, K.; Higaki, Y.; Kawashima, M.; Hidano, A. Decreased level of ceramides in stratum corneum of atopic dermatitis: An etiologic factor in atopic dry skin? *J. Investig. Dermatol.* **1991**, *96*, 523–526. [CrossRef] [PubMed]
42. Akimoto, K.; Yoshikawa, N.; Higaki, Y.; Kawashima, M.; Imokawa, G. Quantitative analysis of stratum corneum lipids in xerosis and asteatotic eczema. *J. Dermatol.* **1993**, *20*, 1–6. [CrossRef] [PubMed]
43. Shimotoyodome, Y.; Tsujimura, H.; Ishikawa, J.; Fujimura, T.; Kitahara, T. Variations of ceramide profile in different regions of the body of Japanese females. *J. Jpn. Cos. Sci. Soc.* **2014**, *38*, 3–8.
44. Takeda, S.; Terazawa, S.; Shimoda, H.; Imokawa, G. β-Sitosterol 3-O-D-glucoside increases ceramide levels in the stratum corneum via the up-regulated expression of ceramide synthase-3 and glucosylceramide synthase in a reconstructed human epidermal keratinization model. *PLoS ONE* **2021**, *16*, e0248150. [CrossRef] [PubMed]
45. Takagi, Y.; Kriehuber, E.; Imokawa, G.; Elias, P.M.; Holleran, W.M. β-Glucocerebrosidase activity in mammalian stratum corneum. *J. Lipid Res.* **1999**, *40*, 861–869. [CrossRef]
46. Tafesse, F.G.; Ternes, P.; Holthuis, J.C. The multigenic sphingomyelin synthase family. *J. Biol. Chem.* **2006**, *281*, 29421–29425. [CrossRef] [PubMed]
47. Jenkins, R.W.; Canals, D.; Hannun, Y.A. Roles and regulation of secretory and lysosomal acid sphingomyelinase. *Cell Signal.* **2009**, *21*, 836–846. [CrossRef]
48. James, Q.; Kimberly, C. Topical corticosteroid application and the structural and functional integrity of the epidermal barrier. *Clin. Aesthet. Dermatol.* **2013**, *6*, 20–27.
49. Yoshikawa, H.; Tasaka, K. Anti-allergic action of glucocorticoids: Comparison with immunosuppressive and anti-inflammatory effects. *Cur. Med. Chem.* **2003**, *2*, 37–50. [CrossRef]
50. Matsuda, H.; Li, Y.; Murakami, T.; Ninomiya, K.; Yamahara, J.; Yoshikawa, M. Effects of escins Ia, Ib, IIa, and IIb from horse chestnut, the seeds of *Aesculus hippocastanum* L., on acute inflammation in animals. *Biol. Pharm. Bull.* **1997**, *20*, 1092–1095. [CrossRef]
51. Shehu, A.; Olurish, T.O.; Zezi, A.U.; Ahmed, A. Saponin and flavonoid-rich fractions of *Laggera aurita* Linn. F. produce central analgesia in murine models of pain. *Niger. J. Pharm. Sci.* **2016**, *15*, 60–69.
52. Leung, K.W.; Cheng, Y.K.; Mak, N.K.; Chan, K.K.; Fan, T.P.; Wong, R.N. Signaling pathway of ginsenoside-Rg1 leading to nitric oxide production in endothelial cells. *FEBS Lett.* **2006**, *580*, 3211–3216. [CrossRef] [PubMed]
53. Lee, Y.J.; Chung, E.; Lee, K.Y.; Lee, Y.H.; Huh, B.; Lee, S.K. Ginsenoside-Rg1, one of the major active molecules from *Panax ginseng*, is a functional ligand of glucocorticoid receptor. *Mol. Cell. Endocrinol.* **1997**, *133*, 135–140. [CrossRef]
54. Yokosuka, A.; Mimaki, Y. Steroidal saponins from the whole plants of *Agave utahensis* and their cytotoxic activity. *Phytochemistry* **2009**, *70*, 807–815. [CrossRef] [PubMed]
55. Lee, Y.Y.; Hashimoto, F.; Yahara, S.; Nohara, T.; Yoshida, N. Steroidal glycosides from *Solanum dulcamara*. *Chem. Pharm. Bull.* **1994**, *42*, 707–709. [CrossRef]
56. Matsuo, Y.; Shinoda, D.; Nakamaru, A.; Kamohara, K.; Sakagami, H.; Mimaki, Y. Steroidal glycosides from *Convallaria majalis* whole plants and their cytotoxic activity. *Int. J. Mol. Sci.* **2017**, *18*, 2358. [CrossRef]
57. Tsvetkov, D.; Dmitrenok, A.; Tsvetkov, Y.; Chizhov, A.; Nifantiev, N. Polyphenol components of the knotwood extracts of *Salix caprea* L. *Russ. Chem. Bull.* **2020**, *69*, 2390–2395. [CrossRef]
58. Wei, Y.; Xie, Q.; Fisher, D.; Sutherland, I.A. Separation of patuletin-3-O-glucoside, astragalin, quercetin, kaempferol and isorhamnetin from *Flaveria bidentis* (L.) Kuntze by elution-pump-out high-performance counter-current chromatography. *J. Chromatogr. A* **2011**, *1218*, 6206–6211. [CrossRef]
59. Nohara, T.; Ito, Y.; Seike, H.; Komori, T.; Moriyama, M.; Gomita, Y.; Kawasaki, T. Study on the constituents of *Paris quadriforia* L. *Chem. Pharm. Bull.* **1982**, *30*, 1851–1856. [CrossRef]
60. Biruk, S.; Kaleab, A.; Raghavendra, Y. Radical scavenging activities of the leaf extracts and a flavonoid glycoside isolated from *Cineraria abyssinica* Sch. Bip. Exa. Rich. *J. Appl. Pharm. Sci.* **2012**, *2*, 44–49.
61. Kobayashi, Y.; Nakano, Y.; Inayama, K.; Sakai, A.; Kamiya, T. Dietary intake of the flower extracts of German chamomile (*Matricaria recutita* L.) inhibited compound 48/80-induced itch-scratch responses in mice. *Phytomedicine* **2003**, *10*, 657–664. [CrossRef]
62. Lee, H.K.; Park, S.B.; Chang, S.Y.; Jung, S.J. Antipruritic effect of curcumin on histamine-induced itching in mice. *Korean J. Physiol. Pharmacol.* **2018**, *22*, 547–554. [CrossRef] [PubMed]
63. Shimoda, H.; Tanaka, J.; Yamada, E.; Morikawa, T.; Kasajima, N.; Yoshikawa, M. Anti type I allergic property of Japanese butterbur extract and its mast cell degranulation inhibitory ingredients. *J. Agric. Food. Chem.* **2006**, *54*, 2915–2920. [CrossRef] [PubMed]

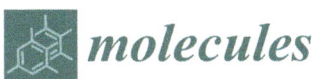

Article

Consumption of Sinlek Rice Drink Improved Red Cell Indices in Anemic Elderly Subjects

Peerasak Lerttrakarnnon [1], Winthana Kusirisin [1], Pimpisid Koonyosying [2], Ben Flemming [2,3], Niramon Utama-ang [4,5], Suthat Fucharoen [6] and Somdet Srichairatanakool [2,*]

1. Department of Family Medicine, Faculty of Medicine, Chiang Mai University, Chiang Mai 50200, Thailand; peerasak.lerttrakarn@cmu.ac.th (P.L.); wkusiris@gmail.com (W.K.)
2. Oxidative Stress Cluster, Department of Biochemistry, Faculty of Medicine, Chiang Mai University, Chiang Mai 50200, Thailand; pimpisid_m@hotmail.com (P.K.); benf9900@gmail.com (B.F.)
3. Department of Earth and Environment, Faculty of Science and Engineering, School of Natural Sciences, University of Manchester, Manchester M13 9PT, UK
4. Cluster of High-Value Products from Thai Rice and Plants for Health, Faculty of Agro-Industry, Chiang Mai University, Chiang Mai 50200, Thailand; niramon.u@cmu.ac.th
5. Department of Product Development Technology, Faculty of Agro-Industry, Chiang Mai University, Chiang Mai 50200, Thailand
6. Thalassemia Research Center, Institute of Molecular Biosciences, Mahidol University Salaya Campus, Nakornpathom 71300, Thailand; suthat.fuc@mahidol.ac.th
* Correspondence: somdet.s@cmu.ac.th; Tel.: +66-53935322

Abstract: Iron fortifications are used for the treatment of iron-deficiency anemia; however, iron dosing may cause oxidative damage to the gut lumen. Thai Sinlek rice is abundant in iron and contains phytochemicals. We aimed at evaluating the effect of an iron-rice (IR) hydrolysate drink (100 mL/serving) on neurological function, red cell indices and iron status in elders. Healthy elderly subjects were divided into three non-anemic groups and one anemic group. The non-anemic groups consumed one WR (2 mg iron/serving) and two IR drinks (15 and 27 mg iron/serving) (groups A, B and D, respectively), while the anemic group consumed one IR drink (15 mg iron serving) (group C) every day for 30 days. There were no significant differences in the MMSE Thai 2002 and PHQ9 test scores for members of all groups, while the nutrition scores and body weight values of group D subjects were significantly increased. Hemoglobin (Hb) and mean corpuscular hemoglobin concentrations increased significantly only in group C. Serum iron and transferrin saturation levels tended to increase in group A, while these levels were decreased in members of group C. Serum antioxidant activity levels were increased in all groups, and were highest in group C. Thus, consumption of an IR drink for 15 days functioned to increase Hb and antioxidant capacity levels in anemic elders.

Keywords: anemia; cognition; elder; hemoglobin; iron; *Oryza sativa*; rice

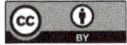

1. Introduction

Anemia is a worldwide public health problem that is caused by a range of factors, including inherited disease, acute blood loss, iron deficiency, end-stage renal disease, pregnancy and aging [1]. Iron-deficiency anemia (IDA) is a common nutritional disease suffered by 1 billion people and must be treated with iron formulations (such as ferrous sulphate, ferric carboxymaltose and Fe_3O_4@Astragalus polysaccharide nanoparticles) [2–4]. Though iron supplementation is an effective therapy, gastrointestinal disturbance and oxidative bowel damage are known to be uncompliant side effects. IDA is diagnosed by measuring biomarkers of iron stores, blood iron parameters and red cell indices. Nutritional anemia in the elderly (about one-third of all those diagnosed with the disease) is important to address because the mortality risk has significantly increased. An adequate energy and protein diet, along with effective iron and vitamin supplementation, have been acknowledged in the prevention and treatment of certain diseases such as anemia [5]. Incidences of iron deficiency have been reported at considerable levels in elderly populations, of which females appear to be at higher risk than males. However, elderly populations of both genders are known to have a similar low dietary iron intake of 10–11 mg/day [6].

Meng and colleagues have reported on the iron content found in different forms of rice (*Oryza sativa* L.), including black rice, red rice, sticky rice and rice millet. A higher degree of iron content was found in black rice when compared with other rice varieties [7]. A previous study has revealed that red blood cell numbers were increased in early weaned piglets after they were fed with high-iron rice [8]. Along with the establishment of iron-fortified foods, the process of agronomic biofortification of rice grains has been increasingly developed in major rice-producing countries for the purposes of addressing micronutrient malnutrition in human populations [9]. Rice beverages are value-added and manufactured by means of enzymatic hydrolysis and bacterial fermentation [10–12]. The effects of temperature, reaction time, raw materials-to-water weight ratio and suitable α-amylase enzyme hydrolysis need to be determined in order to produce high yields of nutrients and bioactive compounds, while sustaining low carbohydrate content in the soluble or concentrated products [12]. However, oxidative mucosal toxicity of ferrous sulphate tablets was found when deglutition disorders were present in elderly patients. Consequently, appropriate iron pharmaceutical formulations (such as syrups and drinks) should be provided to these IDA patients [13]. Red rice grain is concentrated with iron and many phytochemicals (such as phenolics, proanthocyanidins, oryzanol and vitamin E) that are known to exert beneficial effects on human health [14–17]. Hypothetically, Sinlek rice hydrolysate that is abundant in iron together with phytochemicals should be considered a potential nutrient in the treatment of IDA patients. In this study, we focused on evaluating the effects of iron-rice drinks on iron status, red cell indices and brain functions in Thai anemic elderly patients.

2. Results
2.1. Subject Information

Firstly, one hundred and thirty-four elderly volunteers applied for enrolment in this study and twenty-six individuals were excluded. From the relevant calculation, there should be twenty-seven subjects in non-anemic groups A, B and D and in anemic group C at the beginning of the study. However, two subjects in groups A, B and C were excluded due to the occurrence of diseases or related complications. Furthermore, two additional anemic subjects in group C were withdrawn during the course of this study. As is shown in Table 1, a total of one-hundred elderly subjects were enrolled in the study and these subjects were divided into four groups. These groups were then identified as non-anemic groups A ($n = 25$), B ($n = 25$) and D ($n = 27$), and an anemic group C ($n = 23$). The number of female subjects in the anemic group C was lower than in groups B and D, with statistical significance ($p < 0.05$). In addition, the anemic subjects were found to be older than the non-anemic subjects ($p < 0.05$). The average ages of the subjects in groups C, A, B and D were 74.3 ± 7.2, 68.5 ± 5.7, 71.6 ± 7.7 and 68.9 ± 7.9 years respectively, and their height values were 153.4 ± 8.2, 154.1 ± 7.2, 152.1 ± 8.0 and 150.8 ± 6.2 cm, respectively. However, before the study, marital status, education, profession, health behaviors, including exercise, smoking and alcohol drinking, body mass index (BMI) and co-morbidities including chronic diseases, hypertension, diabetic mellitus and hyperlipidemia that were reported in the members of these four groups were not determined to be significantly different among all four groups (Tables 1 and 2).

Table 1. General information of subjects in groups A, B, D and C before the study. Non-anemic elders consumed a WR drink (2 mg iron/100 mL serving) (group A), IR drink (15 mg iron/100 mL serving) (group B) and IR drink (27 mg iron/100 mL serving) (group D), while anemic elders consumed the IR drink (15 mg iron/100 mL serving) (Group C). Data are expressed in absolute numbers and percentages (blanket). * Pearson chi-square test, ** Fisher's exact test ($p < 0.05$) when members of the same group were compared.

Characteristics		Number (Percentage) of Subjects				p-Value When All Groups Were Compared
		Non-Anemic			Anemic	
		Group A	Group B	Group D	Group C	
Gender	Male	7 (28.00)	4 (16.00)	2 (7.41)	12 (52.17)	$p = 0.002$ *
	Female	18 (72.00)	21 (84.00)	25 (92.59)	11 (47.83)	
Age (years)	60–69	13 (52.00)	10 (40.00)	18 (66.67)	5 (21.74)	$p = 0.019$ **
	70–79	11 (44.00)	11 (44.00)	5 (18.52)	12 (52.17)	
	≥80	1 (4.00)	4 (16.00)	4 (14.81)	6 (26.09)	
Marital status	Single	3 (12.00)	3 (12.00)	3 (11.11)	3 (13.04)	$p = 0.491$ **
	Couple	13 (52.00)	11 (44.00)	10 (37.04)	8 (34.78)	
	Divorce/separate	0	0	3 (11.11)	4 (17.39)	
	Widow	9 (36.00)	11 (44.00)	11 (40.74)	8 (34.78)	
Education	Primary school	15 (60.00)	18 (72.00)	17 (62.96)	13 (56.62)	$p = 0.485$ **
	Secondary school	0	1 (4.00)	0	2 (8.70)	
	High school	6 (24.00)	0	5 (18.52)	3 (13.04)	
	Under graduate	2 (8.00)	3 (12.00)	1 (3.70)	2 (8.70)	
	Postgraduate	0	1 (4.00)	1 (3.70)	1 (4.35)	
	Other	2 (8.00)	2 (8.00)	3 (11.11)	2 (8.70)	
Profession	No	16 (64.00)	13 (52.00)	18 (66.67)	10 (43.48)	$p = 0.704$ **
	Agriculture	0	1 (4.00)	0	3 (13.04)	
	Worker	0	2 (8.00)	1 (3.70)	3 (13.04)	
	Merchant	3 (12.00)	3 (12.00)	2 (7.41)	2 (8.70)	
	Pension	2 (8.00)	2 (8.00)	3 (11.11)	1 (4.35)	
	Other	4 (16.00)	4 (16.00)	3 (11.11)	4 (17.39)	

Table 2. Biographic information of subjects in groups A, B, D and C before the study. Non-anemic elders consumed a WR drink (2 mg iron/100 mL serving) (group A), IR drink (15 mg iron/100 mL serving) (group B) and IR drink (27 mg iron/100 mL serving) (group D), while anemic elders consumed the IR drink (15 mg iron/100 mL serving) (Group C). Data are expressed in absolute numbers and percentages (blanket). * Pearson chi-square test, ** Fisher's exact test ($p < 0.05$) when members of the same group were compared.

Health Information		Number (Percentage) of Subjects				p-Value When All Groups Were Compared
		Non-Anemic			Anemic	
		Group A	Group B	Group D	Group C	
BMI (kg/m^2)	<18.5	0	1 (4.00)	0	1 (4.35)	$p = 0.911$ **
	18.5–22.9	9 (36.00)	10 (40.00)	10 (37.04)	7 (30.43)	
	≥23	16 (64.00)	14 (56.00)	17 (62.96)	15 (65.22)	
Chronic diseases		17/25 (68.00)	12/25 (48.00)	18/27 (66.67)	19/23 (82.91)	$p = 0.090$ *
Hypertension		11/25 (44.00)	9/25 (36.00)	13/27 (48.15)	12/23 (52.17)	$p = 0.702$ *
Diabetic mellitus		0/25 (0)	3/25 (12.00)	3/27 (11.11)	3/23 (13.04)	$p = 0.287$ **
Hyperlipidemia		9/25 (36.00)	7/25 (28.00)	12/27 (44.44)	8/23 (34.78)	$p = 0.672$ *
Osteoarthritis		5/25 (20.00)	4/25 (16.00)	4/27 (14.81)	7/23 (30.43)	$p = 0.541$ **
Smoking		1/25 (4.00)	0/25 (0)	1/27 (3.70)	2/23 (3.70)	$p = 0.456$ **
Alcohol drinking		1/25 (4.00)	0/25 (0)	0/27 (0)	2/23 (8.70)	$p = 0.136$ **
Exercise		21/25 (84.00)	19/25 (76.00)	20/27 (74.07)	16/23 (69.57)	$p = 0.693$ *
Drug allergy		4/25 (16.00)	0/25 (0)	5/27 (18.52)	1/23 (4.35)	$p = 0.063$ **

Abbreviations: BMI = body mass index.

Moreover, Barthel activities of daily living (ADL), Mini Mental State Examination (MMSE Thai 2002) and Patient Health Questionnaire 9 (PHQ9) scores were found to be non-significantly different in groups A and B, and between the anemic group and the non-anemic group (Figure 1). The ADL scores for groups A, B, D and C were 19.84 ± 0.80, 19.84 ± 0.37, 19.89 ± 0.42 and 19.83 ± 0.49 points, respectively.

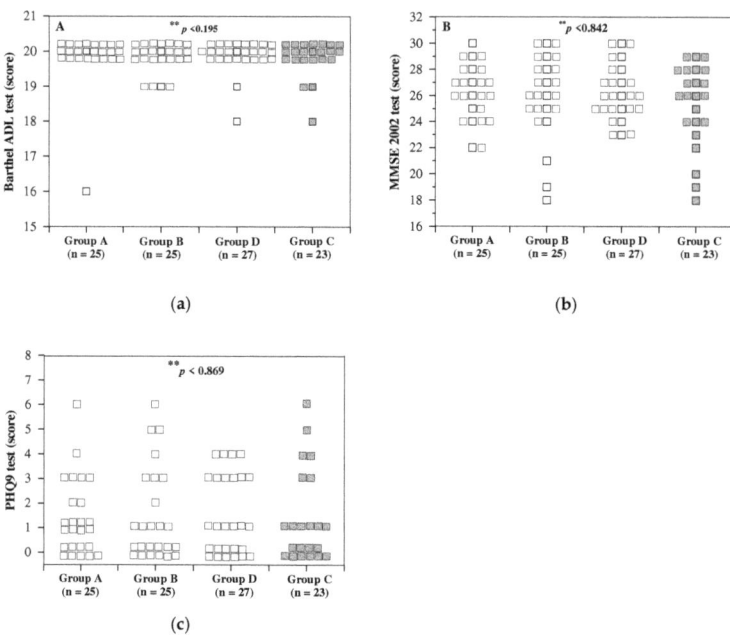

Figure 1. Numbers of subjects in groups A, B, D and C for Barthel ADL (a), MMSE Thai 2002 (b) and PHQ9 (c) tests before the study. Non-anemic elders consumed the WR drink (2 mg iron/100 mL serving) (group A), IR drink (15 mg iron/100 mL serving) (group B) and IR drink (27 mg iron/100 mL serving) (group D), while anemic elders consumed the IR drink (15 mg iron/100 mL serving) (Group C) for 30 days. Data of individual subjects are expressed accordingly. ** Fisher's exact test when members of the same group were compared. Abbreviations: ADL = activities of daily living, MMSE = Mini Mental State Examination, PHQ9 = Patient Health Questionnaire 9.

2.2. Health, Nutritional Scores and Neurological Function

Maintaining and retarding the decline of physical and cognitive function, along with achieving the optimal degree of control of chronic diseases in aging populations, is an important global goal for researchers in the hopes of increasing the life expectancy of humans. Iron supplementation and therapeutic interventions are a nutritional strategy that could be used to prevent IDA and other iron-related disorders in the elderly. As is shown in Figure 2, there were no significant differences in the MMSE Thai 2002 and PHQ9 test scores for members of all groups before and after the study. Surprisingly, the nutrition scores and body weight (BW) values of the subjects in group D were significantly increased from 12.74 ± 0.76 to 13.30 ± 1.03 ($^a p < 0.05$) and 59.50 ± 12.47 kg to 60.37 ± 13.29 kg ($^b p < 0.05$) respectively, during the course of this study. Iron is essential for increase of erythrocyte mass, ribonucleotide reductase-catalyzed cell proliferation and tissue expansion [18]; inversely, primary negative effects associated with IDA include deficits in body weight gain. For instance, pigs fed with a 450–600 mg ferrous sulfate-supplemented basal diet showed significant increases of BW, SI and TIBC values when compared with those fed with the basal diet, suggesting that the iron fortification should improve growth performance [19]. Some studies have reported that excess body mass or obesity was associated with iron excess [20]. Increased iron availability and iron fortification positively affect human growth, and increased growth in humans provided greater amounts of iron 18. In the present study, there was greater BW gain in group D with the IR drink (27 mg iron/serving) than that in group B with the IR drink (15 mg iron/serving) and group A with the WR drink (2 mg iron/serving), possibly due to increased proliferation and expansion of cells (such as adipocytes). Moreover, there were no significant differences in systolic blood pressure (SBP) as well as diastolic blood pressure (DBP) in this study.

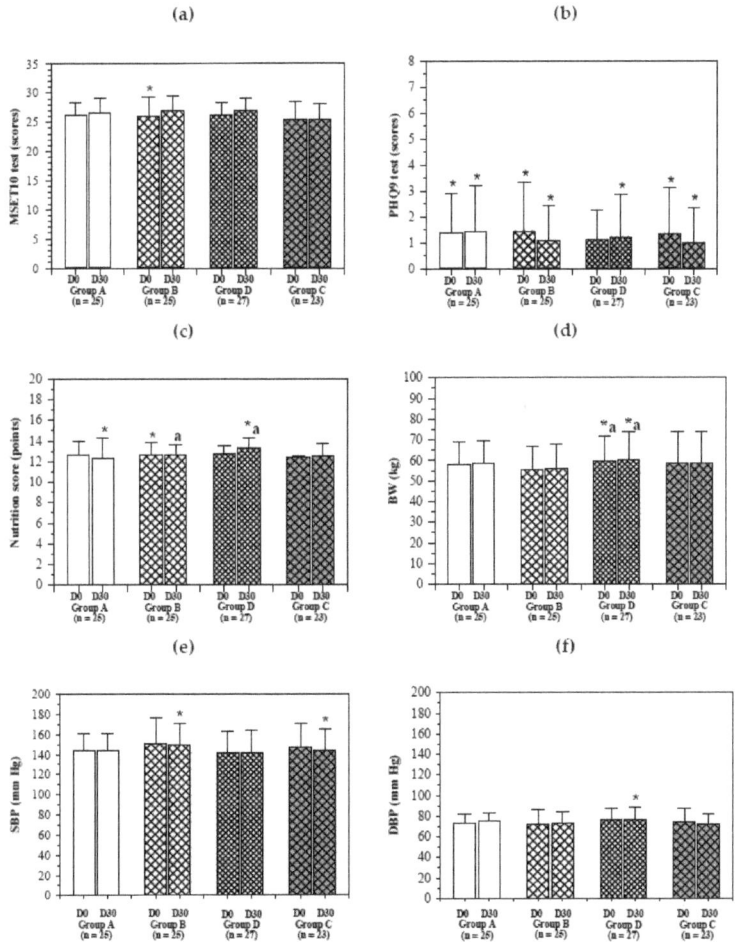

Figure 2. Changes in neurological and nutritional scores, body weight and blood pressure values in elderly subjects. Non-anemic elders consumed the WR drink (2 mg iron/100 mL serving) (group A), IR drink (15 mg iron/100 mL serving) (group B) and the IR drink (27 mg iron/100 mL serving) (group D), while anemic elders (group C) consumed the IR drink (15 mg iron/100 mL serving) for 30 days and reported MMSE Thai 2002 (**a**), PHQ9 (**b**) and nutritional (**c**) scores, BW (**d**) and BP (**e**,**f**) values. Data are expressed as mean ± standard deviation (SD) values. * Shapiro–Wilk W test ($p < 0.05$). [a] Wilcoxon signed rank-sum test $p < 0.05$ when members of the same group were compared before and after the study. Abbreviations: BW = body weight, BP = blood pressure, DBP = diastolic blood pressure, Hg = mercury, IR = iron rice, MMSE Thai 2002 = Mini Mental State Examination Thai 2002, PHQ9 = Patient Health Questionnaire 9, SBP = systolic blood pressure, WR = white rice.

2.3. Hematopoietic Activity

Changes in hematological parameter values for 1, 2 and 3 visits for all groups are shown in Figure 3. Mean blood hemoglobin (Hb) levels of non-anemic subjects in group B were found to have decreased from 13.50 ± 0.92 to 12.97 ± 0.95 g/dL and to 12.83 ± 0.75 g/dL ($p < 0.05$) after receiving the low-dose IR drink for 15 and 30 days, respectively. Remarkably, the Hb level in group C increased from 1 to 2 visits (11.71 ± 0.71 to 11.96 ± 0.95 g/dL) and decreased after 3 visits (11.86 ± 0.86 g/dL). Mean hematocrit (Hct) values of non-anemic subjects in groups B and D were found to have decreased and were statistically significant. Significant differences were recorded in the mean Hct levels in groups B and D, mean white blood cells (WBC) in groups A and D, mean polymorphonuclear cells (PMN) in groups A and B, mean lymphocyte values in group A, mean eosinophil values in groups A, B and D, mean monocyte values in group D, the average mean corpuscular volume (MCV) in group C, the average mean corpuscular hemoglobin (MCH) values in groups A, B and D and the mean platelets in group D. However, no statistically significant differences were observed in the mean RBC values for all groups. Mean changes in Hct values in group A (0.35% ± 0.42%) were found to reveal statistically significant differences when compared with those of group B (−0.72% ± 0.39%) in the last 15 days (−0.07% ± 0.15% and −0.67% ± 0.12%). Using the same low-dose IR drink, the mean change of Hb level variables in group C was found to have increased with statistically significant differences when compared with group B in the first 15 days (0.24 ± 0.13 and −0.53 ± 0.11 g/dL) and 30 days (0.14 ± 0.11 and −0.67 ± 0.12 g/dL). This may be indicative of the effect of the IR drink in increasing Hb levels in anemic subjects when compared to non-anemic subjects. In addition, mean changes in the values of MCV in group C (1.28 ± 0.72 fL) were significantly different when compared with those in groups A, B and D (−0.78 ± 0.39, −2.08 ± 0.87 and −2.75 ± 2.60 fL, respectively) over 30 days. Mean changes in the values of MCH in group C (−0.06 ± 0.14 pg) were significantly different from those in groups A, B and D (−0.17 ± 0.15, −0.77 ± 0.28 and −0.62 ± 0.15 pg, respectively) over 30 days. Changes in the values of mean corpuscular hemoglobin concentration (MCHC) level variables in group C (0.60 ± 0.21 g/dL) revealed significant differences when compared with those of group B (−0.50 ± 0.29 g/dL) in the first 15 days of this study. Nonetheless, mean changes in values of WBC, monocyte and platelets (PLT) were not found to reveal statistically significant differences for all groups.

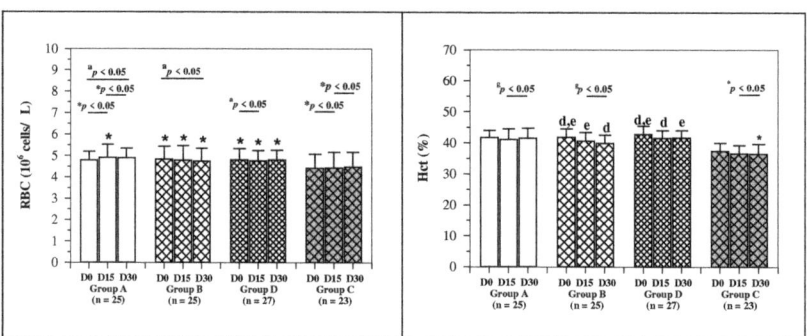

Figure 3. *Cont.*

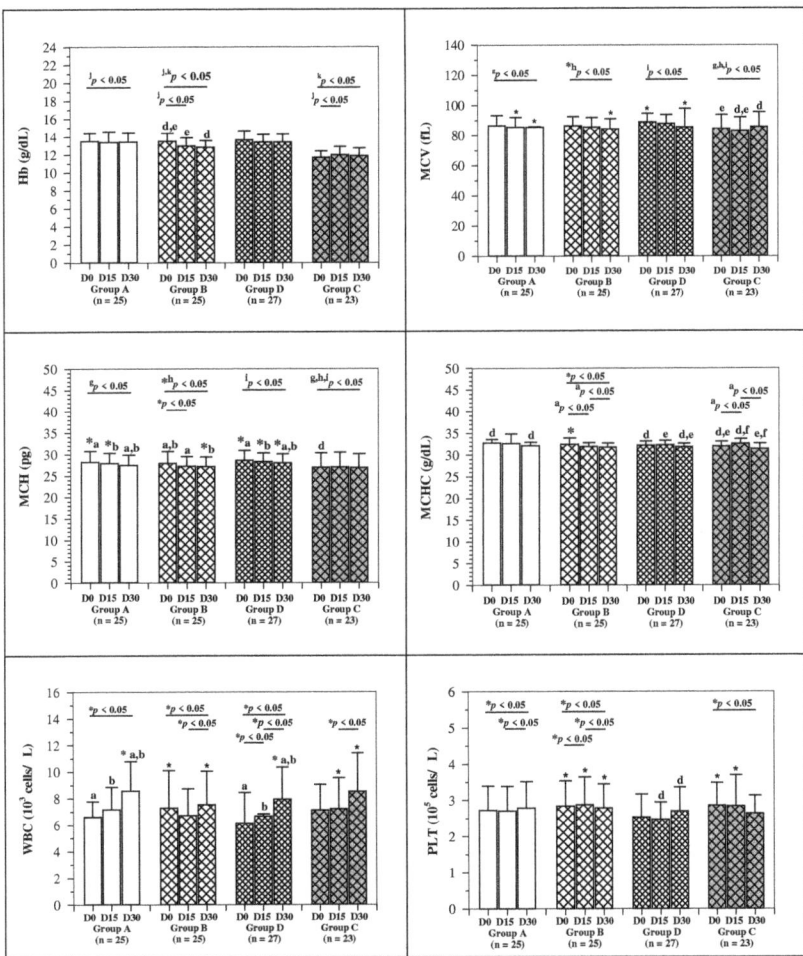

Figure 3. Changes in RBC indices, WBC and platelet numbers of elderly subjects. Non-anemic subjects consumed the WR drink (2 mg iron/100 mL serving) (group A), IR drink (15 mg iron/100 mL serving) (group B) and IR drink (27 mg iron/100 mL serving) (groups D), and anemic subjects consumed the IR drink (15 mg iron/serving) (group C) for 30 days and blood samples were collected for complete blood count analysis. Data are expressed as mean ± SD values. * Comparisons of results of Shapiro–Wilk test ($p < 0.05$). ^{d,e,f} Between D0 and D15, D0 and D30, D15 and D30 for normal distribution by paired Student's t-test ($p < 0.05$) after using repeated analysis of variance (repeated ANOVA) ($p < 0.05$). ^{a,b,c} Comparisons between D0 and D15, D0 and D30 and D15 and D30 for non-normal distribution were performed by the Wilcoxon signed rank test ($p < 0.05$) after using the Friedman test ($p < 0.05$). ^{j,k,l} Bonferroni test ($p < 0.05$) among groups with normal distribution data after using one-way analysis of variance (one-way ANOVA) test. ^{g,h,i} Comparisons of Kruskal–Wallis test ($p < 0.05$) for four groups and Dunn test ($p < 0.05$) between two groups with non-normal distribution data. Abbreviations: EOS = eosinophil, Hb = hemoglobin, Hct = hematocrit, Lym = lymphocyte, MCH = mean corpuscular hemoglobin, MCHC = mean corpuscular hemoglobin, MCV = mean corpuscular volume, Mon = monocytes, PLT = platelet, PMN = polymorphonuclear cell, RBC = red blood cells, WBC = white blood cells.

2.4. Iron Status

The levels of serum Ft concentrations were significantly varied in the subjects of groups A, B and C; however, the Ft levels were not changed by the administration of rice drinks in all groups during the course of this study. Evidently, serum iron (SI) and total iron-binding capacity (TIBC) levels were normal and non-significantly different in all groups, even among anemic subjects (group C). Furthermore, the subjects were not observed to be affected by the IR drinks. Moreover, the administration of rice drinks was found to influence the levels of SI and TIBC significantly in subjects in groups B and D. The rice drink was also found to significantly influence the serum Ft levels of non-anemic subjects, but not in the anemic subjects (Figure 4).

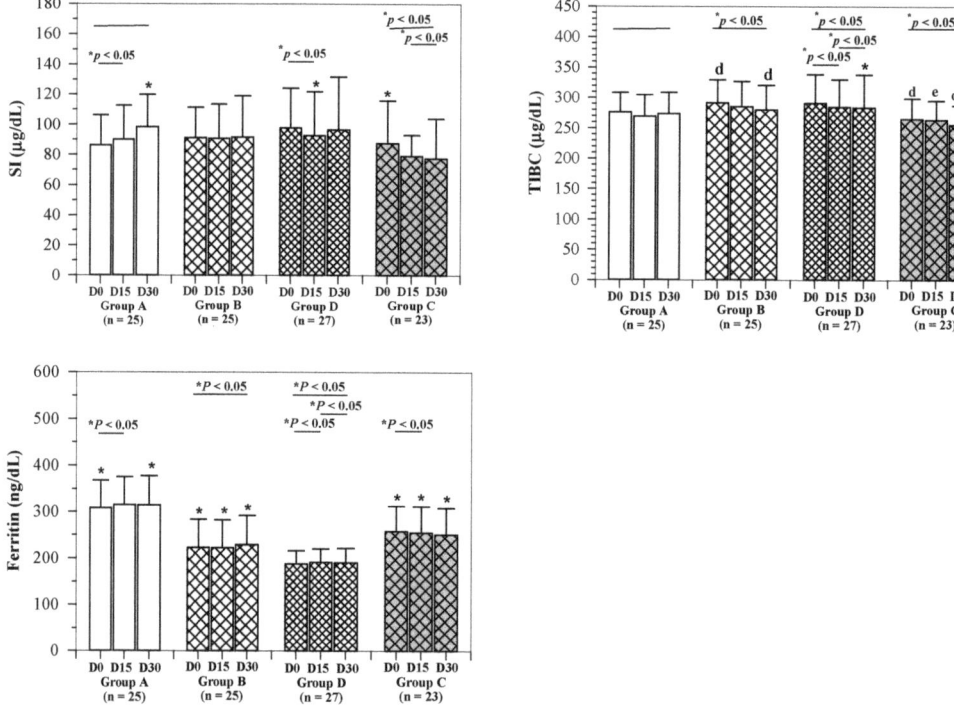

Figure 4. Changes in levels of serum iron, total iron-binding capacity and ferritin of elderly subjects. Non-anemic elders consumed the WR drink (2 mg iron/100 mL serving) (group A), IR drink (15 mg iron/serving) (group B) and IR drink (27 mg iron/100 mL serving) (group D), and anemic elders consumed the IR drink (15 mg iron/100 mL serving) (group C) for 30 days and blood samples were collected for analysis of iron parameters. Data are expressed as mean ± SD values with the exception of ferritin, which is expressed as mean ± SEM values. * Shapiro–Wilk test ($p < 0.05$). [d,e,f] Comparisons between D0 and D15, D0 and D30, D15 and D30 for normal distribution by paired Student's t-test ($p < 0.05$) after using repeated measure ANOVA ($p < 0.05$). Abbreviations: Ft = ferritin, SI = serum iron, TIBC = total iron-binding capacity.

2.5. Serum Antioxidant Capacity

Antioxidant capacity (AC) levels before and after the administration of the rice drink increased significantly in all groups, and the changes in groups A, B, D and C after the administration for 30 days were 31 ± 20, 47 ± 17, 38 ± 13 and 71 ± 19 µg TE/mL, respectively (Figure 5). This finding suggests that the effects of the anti-oxidative phytochemical ingredients were most effective in the anemic elders.

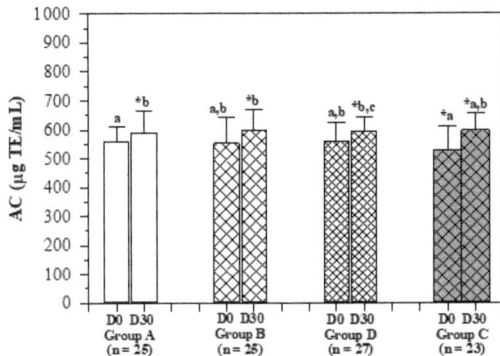

Figure 5. Changes in levels of serum antioxidant capacity of elderly subjects. Non-anemic elders consumed the WR drink (2 mg iron/100 mL serving) (group A), IR drink (15 mg iron/100 mL serving) (group B) and IR drink (27 mg iron/100 mL serving) (group D), while anemic elders consumed the IR drink (15 mg iron/100 mL serving) (group C) for 30 days and blood samples were collected for analysis of antioxidant capacity. Data are expressed as mean ± SD values with the exception of ferritin, which is expressed as mean + standard error of the mean (SEM). * Shapiro–Wilk test ($p < 0.05$). [a,b,c] Comparisons between D0 and D30 for non-normal distribution by Wilcoxon signed rank test ($p < 0.05$) after applying the Friedman test ($p < 0.05$). Abbreviations: AC = antioxidant capacity, TE = Trolox equivalent.

2.6. Blood Biochemical Parameters

The values of all serum biochemical parameters for all groups were generally at the normal levels before and after the study (Tables 3–5). The levels of serum lipids, total protein (TP), albumin (Alb) and FBS were not found to be significantly different when comparisons were made between non-anemic and anemic groups (Table 3). The consumption of WR and IR drinks was found not to influence the levels of these parameters. The levels of blood urea nitrogen (BUN) and serum creatinine (CRE) in anemic subjects seemed to be higher than in non-anemic subjects, but the differences were not determined to be significantly different (Table 4). Similarly, the levels of serum uric acid (UA), sodium ion (Na^+) and potassium ion (K^+) were not significantly different among the groups and were found to be unchanged during the rice drink intervention experiments (Table 4). Likewise, the levels of serum TP, Alb and globulin (Glo) were not significantly different among the groups and during the period of intervention. In contrast, the levels of serum alanine aminotransferase (ALT) and aspartate aminotransferase (AST) activities were different among the groups, for which the levels tended to decrease non-significantly in all groups during the course of the intervention (Table 5).

Table 3. Levels of serum glucose and lipid profiles of elderly subjects. Non-anemic elders consumed the WR drink (2 mg iron/100 mL serving) (group A), IR drink (15 mg iron/100 mL serving) (group B) and IR drink (27 mg iron/100 mL serving) (group D), and anemic elders consumed the IR drink (15 mg iron/100 mL serving) (group C) for 30 days and blood samples were collected for analysis of glucose and lipids. Data are expressed as mean ± SD values. Changes in the mean are shown as mean ± SD values in the brackets.

Parameters	Time	Group A ($n = 25$)	Group B ($n = 25$)	Group D ($n = 27$)	Group C ($n = 23$)
FBS (mg/dL)	D0	82.5 ± 13.2	79.0 ± 14.6 [d,e]	81.0 ± 14.5 [d]	84.4 ± 16.1
	(D0:D15)	(7.3 ± 3.4)	(6.5 ± 2.5)	(7.3 ± 3.1 *)	(1.8 ± 3.2)
	D15	88.8 ± 15.6	85.5 ± 17.7 [d]	87.9 ± 14.0 [d]	86.2 ± 16.4
	(D15:D30)	(4.5 ± 5.0 *)	(−1.4 ± 1.8 *)	(−3.8 ± 2.9 *)	(6.3 ± 3.3 *)
	D30	93.2 ± 26.1 *	84.1 ± 15.6 [e]	85.3 ± 15.2	92.5 ± 21.9
	(D0:D30)	(11.8 ± 6.1 *)	(5.1 ± 2.1)	(3.5 ± 2.9)	(8.1 ± 4.6 *)

Table 3. Cont.

Parameters	Time	Group A (n = 25)	Group B (n = 25)	Group D (n = 27)	Group C (n = 23)
TC (mg/dL)	D0	210 ± 39	209 ± 37 [d]	207 ± 36	193 ± 30
	(D0:D15)	(−11 ± 4 *)	(−8 ± 5)	(−1 ± 5)	(−4 ± 4)
	D15	203 ± 38	202 ± 32	206 ± 39	188 ± 32
	(D15:D30)	(7 ± 5)	(−4 ± 4)	(1 ± 3)	(4 ± 4)
	D30	209 ± 37	198 ± 29 [d]	207 ± 39	192 ± 35
	(D0:D30)	(5 ± 12 *)	(0 ± 8)	(11 ± 7)	(9 ± 13 *)
TG (mg/dL)	D0	120 ± 59	117 ± 54 *	105 ± 36	110 ± 54
	(D0:D15)	(−22 ± 13 *)	(−6 ± 11)	(10 ± 10)	(5 ± 8)
	D15	98 ± 36 [a]	111 ± 62 *	113 ± 50 *	115 ± 52
	(D15:D30)	(27 ± 9)	(6 ± 12 *)	(1 ± 7)	(4 ± 9)
	D30	125 ± 48 *[a]	117 ± 71 *	114 ± 37	119 ± 61 *
	(D0:D30)	(5 ± 12 *)	(0 ± 8)	(11 ± 7)	(9 ± 12 *)
HDL-C (mg/dL)	D0	53 ± 11	54 ± 17 *[a]	55 ± 12 [d]	51 ± 14 [d]
	(D0:D15)	(−5 ± 2 *)	(−3 ± 1)	(−3 ± 1 *)	(−5 ± 1)
	D15	49 ± 13 *[a]	51 ± 15 *[a,b]	53 ± 12 [d]	46 ± 13 [d,e]
	(D15:D30)	(7 ± 2 *)	(4 ± 2)	(3 ± 2 *)	(4 ± 1)
	D30	55 ± 12 [a]	56 ± 17 *[b]	56 ± 15	49 ± 14 [e]
	(D0:D30)	(2 ± 2)	(1 ± 1 *)	(0 ± 2)	(−1 ± 1)
LDL-C (mg/dL)	D0	169 ± 45	159 ± 45 *[a,b]	155 ± 41	146 ± 36 [d]
	(D0:D15)	(−20 ± 7 *)	(−12 ± 5)	(−7 ± 5)	(−5 ± 1)
	D15	153 ± 48	147 ± 37 [a]	148 ± 48 *[a]	134 ± 35 [d,e]
	(D15:D30)	(5 ± 6 *)	(−4 ± 4 *)	(7 ± 4)	(10 ± 4)
	D30	157 ± 45	143 ± 33 [b]	155 ± 46 *[a]	144 ± 42 [e]
	(D0:D30)	(−16 ± 8)	(−16 ± 6)	(−1 ± 4)	(−1 ± 6)

* Comparisons between results for the Shapiro–Wilk test ($p < 0.05$). [d,e,f] Comparison of D0 and D15, D0 and D30 and D15 and D30 for normal distribution by paired Student's t-test ($p < 0.05$) after using repeated ANOVA ($p < 0.05$). [a,b,c] Comparisons between D0 and D15, D0 and D30 and D15 and D30 for non-normal distribution by Wilcoxon signed rank test ($p < 0.05$) after using the Friedman test ($p < 0.05$). Abbreviations: FBS = fasting blood sugar, HDL-C = high-density lipoprotein-cholesterol, LDL-C = low-density lipoprotein-cholesterol, TC = total cholesterol, TG = triglyceride.

Table 4. Levels of blood urea nitrogen, serum creatinine, uric acid and electrolytes of non-anemic subjects who consumed the WR drink (2 mg iron/100 mL serving) (group A), IR drink (15 mg iron/100 mL serving) (group B) and IR drink (27 mg iron/100 mL serving) (group D), and anemic subjects who consumed the IR drink (15 mg iron/100 mL serving) (group C) for 30 days. Data are expressed as mean ± SD values. Changes in the mean are shown as mean ± SD values in the brackets.

Parameters	Time	Group A (n = 25)	Group B (n = 25)	Group D (n = 27)	Group C (n = 23)
BUN (mg/dL)	D0	13.2 ± 2.4 [d]	13.0 ± 3.5	14.0 ± 3.8	15.8 ± 6.9 *
	(D0:D15)	(−1.7 ± 0.4)	(−0.9 ± 0.4)	(−1.1 ± 0.6)	(−0.7 ± 0.8)
	D15	11.6 ± 2.1 [d]	12.1 ± 2.9 *	12.8 ± 2.8	15.1 ± 6.6 *
	(D15:D30)	(0.5 ± 0.4)	(0.8 ± 0.6)	(0.4 ± 0.6)	(0.2 ± 0.6 *)
	D30	12.2 ± 2.2	12.9 ± 2.8	13.0 ± 2.9 *	15.3 ± 5.2 *
	(D0:D30)	(−1.2 ± 0.6 *)	(−0.1 ± 0.7)	(−0.7 ± 0.7)	(−0.4 ± 1.0 *)
CRE (mg/dL)	D0	0.90 ± 0.14	0.87 ± 0.20 *	0.87 ± 0.19 *	1.21 ± 0.61 *
	(D0:D15)	(0.01 ± 0.03)	(0.03 ± 0.03)	(0 ± 0.04)	(0.01 ± 0.04)
	D15	0.91 ± 0.16	0.90 ± 0.19	0.87 ± 0.17 *	1.22 ± 0.62 *
	(D15:D30)	(0 ± 0.04)	(0.05 ± 0.03)	(0.03 ± 0.04)	(0.03 ± 0.04)
	D30	0.94 ± 0.29	0.95 ± 0.21	0.90 ± 0.16	1.25 ± 0.70 *
	(D0:D30)	(0.01 ± 0.06 *)	(0.08 ± 0.04 *)	(0.03 ± 0.05)	(0.04 ± 0.05)

Table 4. Cont.

Parameters	Time	Group A (n = 25)	Group B (n = 25)	Group D (n = 27)	Group C (n = 23)
UA (mg/dL)	D0	6.75 ± 2.07 *	7.35 ± 2.10	6.24 ± 1.86 *	7.63 ± 2.56
	(D0:D15)	(0.07 ± 0.41 *)	(−0.23 ± 0.21)	(0.10 ± 0.46 *)	(0.43 ± 0.55 *)
	D15	6.85 ± 1.90	7.12 ± 1.71 *	6.31 ± 1.36	8.06 ± 2.57
	(D15:D30)	(0.17 ± 0.41)	(0.31 ± 0.21)	(0.16 ± 0.27)	(−0.16 ± 0.37 *)
	D30	7.03 ± 2.03	7.43 ± 1.69	6.43 ± 1.26	7.90 ± 1.75
	(D0:D30)	(0.25 ± 0.50 *)	(0.08 ± 0.25)	(0.26 ± 0.42 *)	(0.27 ± 0.45 *)
Na$^+$ (mmol/L)	D0	142 ± 3 [d,e]	144 ± 3 [*a,b]	143 ± 2	140 ± 3
	(D0:D15)	(−1 ± 1)	(−3 ± 1)	(−2 ± 1 [a])	(−1 ± 1 [a])
	D15	140 ± 2 [d]	141 ± 3 [*a,c]	141 ± 2	139 ± 2
	(D15:D30)	(−0 ± 1)	(−1 ± 1)	(−2 ± 1)	(−0 ± 1)
	D30	140 ± 3 [e]	139 ± 3 [b,c]	140 ± 2	139 ± 3
	(D0:D30)	(−2 ± 1)	(−4 ± 1)	(−3 ± 1 [a])	(−1 ± 1 [a])
K$^+$ (mmol/L)	D0	3.80 ± 0.44	4.03 ± 0.35 [d,e]	4.09 ± 0.80 *	4.27 ± 0.51 [a]
	(D0:D15)	(0 ± 0.08)	(−0.12 ± 0.05)	(−0.24 ± 0.18 *)	(−0.17 ± 0.19 *)
	D15	3.77 ± 0.51	3.91 ± 0.36 [e]	3.92 ± 0.42 *	4.03 ± 0.75 [*a,b]
	(D15:D30)	(−0.05 ± 0.80)	(−0.1 ± 0.05)	(0.01 ± 0.11)	(0.05 ± 0.14 *)
	D30	3.74 ± 0.44	3.81 ± 0.31 [d]	3.95 ± 0.57 *	4.08 ± 0.46 [b]
	(D0:D30)	(−0.04 ± 0.08)	(−0.22 ± 0.06)	(−0.15 ± 0.20 *)	(−0.19 ± 0.10)

* Comparisons of results of the Shapiro–Wilk test ($p < 0.05$). [d,e,f] Between D0 and D15, D0 and D30 and D15 and D30 for normal distribution by paired Student's t-test ($p < 0.05$) after using repeated ANOVA ($p < 0.05$). [a,b,c] Comparisons between D0 and D15, D0 and D30 and D15 and D30 for non-normal distribution by Wilcoxon signed rank test ($p < 0.05$) after using the Friedman test ($p < 0.05$). Abbreviations: BUN = blood urea nitrogen, CRE = creatinine, K$^+$ = potassium ion, Na$^+$ = sodium ion, UA = uric acid.

Table 5. Levels of serum proteins, aspartate aminotransferase and alanine aminotransferase activity of non-anemic subjects who consumed the WR drink (2 mg iron/100 mL serving) (group A), IR drink (15 mg iron/100 mL serving) (group B) and IR drink (27 mg iron/100 mL serving) (group D), while anemic subjects consumed the IR drink (15 mg iron/100 mL serving) (group C) for 30 days. Data are expressed as mean ± SD values. Changes in the mean are shown as mean ± SD values in the brackets.

Parameters	Time	Group A (n = 25)	Group B (n = 25)	Group D (n = 27)	Group C (n = 23)
TP (g/dL)	D0	8.00 ± 0.46	8.14 ± 0.72 [d,e]	7.97 ± 0.40	7.94 ± 0.35 [d]
	(D0:D15)	(−0.24 ± 0.09)	(−0.11 ± 0.15)	(−0.00 ± 0.12)	(−0.24 ± 0.09)
	D15	7.96 ± 0.42 *	7.90 ± 0.56 [e]	7.90 ± 0.54	7.94 ± 0.48 [e]
	(D15:D30)	(−0.09 ± 0.07)	(1.99 ± 0.09)	(−0.34 ± 0.12)	(−0.09 ± 0.07)
	D30	7.82 ± 0.46	7.81 ± 0.52 [d]	7.83 ± 0.53 *	7.60 ± 0.47 [d,e]
	(D0:D30)	(−0.33 ± 0.10)	(−0.11 ± 0.14 *)	(−0.34 ± 0.09)	(−0.33 ± 0.10)
Alb (g/dL)	D0	4.50 ± 0.36	4.55 ± 0.32 *	4.44 ± 0.43 [d]	4.20 ± 0.64 [d]
	(D0:D15)	(−0.15 ± 0.08)	(−0.09 ± 0.10)	(0.00 ± 0.12 *)	(−0.15 ± 0.08)
	D15	4.46 ± 0.51	4.40 ± 0.43 [*a]	4.36 ± 0.52 [e]	4.20 ± 0.60 [e]
	(D15:D30)	(0.21 ± 0.05)	(0.37 ± 0.10)	(0.51 ± 0.14)	(0.21 ± 0.05)
	D30	4.66 ± 0.37	4.62 ± 0.42 [*a]	4.68 ± 0.38 [d,e]	4.71 ± 0.48 [d,e]
	(D0:D30)	(0.06 ± 0.08)	(0.27 ± 0.09)	(0.51 ± 0.17 *)	(0.06 ± 0.08)
Glo (g/dL)	D0	3.56 ± 0.72 [e]	3.57 ± 0.77 [e]	3.53 ± 0.59 [*a]	3.74 ± 0.75 [d]
	(D0:D15)	(−0.05 ± 0.10)	(0.00 ± 0.16 *)	(−0.03 ± 0.14)	(−0.05 ± 0.10)
	D15	3.48 ± 0.63 [d]	3.52 ± 0.80 [d]	3.57 ± 0.64 [b]	3.72 ± 0.84 [e]
	(D15:D30)	(−0.32 ± 0.09 [h])	(−0.39 ± 0.13 [i])	(−0.83 ± 0.17 [g,h,i])	(−0.32 ± 0.09 [h])
	D30	3.16 ± 0.56 [d,e]	3.20 ± 0.71 [d,e]	3.15 ± 0.63 [*a,b]	2.89 ± 0.61 [d,e]
	(D0:D30)	(−0.38 ± 0.09)	(−0.39 ± 0.15)	(−0.86 ± 0.16)	(−0.38 ± 0.09)

Table 5. Cont.

Parameters	Time	Group A (n = 25)	Group B (n = 25)	Group D (n = 27)	Group C (n = 23)
AST (U/L)	D0	19 ± 6	19 ± 4	20 ± 10 *	18 ± 4
	(D0:D15)	(−1 ± 1)	(−1 ± 2 *)	(−1 ± 1)	(−1 ± 1)
	D15	18 ± 4	18 ± 3	20 ± 8	18 ± 4
	(D15:D30)	(0 ± 1)	(−1 ± 1)	(−0 ± 1)	(0 ± 1)
	D30	18 ± 5	18 ± 4	19 ± 7 *	17 ± 4
	(D0:D30)	(−1 ± 1)	(−2 ± 2 *)	(−1 ± 1)	(−1 ± 1)
ALT (U/L)	D0	19 ± 9 *a,b	20 ± 5 d,e	21 ± 12 *a,b	19 ± 8 d,e
	(D0:D15)	(−4 ± 1)	(−4 ± 1)	(−4 ± 1 *)	(−4 ± 1)
	D15	15 ± 5 a	15 ± 3 e	17 ± 9 *a	15 ± 6 d
	(D15:D30)	(−0 ± 1)	(−0 ± 1)	(−1 ± 1)	(−0 ± 1)
	D30	15 ± 4 b	15 ± 5 d	17 ± 10 *b	14 ± 5 e
	(D0:D30)	(−5 ± 1)	(−4 ± 1)	(−5 ± 1 *)	(−5 ± 1)

* Comparisons of results of the Shapiro–Wilk test ($p < 0.05$). d,e,f Between D0 and D15, D0 and D30 and D15 and D30 for normal distribution by paired Student's t-test ($p < 0.05$) after using repeated ANOVA ($p < 0.05$), a,b,c Comparisons between D0 and D15, D0 and D30 and D15 and D30 for non-normal distribution by Wilcoxon signed rank test ($p < 0.05$) after using the Friedman test ($p < 0.05$). g,h,i Comparisons of Kruskal–Wallis test ($p < 0.05$) for four groups and Dunn test ($p < 0.05$) between two groups with non-normal distribution data. Abbreviations: Alb = albumin, ALT = alanine aminotransferase, AST = aspartate aminotransferase, Glo = globulin, TP = total protein.

3. Discussion

With regard to a global IDA, rice fortification could increase the intake of micronutrients, particularly iron. The World Health Organization (WHO) has recommended to fortify polished rice with iron to achieve intake that meets the average requirement (150–300 g rice/cap/day (7 mg iron/100 g)) of adults [21]. The iron fortification of rice is a promising strategy that can be applied to improve iron nutrition in order to treat and prevent iron deficiency. With regard to iron bioavailability, fractional iron absorption in young women was found to be significantly higher in subjects who consumed ferric pyrophosphate (FPP) and citrate-fortified rice (4 mg iron/meal) when compared with those who consumed FPP-fortified rice and a citrate solution. However, no differences were observed in those who consumed the ferrous sulfate (FS)-fortified rice reference meal [22]. In Thailand, Chitpan and coworkers had previously fortified dried broken rice with ferrous sulfate, ferrous lactate or ferric ethylenediaminetetraacetic acid (FeEDTA) at 5.3 mg of iron/20 g serving. It was found that FeEDTA fortification was the most suitable option and was revealed to be the most stable over time [23]. In addition, the fortification of FeEDTA (5–10 mg of iron/day) in phyto-diets containing phytates and polyphenolics did not produce any direct toxic effects but did increase zinc and copper absorption [24]. Nonetheless, iron fortification must follow the WHO guidelines in order to achieve the highest degree of iron bioavailability and efficacy [25]. In this study, we used cross-bred Sinlek rice in the iron-rice drink (27 mg of iron/100 mL serving) that contained anti-oxidative phenolic compounds and γ-oryzanol. Importantly, this specific iron-rice drink received a high degree of acceptance among tested consumers. Vitamin C is an important factor in the enhancement of iron bioavailability [26,27], so it has to be taken into consideration for oral iron intervention. A previous study has reported original vitamin C levels of 29.7 and 36.6 mg in 100 g of wet Riceberry and Sinlek rice grains, respectively (Oraphan Srichuenchom B.Sc. Special Problem Study, Kasetsart University 2014). Herein, we have detected very low vitamin C contents in all rice drinks, which was probably due to the losses incurred during hydrolysis and heat lability. The limitations of this study include small serum volumes and an absence of determination of vitamin C concentrations in the sera. Vitamin C is abundant in citrus fruit and functions to convert dietary Fe^{3+} to more soluble Fe^{2+}, which can be readily absorbed into the intestinal epithelial membrane via the divalent metal iron transporter 1. With this in mind, commercial citric acid, which is a weak tridentate iron (Fe^{2+} and Fe^{3+})-chelating chelator [28,29], was added as a food-flavoring and iron-stabilizing agent to the drinks. For the satisfaction of consumers, 0.1% citric acid chelator (food grade) was added as an ingredient to soya sauces that had been fortified with ferrous sulfate, sodium FeEDTA, ferric ammonium citrate, ferrous lactate and ferrous gluconate [30], which was consistent with our recent study [31]. Hepcidin is an important iron-regulatory hormone, for which the suppression under anemic condition allows for more dietary iron to be absorbed during upregulation by oral administration of high-dose iron. This can limit the efficiency of iron absorption [32].

Interestingly, Indian school children who had been fed a high iron (12.5 mg)-fortified meal for 6 months significantly improved their physical performance, but the intervention did not influence blood Hb concentrations, biochemical parameters and cognitive function. However, a prevalence of anemia was observed to have decreased in children who were fed with a low iron (6.25 mg)-fortified meal [33]. One report has supported the contention that interventions of iron-biofortified food significantly improved the cognitive performance of subjects with regard to attention and memory domains, but did not have an effect on iron deficiency or anemia [15]. In addition, Cambodian school children who were infected with hookworm were associated with low body iron levels and potentially low cognitive performance; however, hook worm infection was found to be more prevalent in the subjects who consumed iron-fortified rice [34,35]. Moreover, consumption of regular Indian rice (1 kg) fortified with FPP (20 mg iron), folic acid (1.3 mg) and vitamin B1, B6 and B12 complexes for 8 months significantly improved the average cognitive performance scores when evaluating subjects with the Annual Status of Education Report of the Pratham Resource Center. These fortifications also increased blood Hb levels in Indian school children [36]. On the other hand, iron deficiency can result in impaired psychomotor development and cognitive function in infants and preschoolers, defective work performance in adults and low birth weights among pregnant women. With regard to neuro-protective properties, tocopherols, such as vitamin E (α-tocopherol), and tocotrienols that are major lipid-soluble chain-breaking antioxidants abundant in rice, have been reported to protect membrane integrity and lipid peroxidation, as well as to inhibit histamine 1 receptor neuronal cells [31,37–39]. Additionally, higher iron intakes associated with many foods have been assessed in elderly populations using dietary pattern studies based on the Reduced Rank Regression or the Food Frequency Questionnaire. It was determined that higher iron intake was associated with a high risk of type 2 diabetes, cognitive impairment, Parkinson's disease and Alzheimer's disease (AD) [40–44]. Specifically, a higher intake of dietary heme-iron, but neither non-heme-iron nor supplemental iron, could result in an increase in an accumulation of iron in the body and brain, along with a risk of iron-related disorders in the elderly. Moreover, cognitive improvement may be associated with the anti-oxidation capabilities of iron-rice drinks, as will be explained in the next section.

It has been reported that weekly consumption of micronized FPP-fortified rice (56.4 mg iron/50 g) for 18 weeks decreased the prevalence of anemia (from 31% to 19%) but did not improve blood Hb levels (before intervention: 11.4 g/dL and after intervention: 11.7 g/dL) in Brazilian infants [45]. However, polished rice that had been fortified with micronized FPP, zinc oxide, thiamin mononitrate and folic acid (50 g serving/day) was found to improve the levels of zinc, thiamine, folic acid, MCH and MCHC significantly within 4 months in Indian preschool children [46]. Likewise, twice-weekly supplementation of iron (30 mg) and folic acid (300 µg) for 20.5 weeks significantly increased blood Hb and serum Ft levels in young Cambodian children with HbA, as well as those with HbE, in which watery stool and restlessness were significantly more prevalent than in the placebo group [47]. More importantly, the treatment of Wistar rats with IR hydrolysate (50 mg/kg) for 90 days significantly increased levels of RBC, Hb, Hct and MCV when compared to the DI control group. This outcome suggests that certain active components, such as high iron content and phytochemicals in the hydrolysate, could effectively enhance erythropoiesis [48]. As is shown in Table 1, the numbers of anemic male and female subjects in group C are nearly the same, whereas there were more non-anemic female subjects in groups A, B and D than male subjects ($p < 0.05$). However, group C had the largest number of 80-year-old subjects ($p < 0.05$). Thus, increased Hb levels among the anemic elders (group G) on the first

15 days resulted from the oral intervention of the Sinlek IR rice beverage, which accelerated the duodenal absorption of dietary iron. In previous studies, women of childbearing age have been known to become anemic during pregnancy due to the massive loss of menstrual blood. In addition, around 22% of Mexican women were found to be anemic as a consequence of their level of iron deficiency (80.8% of the total population). These subjects were also reported to have a low intake of vegetables and citrus fruit that would enhance their levels of iron absorption [49]. All female subjects enrolled in this study had already undergone menopause and were not deficient in iron; therefore, gender was not a confounding factor that contributed to the increased level of hemopoietic activity in group C. During the course of aging, inflammation can have a deleterious effect on hematopoietic stem cell function, self-renewal capacity and RBC membrane integrity, all of which can lead to anemia [50,51]. Results of this study confirm that the blood hemoglobin levels of anemic elders (group C) were increased by oral administration of the iron-rice drink, but this was not the case for female subjects nor those that were of advanced age.

The consumption of FPP-premixed rice significantly increased serum ferritin levels and reduced IDA among Filipino schoolchildren when compared to non-fortified rice used as a control [52]. Furthermore, this supplemented rice diet also increased body iron stores among Indian children [46]. In a current study, healthy women revealed a fractional degree of iron absorption from iron-fortified bouillon cubes in the following order of fortification: ferrous sulfate > *Aspergillus oryzae* grown in FPP > FPP in a positively correlated manner ($p < 0.05$) [53]. Unfortunately, it has been reported that hookworm prevalence was significantly increased from 18.4% by micronutrient-fortified rice formula I (7.55 mg of iron/g) to 22.7% by micronutrient-fortified rice formula II (10.67 mg of iron/g) in Cambodian children, especially in those who live in environments with high-infection areas [35]. Notably, all elderly subjects enrolled in this study lived in the city of Chiang Mai, which is far away from the known prevalent and/or endemic areas of hookworm. Hence, the subjects were not necessarily affected by iron deficiency caused by hookworm infection. This was particularly true for the members of group C, who reported decreased SI levels when compared to the members of the other three groups. Our findings with regard to luminal absorptive iron have revealed an increase in SI and transferrin saturation at 5 h and maximal levels at 15 h in rats that consumed a single IR hydrolysate (500 mg/kg) [48]. Similar to our results, the feeding of rice containing iron-saturated lactoferrin (Lf) at doses of 100–500 mg Lf/kg BW to Wistar rats for 28 days increased RBC numbers ($p < 0.05$) and Hb values, while decreasing SI, increasing TIBC ($p < 0.05$) and unchanging Ft values in the serum when compared with normal saline feeding [54]. It is possible that the iron present in the IR drinks was used as a substrate for de novo synthesis of heme, leading to increases of Hb and RBC production and a decrease in SI. When compared with the other three groups, SI and TIBC levels in group C anemic individuals who consumed the low-dose IR drink tended to decrease during the course of this study; however, there was neither a significant decrease in TIBC (an indirect measure of Tf level) nor a decrease in SI.

Consistent with the increased serum antioxidant capacity, IR hydrolysate exerted higher antioxidant and anti-RBC hemolysis properties in vitro than the WR hydrolysate in a concentration-dependent manner [48]. This outcome was possibly due to the presence of phenolic compounds (e.g., cyanidin, ferulic acid, chlorogenic acid and so on) and γ-oryzanol [31]. In addition, treatments with Thai brown rice (var. Khao Dawk Mali 105) have revealed anti-oxidative protection against carbon tetrachloride-induced hepatotoxicity by inhibiting liver injury, lipid peroxidation, protein oxidation and DNA damage, while decreasing cytochrome P450 (CYP2E isozyme), glutathione S-transferase, glutathione peroxidase, superoxide dismutase and catalase activities. Furthermore, these treatments ultimately reduced the glutathione contents in the livers of laboratory rats. Notably, germinated rice was more significantly effective than un-germinated rice and white rice, respectively. This was possibly due to the existence of phenolic acids, α-oryzanol, tocotrienol and γ-amino butyric acid [54]. Moreover, antioxidant polyphenolic compounds, especially flavonoids, excluding anthocyanin, present in plant-based foods were found to exhibit certain cognitive benefits and protective effects against neurodegenerative diseases, possibly by inhibiting neuroinflammation, improving cerebrovascular blood flow and neuronal synaptic plasticity, inducing angiogenesis and neurogenesis and scavenging neurotoxins in the brain [55–57]. Furthermore, the consumption of polyphenolic-rich diets was found to inhibit neuro-inflammatory processes that are associated with aging people and AD patients via systemic inflammation and human gut microbiome, and may further improve their cognitive decline [58]. Hence, the major active compounds, particularly bioiron and phenolic compounds, that are present in Sinlek iron rice could effectively exert neuro- and erythropoiesis-modulating properties. Consistently, feeding black rice and brown rice (dewaxed and germinated forms) significantly lowered the plasma levels of AST and ALT activities in animals [59–61]. Likewise, ethyl acetate extracts of rice bran and purple rice, predominantly containing ferulic acid and quercetin, significantly decreased levels of plasma TC and LDL-C, along with hepatic lipid in mice and patients with polygenic hypercholesterolemia [62–64]. More importantly, the feeding of red yeast rice together with a Mediterranean diet was more effective in decreasing ($p < 0.05$) serum LDL-C levels in diabetic and dyslipidemic patients than in subjects fed with the diet alone. However, these supplemented diets did not change serum AST and ALT activities [65]. Apparently, the IR drink influenced the levels of serum lipids and liver function enzymes in elderly subjects during the course of this study, suggesting hypolipidemic and hepato-modulating effects.

Study limitations: We assessed the efficacy of the natural IR drink per se in improvement of iron deficiency and IDA in elderly subjects, but did not fortify the drinks with iron compounds or folic acid. In addition, folic acid was not added to the iron rice as a coenzyme for heme synthesis, but it may be persistent in sufficient amounts in the rice or could be derived from luminal normal flora synthesis. The intervention time was only 30 days, which is very short when compared to other clinical trials. Additionally, the responses of erythropoiesis and brain function to the iron-rich food were noticeably slower in the elderly population than in developing children and adolescents. Together, the elders who enrolled in this study did not report a reduction in iron deficiency status and may require a longer period of time to adjust their erythropoietic activity in response to the iron intervention.

4. Materials and Methods

4.1. Materials

4.1.1. Chemicals and Reagents

6-Hydroxy−2,5,7,8-tetramethylchroman−2-carboxylic acid (Trolox) was purchased from Sigma-Aldrich Chemicals, St. Louis, MO, USA. Reagents and calibrators for the analyses of serum cholesterol, triglyceride, glucose, protein and albumin were purchased from Randox Laboratories, Crumin, United Kingdom. Reagents and calibrators for the analysis of SI, TIBC and serum Ft were purchased from Roche Diagnostics Corporation, Indianapolis, IN, United States. All other materials and solvents were of the highest purity or HPLC grade.

4.1.2. Food Ingredients

Sinlek iron rice and Jasmin white rice were purchased from a private organic rice farm located in Doi Saked District, Chiang Mai Province, Thailand. Citric acid monohydrate (food additive, Special Food Supplier, Samuthpakarn, Thailand) without detectable levels of iron, mercury and lead was purchased from Tesco Supermarket in Chiang Mai Province, Thailand. Polyflora bee honey (Food-grade, Eurngluang Brand) was obtained from Polyplus Company Limited, Muang Chiang Mai, Thailand, for which 100 g contained 1.12 g protein, 0 g fats, 8.89 g carbohydrates, 72.28 g natural sugars, 0.75 g dietary fiber, 1.06 mg sodium, 0.33 mg vitamin C, 4.3 mg calcium and 0.21 mg iron. A heat-stable α-amylase (Termamyl®, Novozymes™) obtained from *Bacillus* spp. was purchased from Sigma-Aldrich Chemicals, St. Louis, MO, USA.

4.2. Production of Rice Drink

The rice drink was produced, and chemical compositions were analyzed using the recently published method established by Koonyosying and colleagues [31]. Briefly, rice grains were polished, ground, filtered on nylon 300-µm mesh fabric (Hebei Shangshai Bolting Cloth Manufacturing Company Limited, Shandon, People' Republic of China) and boiled in hot water (6 kg/60 L) at 80 °C for 10 min. After cooling, the rice slurry was incubated with the α-amylase (Termamyl®) at 80 °C for 120 min and digestion was stopped by the immediate heating of the hydrolysate at 100 °C for 10 min. We then used the Design Expert version 6.2.10 Program, Product- and Consumer-Oriented tests, to optimize the ingredient composition and obtain the most suitable products. Rice hydrolysate was filtered, concentrated to 20-Brig dryness, using a freeze-dry lyophilizing machine, acidified to a pH value of 4.0 with 1% (v/v) citric acid, flavored with bee honey, poured into 100 mL glass bottles and sterilized at standard temperature and pressure values. From the inductively coupled plasma mass spectrometric analysis, WR (2 mg iron/100 mL serving), low-dose IR (15 mg iron/100 mL serving) and high-dose IR (27 mg iron/100 mL serving) were provided to each group of the subjects throughout the course of the study [66]. In addition, carbohydrates, protein, fat and the bioactive compounds, including total phenolic (1.15, 1.33 and 2.08 mg gallic acid equivalent, respectively), γ-oryzanol (54, 193 and 316 mg, respectively) and antioxidant capacity (111, 856 and 1400 mg Trolox equivalent, respectively), were comprised in the drinks [31]. Using liquid chromatographic/mass spectrometric analysis, the IR drink has shown the presence of several phenolic compounds, *p*-protocatechuoyl-*O*-glucoside and kaempferol, which were not found in the WR drink [31]. Vitamin C or L-ascorbic acid was analyzed using the high-performance liquid chromatography-diode array detection (HPLC-DAD) method established by Lakshanasomya [67]. Briefly, WR and IR drinks and standard vitamin C (2.5–30 µg/mL) were prepared in 3% meta-phosphoric acid, and the samples (20 µL) were subsequently injected into the HPLC-DAD system (Agilent Series 1100, Agilent Technologies Inc., Santa Clara, CA, USA) connected to a reverse-phase column (C18 type, 125 × 4 mm, 5 µm particle size, Lichrocard, Lichrospher 100, Merck Millipore, Merck KGaA, Darmstadt, Germany). Both were then isocratic eluted with the mobile-phase solvent (3 mM phosphate buffer, pH 3.3 in 0.35% (v/v) 3% meta-phosphoric acid at a flow rate of 0.5 mL/min), while the OD of the eluents was detected at 248 nm. The vitamin C peak of the rice drinks was compared with that of authentic vitamin C at the same retention time and used for the quantification standard established from the calibration curve. In the analysis, the WR drink contained 0.04 mg vitamin C/100 mL per serving, while the low-dose and high-dose IR drinks contained 0.13 and 0.38 mg vitamin C/100 mL per serving, respectively. Essentially, 3.7% (v/v) bee honey as a flavoring agent and 1% citric acid as a stabilizing agent were added to the drinks.

4.3. Subject Recruitment

According to the inclusion criteria, elderly subjects enrolled in this study were aged >60 years living in Chiang Mai and were able to communicate in Thai. The exclusion criteria included the following: ADL score ≤ 11, history of thalassemia, uncontrolled diabetes with FBS > 130 mg/dL or postprandial blood sugar > 180 mg/dL, abnormal bleeding within 3 m, cancer of colon, esophagus, stomach, small intestine, or ampullary, angiodysplasia, celiac disease, gastric antral vascular ectasia, blood donation less than 3 months, *Helicobacter pylori*-infected gastritis, esophagitis, gastrectomy/colectomy, or a period of treatment with proton-pump inhibitors, iron formulations or folic acid.

The sample size (n) was calculated using the following Formula (1):

$$N = (Z_1 - \alpha/2 + Z_1 - \beta)^2 \, [\sigma^2_{treatment} + \sigma^2_{control}/r]/\Delta^2 \tag{1}$$

where $r = n_{control}/n_{treatment}$, $\Delta = \mu_{treatment} - \mu_{control}$, $\alpha = 0.01$, $\beta = 0.2$, $\mu_{treatment} = 11$, $\mu_{control} = 10$ and SD = 1. According to this calculation, 25 volunteers were placed in each group and a value of 10% was then added as a calculated number for the purpose of loss during follow-up. Ultimately, 27 subjects in each group were recruited for this study. We

52. Angeles-Agdeppa, I.; Capanzana, M.V.; Barba, C.V.; Florentino, R.F.; Takanashi, K. Efficacy of iron-fortified rice in reducing anemia among schoolchildren in the Philippines. *Int. J. Vitam. Nutr. Res.* **2008**, *78*, 74–86. [CrossRef]
53. Bries, A.E.; Hurrell, R.F.; Reddy, M.B. Iron absorption from bouillon fortified with iron-enriched *Aspergillus oryzae* Is higher than that fortified with ferric pyrophosphate in young women. *J. Nutr.* **2020**, *150*, 1109–1115. [CrossRef]
54. Cerven, D.; DeGeorge, G.; Bethell, D. 28-Day repeated dose oral toxicity of recombinant human apo-lactoferrin or recombinant human lysozyme in rats. *Regul. Toxicol. Pharmacol.* **2008**, *51*, 162–167. [CrossRef]
55. Commenges, D.; Scotet, V.; Renaud, S.; Jacqmin-Gadda, H.; Barberger-Gateau, P.; Dartigues, J.F. Intake of flavonoids and risk of dementia. *Eur. J. Epidemiol.* **2000**, *16*, 357–363. [CrossRef] [PubMed]
56. Vauzour, D.; Vafeiadou, K.; Rodriguez-Mateos, A.; Rendeiro, C.; Spencer, J.P. The neuroprotective potential of flavonoids: A multiplicity of effects. *Genes Nutr.* **2008**, *3*, 115–126. [CrossRef] [PubMed]
57. Caldwell, K.; Charlton, K.E.; Roodenrys, S.; Jenner, A. Anthocyanin-rich cherry juice does not improve acute cognitive performance on RAVLT. *Nutr. Neurosci.* **2015**, *19*, 423–424. [CrossRef] [PubMed]
58. McGrattan, A.M.; McGuinness, B.; McKinley, M.C.; Kee, F.; Passmore, P.; Woodside, J.V.; McEvoy, C.T. Diet and inflammation in cognitive ageing and Alzheimer's disease. *Curr. Nutr. Rep.* **2019**, *8*, 53–65. [CrossRef]
59. Inagawa, H.; Saika, T.; Nishiyama, N.; Nisizawa, T.; Kohchi, C.; Uenobe, M.; Soma, G.I. Dewaxed brown rice feed improves fatty liver in obese and diabetic model mice. *Anticancer Res.* **2018**, *38*, 4339–4345. [CrossRef]
60. Hou, Z.; Qin, P.; Ren, G. Effect of anthocyanin-rich extract from black rice (*Oryza sativa* L. Japonica) on chronically alcohol-induced liver damage in rats. *J. Agric. Food Chem.* **2010**, *58*, 3191–3196. [CrossRef]
61. Mohd Esa, N.; Abdul Kadir, K.K.; Amom, Z.; Azlan, A. Antioxidant activity of white rice, brown rice and germinated brown rice (in vivo and in vitro) and the effects on lipid peroxidation and liver enzymes in hyperlipidaemic rabbits. *Food Chem.* **2013**, *141*, 1306–1312. [CrossRef] [PubMed]
62. Jung, E.H.; Kim, S.R.; Hwang, I.K.; Ha, T.Y. Hypoglycemic effects of a phenolic acid fraction of rice bran and ferulic acid in C57BL/KsJ-db/db mice. *J. Agric. Food Chem.* **2007**, *55*, 9800–9804. [CrossRef] [PubMed]
63. Shen, Y.; Chen, L.; Zhang, H.; Zhang, Y.; Wang, L.; Qian, H.; Qi, X. In vitro and in vivo antioxidant activity of ethyl acetate extraction of purple rice. *Cell Mol. Biol. (Noisy-le-grand)* **2016**, *62*, 96–103.
64. Cicero, A.F.G.; Fogacci, F.; Bove, M.; Veronesi, M.; Rizzo, M.; Giovannini, M.; Borghi, C. Short-term effects of a combined nutraceutical on lipid level, fatty liver biomarkers, hemodynamic parameters, and estimated cardiovascular disease risk: A double-blind, placebo-controlled randomized clinical trial. *Adv. Ther.* **2017**, *34*, 1966–1975. [CrossRef] [PubMed]
65. Sartore, G.; Seraglia, R.; Burlina, S.; Bolis, A.; Marin, R.; Manzato, E.; Ragazzi, E.; Traldi, P.; Lapolla, A. High-density lipoprotein oxidation in type 2 diabetic patients and young patients with premature myocardial infarction. *Nutr. Metab. Cardiovasc. Dis.* **2014**, *25*, 418–425. [CrossRef]
66. Nuttall, K.L.; Gordon, W.H.; Ash, K.O. Inductively coupled plasma mass spectrometry for trace element analysis in the clinical laboratory. *Ann. Clin. Lab. Sci.* **1995**, *25*, 264–271.
67. *Compendium of Methods for Food Analysis/cDepartment of Medical Sciences and National Bureau of Agriculture Commodity and Food Standards*; Department of Medical Sciences and National Bureau of Agriculture Commodity and Food Standards, Ministry of Public Health: Nonthaburi, Thailand, 2003.
68. Boonvisudhi, T.; Kuladee, S. Association between internet addiction and depression in Thai medical students at Faculty of Medicine, Ramathibodi Hospital. *PLoS One* **2017**, *12*, e0174209. [CrossRef]
69. Senanarong, V.; Vannasaeng, S.; Poungvarin, N.; Ploybutr, S.; Udompunthurak, S.; Jamjumras, P.; Fairbanks, L.; Cummings, J.L. Endogenous estradiol in elderly individuals: Cognitive and noncognitive associations. *Arch. Neurol.* **2002**, *59*, 385–389. [CrossRef]
70. Trongsakul, S.; Lambert, R.; Clark, A.; Wongpakaran, N.; Cross, J. Development of the Thai version of Mini-Cog, a brief cognitive screening test. *Geriatr. Gerontol. Int.* **2014**, *15*, 594–600. [CrossRef]
71. Velasco-Rodriguez, R.; Perez-Hernandez, M.G.; Mora-Brambila, A.B.; Bazan-Arellano, D.A.; Vasquez, C. Serum ferritin and nutritional status in older adults at eldercare facilities. *J. Nutr. Health Aging* **2012**, *16*, 525–528. [CrossRef]
72. Schlosnagle, D.C.; Hutton, P.S.; Conn, R.B. Ferrozine assay of serum iron and total iron-binding capacity adapted to the COBAS BIO centrifugal analyzer. *Clin. Chem.* **1982**, *28*, 1730–1732. [CrossRef] [PubMed]

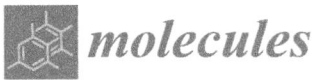

Article

Stress-Relieving Effects of Sesame Oil Aroma and Identification of the Active Components

Hiroaki Takemoto [1,*], Yuki Saito [2], Kei Misumi [2], Masaki Nagasaki [2] and Yoshinori Masuo [2,*]

1. Department of Molecular Toxicology, Faculty of Pharmaceutical Sciences, Toho University, 2-2-1 Miyama, Funabashi, Chiba 274-8510, Japan
2. Laboratory of Neuroscience, Department of Biology, Faculty of Science, Toho University, 2-2-1 Miyama, Funabashi, Chiba 274-8510, Japan; 5218033s@st.toho-u.ac.jp (Y.S.); 5218077m@st.toho-u.ac.jp (K.M.); 5218056n@st.toho-u.ac.jp (M.N.)
* Correspondence: hiroaki.takemoto@phar.toho-u.ac.jp (H.T.); yoshinori.masuo@bio.sci.toho-u.ac.jp (Y.M.); Tel.: +81-47-472-2539 (H.T.); +81-47-472-5257 (Y.M.)

Abstract: (1) Sesame oil aroma has stress-relieving properties, but there is little information on its effective use and active ingredients. (2) Methods: ICR male mice were housed under water-immersion stress for 24 h. Then, the scent of sesame oil or a typical ingredient was inhaled to the stress groups for 30, 60, or 90 min. We investigated the effects of sesame oil aroma on mice behavior and the expression of the dual specificity phosphatase 1 (*DUSP1*) gene, a candidate stress marker gene in the brain. (3) Results: In an elevated plus-maze test, the rate of entering into the open arm of a maze and the staying time were increased to a maximum after 60 min of inhalation, but these effects decreased 90 min after inhalation. As for the single component, anxiolytic effects were observed in the 2,5-dimethylpyrazine and 2-methoxy phenol group, but the effect was weakened in the furfuryl mercaptan group. The expression levels of *DUSP1* in the hippocampus and striatum were significantly decreased in 2,5-dimethylpyrazine and 2-methoxy phenol groups. (4) Conclusions: We clarified the active ingredients and optimal concentrations of sesame oil for its sedative effect. In particular, 2,5-dimethylpyrazine and 2-methoxy phenol significantly suppressed the stress-induced changes in the expression of *DUSP1*, which are strong anti-stress agents. Our results suggest that these molecules may be powerful anti-stress agents.

Keywords: sesame oil aroma; 2,5-dimethylpyrazine; 2-methoxy phenol; water-immersion stress; antianxiety; elevated plus-maze test; dual specificity phosphatase 1

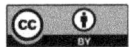

1. Introduction

Central nervous system disorders have a great impact on society due to the general aging process of the population and lifestyle factors. Stress is one of the most prevalent psychological disorders in developed countries and leads to other clinical concerns, such as anxiety, insomnia, or depression [1]. Prolonged periods of stress produce deleterious effects that might become chronic and/or life-threatening. These effects are related to its involvement in medical conditions such as metabolic syndrome, cardiovascular disease, type 2 diabetes mellitus, allergies, and autoimmune diseases. Furthermore, brain disorders and functions are notably influenced by stress. Its role in precipitating psychiatric pathologies is either suggested or demonstrated for conditions such as mood disorders, anxiety disorders, and post-traumatic stress disorder [2].

Benzodiazepines (BZD) and selective serotonin reuptake inhibitors (SSRIs) are highly prescribed as anxiolytic and antidepressant drugs, respectively. BZD, such as diazepam, lorazepam, or alprazolam, produces calming effects via binding to $GABA_A$ receptors but may also produce somnolence, cognitive impairment, and ataxia as adverse drug reactions [3]. SSRIs (e.g., fluoxetine, paroxetine, and citalopram) are prescribed as antidepressants because they are able to selectively block the serotonin transporter, but side effects include sexual dysfunction, sleep disturbance, and suicidal tendencies [4]. Both groups of medicines can produce withdrawal and rebound effects when their use discontinues.

Phytotherapy has recently attracted much attention for reducing daily stress and preventing central disorders. Particularly, essential oils have a long tradition in pharmaceutical sciences as natural products with pharmacological, cosmetic, and nutritional applications [5]. The use of essential oil in the form of aromatherapy is widely extended, with some of them being used as agents to relieve anxiety and stress [6]. For example, lavender essential oil is traditionally used and approved by the European Medicines Agency as herbal medicine to relieve stress and anxiety [1].

Previously, we investigated the anti-stress effect of sesame oil aroma [7]. Various kinds of foods have drawn attention in recent years due to their stress relaxation effects. Sesame seeds have been a popular healthy food product in Japan since ancient times, and Japan imports the second-largest amount as a nation, following the US and Europe [8]. Sesame lignans, which show antioxidant effects, are known as the most popular active ingredient in sesame, while sesame seeds have a characteristic aroma. When mice were subjected to 24 h of water-immersion stress as a sleep-disordered stress, the number of entries into the open arm of the maze decreased, and anxiety-like behavior was observed in the elevated plus-maze test. However, the inhalation of sesame oil aroma for 90 min after water-immersion stress attenuated the anxiety-like behavior.

Furthermore, the expression of *DUSP1* (dual specificity phosphatase 1) gene was investigated. *DUSP* is known to be negative regulators of the mitogen-activated protein kinase cascade and modulate diverse neural functions, such as neurogenesis, differentiation, and apoptosis. *DUSP* genes have furthermore been associated with mental disorders such as depression and neurological disorders [9]. Although the expression of *DUSP1* in the brain was increased by water-immersion stress, the increased level was significantly attenuated by the sesame oil aroma.

The unique fragrance ingredients of roasted sesame seeds are composed of several molecules. Xiao Jia et al. reported that fifteen volatile compounds with the highest odor activity values were selected as the key odors contributing to the flavor profile of sesame oil aroma, including 2-methyl-propanal, 2-methyl-butanal, furaneol, 1-octen-3-one, 4-methyl-3-penten-2-one, 1-nonanol, 2-methyl-phenol, 2-methoxy phenol, 2-methoxy-4-vinylphenol, 2,5-dimethylpyrazine, 2-furfuryl mercaptan, 2-thiophenemethanethiol, methanethiol, methional, and dimethyl trisulfide [10]. Generally, sulfur-containing compounds, pyrroles, and pyrazines seem to play important roles in the characteristic odor of sesame oil. Furthermore, among these compounds, pyrazines are major volatiles in sesame oil [11]. They are commonly found in the aroma of roasted coffee [12], and it has been reported that coffee bean volatiles have anxiolytic and hypnotic effects in mice [13].

In the present study, we analyzed the effect of sesame oil aroma in more detail. Fragrance inhalation has primary effects and toxic effects, so the optimal duration of inhalation administration was determined. Furthermore, we identified the active components of sesame oil aroma. Previously, pyrazines, methoxyphenols, and sulfur compounds were detected from sesame oil aroma by GC-MS analysis. We investigated the anxiolytic effect of 2,5-dimethylpyrazine, 2-methoxy phenol, and furfuryl mercaptan (Figure 1). In this study, to obtain the data for the effective use of sesame oil scent, an analysis was conducted of the anti-stress effects of sesame oil at different inhalation times, and the effects of typical compounds contained in sesame oil were evaluated from the elevated plus-maze test and analysis of genetic variation by real-time PCR.

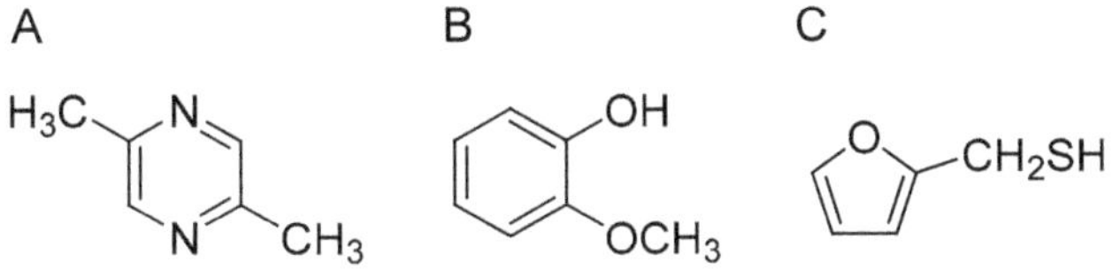

Figure 1. Chemical structures of 2,5-dimethylpyrazine (**A**), 2-methoxy phenol (**B**), and furfuryl mercaptan (**C**).

2. Results

2.1. Anxiolytic Effect of Sesame Oil Aroma

After 24 h of stress-loading, the mice inhaled sesame oil aroma for 0 min, 30 min, 60 min, or 90 min. In an elevated plus-maze test, the number of entries into each of the open arms of the maze and the closed arm was measured, and a ratio of the open arm entry number per entry number to the open and closed arms was calculated as the open arm entry rate (Figure 2A). Figure 2B shows the staying time in the open arm. The average value of the open arm entry rate of the 0 min group was 23.6%, while it was 65.8% for the 30 min group and 90.2% for the 60 min group (Figure 2A). The ratio of the open arm entry increase was dependent on the inhalation time. However, the 90 min group value was 62.8%, indicating a decrease in the anxiolytic effect. The result of the staying time in the open arm was similar to that of the open arm entry rate. The average value of the staying time in the open arm of the 0 min group was 128.8 s, while it was 312.7 s for the 30 min group and 391.0 s for the 60 min group (Figure 2B). However, the value in the 90 min group was 253.3 s. These results suggest that the odor of sesame oil may have an anxiety-depressing action. A significant stress-reducing effect was found to appear 30 min after inhalation administration, and it was found that the greatest effect was observed 60 min after inhalation administration.

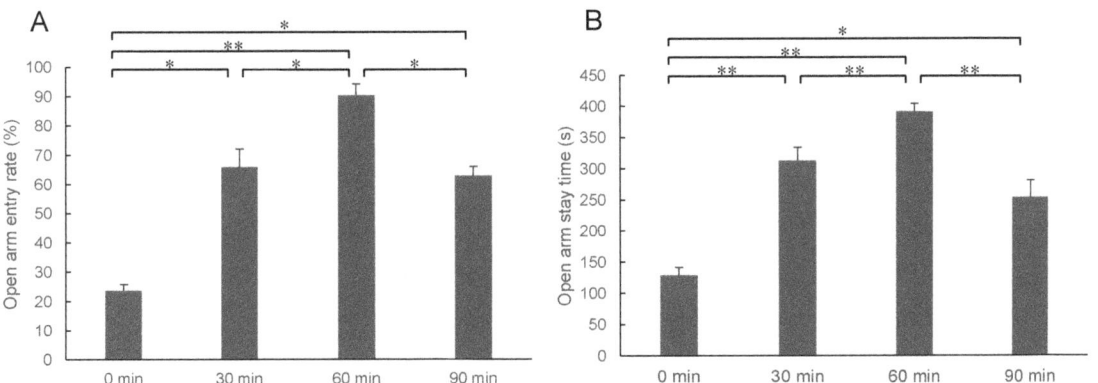

Figure 2. Elevated plus-maze test. (**A**) Open arm entry rate (%), (**B**) open arm stay time (s). Results represent mean ± SEM (n = 6). * $p < 0.05$, ** $p < 0.01$ (Two-way ANOVA followed by Tukey's test or Student's *t*-test).

2.2. Anxiolytic Effect of Constituents of Sesame Oil Aroma

After 24 h of stress-loading, the mice inhaled 2,5-dimethylpyrazine, 2-methoxy phenol, or furfuryl mercaptan, a constituent of sesame oil aroma, for 30 min. The open arm entry rate and the staying time in the open arm are shown in Figure 3. The open arm entry rate of the sesame oil group was 65.8%, while that of the 2,5-dimethylpyrazine group was 83.3%, and that of the 2-methoxy phenol group was 88.2%. However, the effect of furfuryl mercaptan was weakened, and the open arm entry rate was only 22.6% (Figure 3A). Similarly, the staying time in the open arm of the 2,5-dimethylpyrazine (479.7 s) and 2-methoxy phenol groups (519.4 s) were longer than that of sesame oil (312.7 s), while that of the furfuryl mercaptan group (118.3 s) was significantly shorter than that of sesame oil (312.7 s) (Figure 3B). These results suggested that 2,5-dimethylpyrazine and 2-methoxy phenol are the active ingredients involved in the stress-relieving effect of sesame oil.

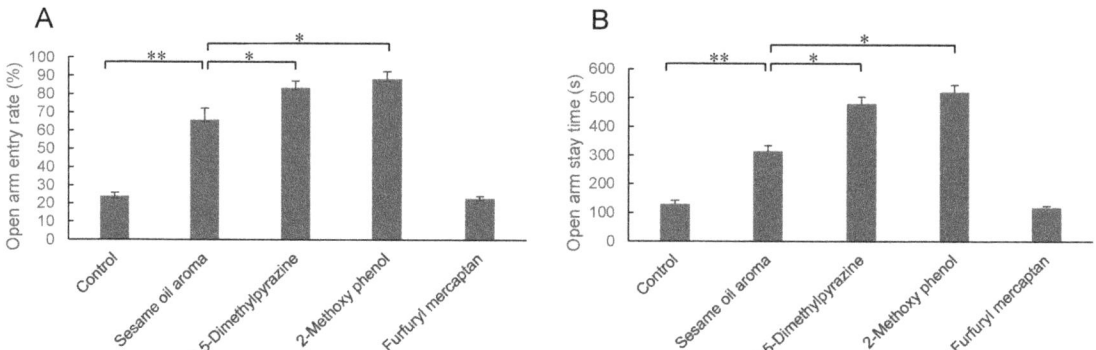

Figure 3. Elevated plus-maze test. (**A**): open arm entry rate (%), (**B**): open arm stay time (s). Results represent mean ± SEM (n = 6). * $p < 0.05$, ** $p < 0.01$ (Two-way ANOVA followed by Tukey's test or Student's t-test).

2.3. DUSP1 Expression after Sesame Oil Aroma Inhalation

After 24 h of stress-loading, the mice inhaled sesame oil aroma for 0 min, 30 min, 60 min, or 90 min. The expression levels of *DUSP1* gene were measured at the end of inhalation administration (Figure 4). The expression level of *DUSP1* in the hippocampus was significantly increased in the 30 min inhalation group ($p < 0.05$, two-way ANOVA). However, the expression levels in the 60 and 90 min inhalation groups decreased (Figure 4A). On the other hand, in the striatum, the expression level significantly decreased after 30 min and 60 min inhalation, and this tendency was also observed in 90 min inhalation group (Figure 4B).

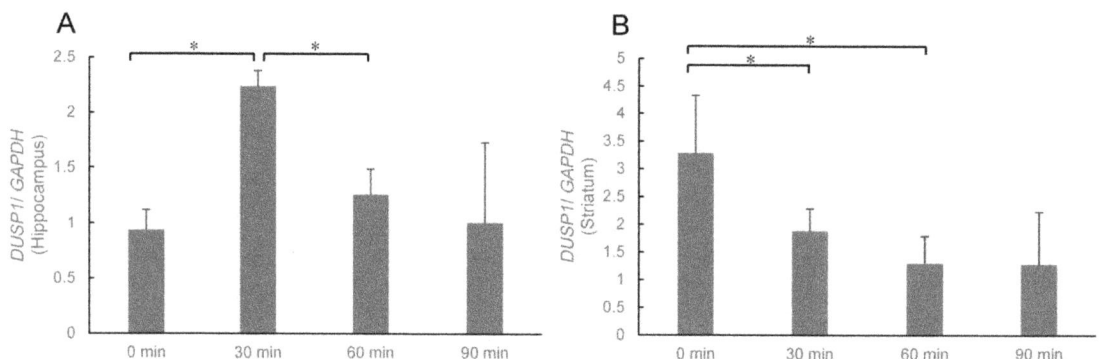

Figure 4. Expression level of *DUSP1* in the hippocampus (**A**) and striatum (**B**). Results show means ± SEM (control/saline, stress/saline, control/sesame, stress/sesame, n = 6). * $p < 0.05$ (two-way ANOVA followed by Tukey's test or Student's t-test).

2.4. DUSP1 Expression after Inhalation of Constituents of Sesame Oil Aroma

After 24 h of stress-loading, the mice inhaled 2,5-dimethylpyrazine, 2-methoxy phenol, or furfuryl mercaptan for 90 min (Figure 5). The expression level in both the striatum and hippocampus significantly decreased in the 2,5-dimethylpyrazine and 2-methoxy phenol groups ($p < 0.05$, two-way ANOVA). The effect of furfuryl mercaptan was lower than the other two compounds, and the expression level tended to decrease; however, there were no significant differences.

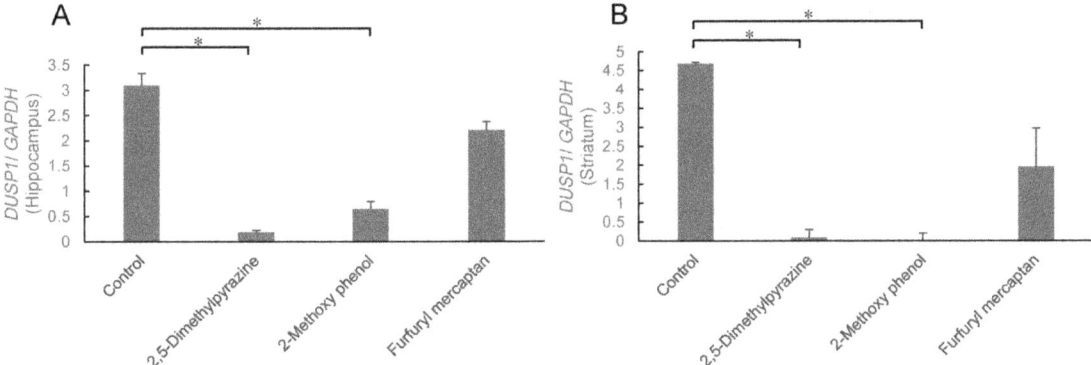

Figure 5. Expression level of *DUSP1* in the hippocampus (**A**) and striatum (**B**). Results show means ± SEM (control/saline, stress/saline, control/sesame, stress/sesame, n = 6). * $p < 0.05$ (two-way ANOVA followed by Tukey's test or Student's *t*-test).

3. Discussion

We have previously reported that sesame oil aroma has an anti-stress effect [7]. In the present study, we performed a detailed analysis of the functionality of sesame oil aroma. Firstly, the effect of inhalation time on the anti-stress effect was analyzed. To evaluate the effect of anti-stress on behavior, we conducted an elevated plus-maze test. The water-immersion stress has been shown to reduce the penetration rate to the open arm and the staying time in the open arms [7]. The anti-stress effect of sesame oil aroma appeared 30 min after inhalation, and the effect was even stronger 60 min after inhalation (Figure 2). On the other hand, the anti-stress effect weakened after 90 min of inhalation. It is known that the inhaled volatile constituents act on the central nervous system through olfactory nerves and the bloodstream [14]. It was suggested that the increased blood levels of the active ingredient in sesame oil may cause toxicity after 90 min of inhalation.

Lavender oil mainly includes linalool and linalyl acetate, and it has been reported that linalool has a sedative effect on humans by vapor inhalation at low doses [15]. However, it also has nerve toxicity, and the LC_{50} for mammals is 2740 mg/m^3 [16]. We previously investigated the relationship between blood concentration of fragrance components and onset of the sedative effect by intravenous administration test. Valerena-4,7(11)-diene, a component of *Valeriana officinalis* oil, was administered intravenously at doses of 10, 100, and 1000 μg/kg, and open field tests were performed. Sedative effects were greater in the 100 μg/kg group than in the 10 μg/kg group; however, treatment with 1000 μg/kg caused a decreasing effect, suggesting an overdose. It was suggested that prolonged inhalation of sesame oil flavor weakened anti-stress effects.

We then examined *DUSP1* gene expressions in the hippocampus and striatum. The hippocampus plays an important role in stress regulation. It exerts inhibitory control over hypothalamic-pituitary-adrenal-axis activity and is also more broadly involved in cognitive and affective processing via its widespread connections with other limbic prefrontal regions [17]. The striatum is classically described as playing a key role in motor function and is a part of the basal ganglia, which is important for adjusting the execution of motor habits. Thus, deficits in motor automaticity are a characteristic of basal ganglia-related illnesses, such as Parkinson's disease.

Furthermore, anxiety, one of the main symptoms of depression, may be regulated by the striatum. As one of the striatum-related circuit mechanisms underlying anxiety, the striatal–prefrontal pathway is involved and becomes less connected, the cortico-striatal connections are also impaired, and anxiety is expressed [18]. It is known that the expression level of *DUSP1* is elevated in the rat brain experiencing chronic stress [19] and decreased by treatment with antidepressants [20]. *DUSP1* gene may be a representative of a promising new drug target for the treatment of depression and other mood disorders. The present study demonstrated that the scent of sesame oil significantly inhibited the expression level of *DUSP1* in the striatum. On the other hand, the level in the hippocampus was increased instantaneously in 30 min inhalation group (Figure 4).

In the present study, we further analyzed the anti-stress effects of typical aromatic components of sesame oil by inhalation administration. 2,5-Dimethylpyrazine and 2-methoxy phenol showed stronger anti-stress effects than sesame oil, while furfuryl mercaptan had no effect (Figure 3). Pyrazines and phenols are also commonly found in the roasted aroma of coffee and tea. These compounds have been suggested to have a stress-reducing effect [21] 2,5-Dimethylpyrazine 2-methoxy phenol, roasted aroma contained in sesame oil, seems to be an active ingredient involved in its stress-reducing effects. It is reported the effect of alkylpyrazine derivatives on pentobarbital-induced sleeping time, picrotoxin-induced convulsion, and γ-aminobutyric acid levels in mouse brain [21]. These results suggest that alkylpyrazine derivatives may strengthen the GABAnergic system in the brain.

On the other hand, sulfur compounds such as furfuryl mercaptan have also been identified as the characteristic aroma component in roasted coffee, wheat bread, and popcorn, and these compounds were confirmed as key contributors to the flavor of sesame seeds [22]. Furfuryl mercaptan did not show anti-stress effects in the elevated plus-maze test, and the expression level of *DUSP1* tended to decrease but did not differ from the control. Unpleasant smelling gases such as halitosis are caused by volatile sulphur compounds such as hydrogen sulphide, methyl mercaptan, and dimethyl sulphide [23]. Furfuryl mercaptan may also exhibit anti-stress effects, although the concentration used in this experiment is considered to be the borderline concentration at which both pleasant and unpleasant effects appear. Therefore, it is necessary to verify the effect of low concentrations of furfuryl mercaptan in the future. *DUSP1* in the hippocampus was elevated 30 min after sesame oil administration, but this may be due to an unpleasant odor. However, the level of *DUSP1* decreased after 60 min of sesame oil administration, which may reflect the anti-stress effects of the compounds found in this study. The anti-stress effects of sesame oil may be maximized with 60 min of inhalation.

The safety of sesame oil has been tested for lignans [24]. A single-blind, placebo-controlled, parallel-group, and multiple oral dose study was conducted on 48 healthy subjects to investigate the pharmacokinetics and safety of multiple oral doses of sesame lignans (sesamin and episesamin). No serious adverse events were observed in this study. The pharmacokinetic study results demonstrate that no accumulation was observed following multiple 50 mg doses of sesame lignans. Therefore, the use of fragrances, especially for their anti-stress effects, is considered safe to use.

Recently, aromatherapy has attracted much attention as an alternative medicine, especially for psychosomatic diseases caused by stress. We have studied the effects of the odor of sesame oil and clarified the optimal time for inhalation of sesame oil, which has a sedative effect. Furthermore, we found that the sesame odor components, 2,5-dimethylpyrazine and 2-methoxy phenol, significantly suppressed stress-induced changes in the expression of *DUSP1*, a candidate stress marker gene in the striatum and hippocampus.

4. Materials and Methods
4.1. Materials

Aromatic sesame oil used in this study was purchased from Kuki Sangyo Co., Ltd. (Mie, Japan). This oil was produced by pressing and extracting white sesame seeds from Guatemala, followed by a cooling process. 2,5-Dimethylpyrazine (purity > 98%, GC), 2-methoxy phenol (purity > 98%, GC) and furfuryl mercaptan (purity > 98%, GC) were purchased from Tokyo Chemical Industry Co., Ltd. (Tokyo, Japan).

4.2. Animal Experiment

This study was carried out according to the animal experiment handling provisions of Toho University's Animal Experiment Committee. The committee approved the animal experiment design plan. ICR male mice at 5 weeks of age purchased from Clea Japan (Tokyo, Japan) were housed in an acrylic cage, three animals per cage, and kept under the 12 h light/dark cycle (light period 08:00–20:00) at 24 ± 2 °C. Food and water were allowed ad libitum. After adapting to the rearing environment for over a week, mice were randomly divided into groups of four mice per group. All groups of mice were bred for 24 h in a cage with water to the extent to which the limb of the mouse is immersed (water depth of about 1 cm), whereby the mice experience a stress response due to the induced discomfort and insomnia [25]. The inhalation commenced at 10:30, just after 24 h of stress-loading. The odor was placed in a glass box in which a piece of filter paper was impregnated with 50 µL of sesame oil, or 5 µL of 2,5-dimethylpyrazine, 2-methoxy phenol, or furfuryl mercaptan was adhered to the inside, and mice inhaled for 30, 60, or 90 min. Physiological saline was used as a control. After completing the inhalation administration, behavioral tests and dissections were performed as follows. This study was carried out according to the animal experiment handling provision by Toho University Animal Experiment Committee. The animal experiment design plan has been approved by the committee (approval number: 21-31-476, date: 1 April 2021).

4.3. Behavioral Analysis

The evaluation of anxiety-like behavior was performed by the elevated plus-maze test for 10 min just after completion of the inhalation of the aroma. The maze consists of an arm length of 30 cm, an arm width of 5 cm, a height from the floor of 60 cm, and a closed arm wall height of 20 cm. Immediately after putting the mouse in the center of the maze, the behavior of the animals was recorded with a video camera. The number of entering the open arm and the staying time and the number of entering into the closed arm and the staying time, were automatically recorded using the behavioral tracking software ANY-maze (Muromachi Kikai, Tokyo, Japan) [7].

4.4. Total RNA Extraction

The mice were decapitated, and the whole brains were collected. The whole brain was dissected on ice, and the striatum and hippocampus were sampled. The brain tissue was immediately frozen in liquid nitrogen, and the frozen tissue was pulverized in liquid nitrogen to convert it into powder form. One milliliter of Qiazol (Qiagen, Hilden, Germany) was added to each brain tissue sample and stirred until the sample was completely dissolved. The total RNA was extracted with RNeasy Mini Kit (Qiagen) and RNase-Free DNase set (Qiagen) as per the manufacturer's protocols. The RNA was dissolved in RNase-free water, and the concentration and the purity of the obtained total RNA were measured using NanoDrop (Thermo Fisher Scientific, Waltham, MA, USA). Samples with a low purity were ethanol-precipitated with Ethachinmate (Nippon Jean, Tokyo, Japan). The total RNA was stored at -80 °C [7].

4.5. cDNA Synthesis

Reverse transcription was performed from the obtained RNA to synthesize cDNA using ReverTra Ace® qPCR RT Master Mix (Toyobo, Osaka, Japan). First, the amount of sample was calculated so that the RNA concentration of each sample was 1 pg/µL to 1 µg/µL in 10 µL. A total of 6 µL of nuclease-free water was added to 2 µL of each sample, and 2 µL of 2 × RT Master Mix (ReverTra Ace® qPCR RT Master Mix, Toyobo) was added. cDNA was synthesized by reverse transcription using GeneAmp PCR System 9700 (Applied Biosystems, Thermo Fisher Scientific). The conditions for cDNA synthesis were 15 min at 37 °C, 5 min at 50 °C, and 5 min at 98 °C. The synthesized cDNA was stored at -20 °C [7].

4.6. Real-Time Reverse Transcription-Polymerase Chain Reaction (Real-Time RT-PCR)

For real-time RT-PCR, we used a TB Green Premix Ex Taq II (Takara Bio, Shiga, Japan). For each 2 µL of the cDNA sample, 1.6 µL of primer (Forward and Reverse, 0.8 µL each) (Table 1) (Takara Bio) was added, and 8.5 µL of RNase free water, 12.5 µL of TB Green Premix Ex Taq II and 0.4 µL of Rox Reference Dye was added to make a total of 25 µL. The expression level of cDNA was measured using an Applied Biosystems® 7500 real-time PCR system (Thermo Fisher Scientific). The holding stage was at 50 °C for 2 min and 95 °C for 10 min. The cycling stage for 40 cycles was at 95 °C for 15 s, and 60 °C for 1 min. The melt curve stage was at 95 °C for 15 s, 60 °C for 1 min, 95 °C for 30 s, and 60 °C for 15 s. The analysis of the gene expression level of each sample was carried out in comparison with the expression level of glyceraldehyde 3-phosphate dehydrogenase (*GAPDH*), which is a housekeeping gene. The expression levels of *DUSP1* were calculated as correction values divided by the expression level of *GAPDH*. The primer sequences of each gene used in this study were the same as in the previous report [7].

Table 1. The primer sequence of each gene measured in the present study.

Gene	Primer
GAPDH	Forward: 5′-GGGTCCCAGCTTAGGTTCATCA-3′
	Reverse: 5′-GTTCACACCCACCTTCACCATT-3′
DUSP1	Forward: 5′-CGCAGTGCCTGTTGTTGGA-3′
	Reverse: 5′-TGAAGCGCACGTTCACTGAG-3′

4.7. Statistical Analysis

The results were expressed as mean ± SEM. ANOVA analysis was performed for the significance among four groups, and further analysis was conducted using the Tukey method. In some cases, the results were analyzed by a Student's *t*-test to determine the significant difference between the two groups. $p < 0.05$ was considered to be statistically significant. Analyses were performed with BellCurve for Excel (Social Survey Research Information Co., Ltd. Tokyo, Japan).

5. Conclusions

The effect of sesame oil aroma and its associated typical ingredients on behavior and stress-related biomarkers was investigated. In an elevated plus-maze test, the anxiolytic effect of sesame oil aroma was observed to maximum after 60 min inhalation, but the effect was decreased 90 min after inhalation. As for the single component, anxiolytic effects were observed in the 2,5-dimethylpyrazine and 2-methoxy phenol groups, but the effect was weakened in the furfuryl mercaptan group. The expression of *DUSP1* also showed similar results to an elevated plus-maze test. We clarified the sesame oil's active ingredients and optimal concentrations for its sedative effects. 2,5-Dimethylpyrazine and 2-methoxy phenol significantly suppressed the stress-induced changes in the expression of *DUSP1*, a candidate stress marker gene in the striatum and hippocampus.

Author Contributions: H.T. and Y.M. designed the experiments and analyzed the data; H.T., Y.S., K.M. and M.N. performed the experiments; Y.M. conceptualized and oversaw the project; H.T. and Y.M. co-wrote the manuscript. All authors have read and agreed to the published version of the manuscript.

Funding: This research was supported by the Grant-in-Aid for Young Scientists (19K16400) of the Japan Science and Technology Agency (JST), Japan donated to H.T.

Institutional Review Board Statement: This study was carried out according to the animal experiment handling provision by Toho University Animal Experiment Committee. The animal experiment design plan has been approved by the committee (approval number: 21-31-476, date: 1 April 2021).

Informed Consent Statement: Not applicable.

Data Availability Statement: The data presented in this study are available on request from the corresponding author.

Acknowledgments: The authors are grateful to Kazuo Koike (Toho University) and Tadaaki Sato (International University of Health and Welfare). This research was conducted in collaboration with the Research and Development department of the Kewpie Corporation.

Conflicts of Interest: The authors declare no conflict of interest.

References

1. López, V.; Nielsen, B.; Solas, M.; Ramírez, M.J.; Jäger, A.K. Exploring Pharmacological Mechanisms of Lavender (*Lavandula angustifolia*) Essential Oil on Central Nervous System Targets. *Front. Pharmacol.* **2017**, *19*, 280. [CrossRef]
2. Moreno-Rius, J. The cerebellum under stress. *Front. Neuroendocrinol.* **2019**, *54*, 100774. [CrossRef]
3. Atkin, T.; Comai, S.; Gobbi, G. Drugs for Insomnia beyond Benzodiazepines: Pharmacology, Clinical Applications, and Discovery. *Pharmacol. Rev.* **2018**, *70*, 197–245. [CrossRef]
4. Papakostas, G.I. Tolerability of modern antidepressants. *J. Clin. Psychiatry* **2008**, *69*, 8–13.
5. Bakkali, F.; Averbeck, S.; Averbeck, D.; Waomar, M. Biological effects of essential oils—A review. *Food Chem. Toxicol.* **2007**, *46*, 446–475. [CrossRef]
6. Setzer, W.N. Essential oils and anxiolytic aromatherapy. *Nat. Prod. Commun.* **2009**, *4*, 1305–1316. [CrossRef]
7. Takemoto, H.; Take, C.; Kojima, K.; Kuga, Y.; Hamada, T.; Yasugi, T.; Kato, N.; Koike, K.; Masuo, Y. Effects of Sesame Oil Aroma on Mice after Exposure to Water Immersion Stress: Analysis of Behavior and Gene Expression in the Brain. *Molecules* **2020**, *24*, 5915. [CrossRef]
8. Morris, J.B. Food, industrial, nutraceutical, and pharmaceutical uses of sesame genetic resources. In *Trends in New Crops and New Uses*; Janick, J., Whipkey, A., Eds.; ASHS Press: Alexandria, VA, USA, 2002; pp. 153–156.
9. An, N.; Bassil, K.; Al Jowf, G.I.; Steinbusch, H.W.M.; Rothermel, M.; de Nijs, L.; Rutten, B.P.F. Dual-specificity phosphatases in mental and neurological disorders. *Prog. Neurobiol.* **2021**, *198*, 101906.
10. Jia, X.; Zhou, Q.; Wang, J.; Liu, C.; Huang, F.; Huang, Y. Identification of key aroma-active compounds in sesame oil from microwaved seeds using E-nose and HS-SPME-GC×GC-TOF/MS. *J. Food Biochem.* **2019**, *43*, e12786.
11. Park, M.H.; Jeong, M.K.; Yeo, J.; Son, H.J.; Lim, C.L.; Hong, E.J.; Noh, B.S.; Lee, J. Application of solid phase-microextraction (SPME) and electronic nose techniques to differentiate volatiles of sesame oils prepared with diverse roasting conditions. *J. Food Sci.* **2011**, *76*, 80–88.
12. Chin, S.T.; Eyres, G.T.; Marriott, P.J. Identification of potent odorants in wine and brewed coffee using gas chromatography-olfactometry and comprehensive two-dimensional gas chromatography. *J. Chromatogr. A* **2011**, *1218*, 7487–7498. [CrossRef]
13. Hayashi, Y.; Sogabe, S.; Hattori, Y.; Tanaka, J. Anxiolytic and hypnotic effects in mice of roasted coffee bean volatile compounds. *Neurosci. Lett.* **2012**, *531*, 166–169. [CrossRef]
14. Satou, T.; Matsuura, M.; Takahashi, M.; Umezu, T.; Hayashi, S.; Sadamoto, K.; Koike, K. Anxiolytic-like effect of essential oil extracted from *Abies sachalinensis*. *Flavour Fragr. J.* **2011**, *26*, 416–420. [CrossRef]
15. Sugawara, Y.; Hara, C.; Tamura, K.; Fujii, T.; Nakamura, T.; Aoki, T. Sedative effect on humans of inhalation of essential oil of linalool: Sensory evaluation and physiological measurements using optically active linalools. *Anal. Chim. Acta* **1998**, *365*, 293–299. [CrossRef]
16. Takemoto, H.; Ito, M.; Shiraki, T.; Yagura, T.; Honda, G. Sedative effects of vapor inhalation of agarwood oil and spikenard extract and identification of their active components. *J. Nat. Med.* **2008**, *62*, 41–46. [CrossRef]
17. Gujral, S.; Aizenstein, H.; Reynolds, C.F.; Butters, M.A.; Erickson, K.I. Exercise effects on depression: Possible neural mechanisms. *Gen. Hosp. Psychiatry* **2017**, *49*, 2–10. [CrossRef]
18. Miyanishi, H.; Nitta, A. A Role of BDNF in the Depression Pathogenesis and a Potential Target as Antidepressant: The Modulator of Stress Sensitivity "Shati/Nat8l-BDNF System" in the Dorsal Striatum. *Pharmaceuticals* **2021**, *14*, 889. [CrossRef]
19. Iio, W.; Matsukawa, N.; Tsukahara, T.; Kohari, D.; Toyoda, A. Effects of chronic social defeat stress on MAP kinase cascade. *Neurosci. Lett.* **2011**, *504*, 281–284. [CrossRef]
20. Déry, N.; Goldstein, A.; Becker, S. A role for adult hippocampal neurogenesis at multiple time scales: A study of recent and remote memory in humans. *Behav. Neurosci.* **2015**, *129*, 435–449. [CrossRef]
21. Yamada, K.; Watanabe, Y.; Aoyagi, Y.; Ohta, A. Effect of alkylpyrazine derivatives on the duration of pentobarbital-induced sleep, picrotoxin-induced convulsion and gamma-aminobutyric acid (GABA) levels in the mouse brain. *Biol. Pharm. Bull.* **2001**, *24*, 1068–1071. [CrossRef]
22. Sha, S.; Chen, S.; Qian, M.; Wang, C.; Xu, Y. Characterization of the Typical Potent Odorants in Chinese Roasted Sesame-like Flavor Type Liquor by Headspace Solid Phase Microextraction-Aroma Extract Dilution Analysis, with Special Emphasis on Sulfur-Containing Odorants. *J. Agric. Food Chem.* **2017**, *65*, 123–131. [CrossRef]
23. Mitsubayashi, K.; Minamide, T.; Otsuka, K.; Kudo, H.; Saito, H. Optical bio-sniffer for methyl mercaptan in halitosis. *Anal. Chim. Acta* **2006**, *28*, 75–80. [CrossRef]

24. Tomimori, N.; Tanaka, Y.; Kitagawa, Y.; Fujii, W.; Sakakibara, Y.; Shibata, H. Pharmacokinetics and safety of the sesame lignans, sesamin and episesamin, in healthy subjects. *Biopharm. Drug. Dispos.* **2013**, *34*, 462–473. [CrossRef]
25. Seo, H.-S.; Hirano, M.; Shibato, J.; Rakwal, R.; Hwang, I.K.; Masuo, Y. Effects of Coffee Bean Aroma on the Rat Brain Stressed by Sleep Deprivation: A Selected Transcript- and 2D Gel-Based Proteome Analysis. *J. Agric. Food Chem.* **2008**, *56*, 4665–4673. [CrossRef]

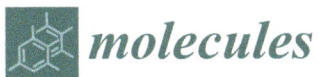

Review

Natural Ingredients from Medicine Food Homology as Chemopreventive Reagents against Type 2 Diabetes Mellitus by Modulating Gut Microbiota Homoeostasis

Xiaoyan Xia [1] and Jiao Xiao [2,*]

1. School of Traditional Chinese Medicine, Shanxi Datong University, Datong 037009, China; xiaoyanxia1202@163.com
2. Wuya College of Innovation, Shenyang Pharmaceutical University, Shenyang 110016, China
* Correspondence: 109160001@syphu.edu.cn; Tel.: +86-24-43520739

Abstract: Type 2 diabetes mellitus (T2DM) is a noteworthy worldwide public health problem. It represents a complex metabolic disorder, mainly characterized as hyperglycemia and lipid dysfunction. The gut microbiota dysbiosis has been proposed to play a role in the development of diabetes. Recently, there has been considerable interest in the use of medicine food homology (MFH) and functional food herbs (FF) to ameliorate diabetes and lead to a natural and healthy life. Hence, this review compiles some reports and findings to demonstrate that the practical use of the MFH/FF can modulate the homoeostasis of gut microbiota, thereby ameliorating the development of T2DM. The results provided useful data to support further investigation of the functional basis and application of MFH/FF to treat T2DM through maintaining intestinal homeostasis.

Keywords: medicine food homology; functional food herbs; type 2 diabetes mellitus; gut microbiota

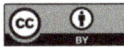

1. Introduction

Diabetes mellitus is one of the major public health problems and has become a health global burden. Based on the data of IDF, there were approximately 451 million diabetic patients aged 18 to 99 in the world in 2017. By 2045, this figure is expected to increase to 693 million [1]. Diabetes mainly includes Type-1 (T1DM) and Type-2 Diabetes Mellitus (T2DM), of which T2DM accounts for roughly 90–95% [2]. T2DM is a complex metabolic disorder, which is chiefly characterized by hyperglycemia, with glycolipid dysfunction, progressive loss and dysfunction of islet β-cell, and insulin resistance. T2DM is usually accompanied by oxidative stress and inflammation, and long-term hyperglycemia may lead to diverse diabetic complications [3].

One of the main reasons for the sharp increase in the incidence of T2DM is the significant changes in human behavior and lifestyle. Through diet modification, regular exercise, weight control, and patient education, T2DM can be managed and medications can be avoided. Diabetes is characterized by "leaky gut" syndrome, where bacterial cell wall components enter the blood circulation of the animal host in a large amount, which may cause metabolic endotoxemia and systemic low-grade inflammation [4]. Gut microbiota acts an important role in modulating the systemic and intestinal immunity and metabolic homeostasis [5]. Studies have shown that the consortium of gut microbiota is closely related to host genetics and other diverse conditions, such as food habits, stresses, exposure to drugs or toxins [5]. It was reported that the gut microbiota in healthy people is diversified, achieving more short chain fatty acids (SCFA) and producing more branched amino acids, while the intestinal flora of diabetes is more likely to produce compounds that affects glucose metabolism. The intestinal microbiota can digest diverse dietary fibers that cannot be digested by the host, and produce SCFAs as its metabolites, such as acetate, butyrate and propionate [6]. Propionate can maintain gluconeogenesis in the intestinal tract, thereby making better use of energy, while butyrate, with anti-inflammatory activity, can reduce the permeability of the intestine [6]. In T2DM patients, butyrate producing microbiota are significantly reduced, specifically the Clostridiales order, including the genera *Ruminococcus* and *Subdoligranulum*, and species such as *Roseburia intestinalis* and *Roseburia inulinivorans* [7,8].

In ancient China, diabetes was called 'Xiao Ke', manifested as persistent thirst and hunger, excessive urination, and weight loss. For thousands of years, Chinese herbal prescriptions and traditional Chinese medicine (TCM) medicinal materials have been commonly used to intervene in 'Xiaoke' disease. Historically, many of the formulations and medicinal herbs have been used as food for safe and effective long-term consumption [9]. Natural plants are essential for the management of many human diseases, such as diabetes [10]. Numerous herbal medicinal plants are natural sources of antioxidants, which can reduce the oxidative stress generated by STZ in β-cells. World Health Organization (WHO) has recommended the evaluation and application of traditional botanical treatments for diabetes because they are effective and non-toxic, have fewer side effects or have no side effects, and are considered excellent candidates for oral therapy [11]. In recent years, more and more researchers have been paying attention to natural products from traditional herbs and foods for their safety, efficacy, and potency in treating diabetes [12].

The concept of 'medicine and food homology' was proposed in the *Huang Di Nei Jing Su Wen*: 'Eating on an empty stomach as food, and administering to the patient as medication' embodies the theory of medicine food homology (MFH); that is, some food classes can also be used as drugs. Functional food (FF), also known as health food, refers to a specific type of food that is not aimed at curing diseases but can modulate human body functions. "Notice on Further Regulating the Management of Raw Materials for Health Foods" was issued in 2012 by the Ministry of Health, which covers both foods and medicines [9]. In addition, 110 MHF and 114 FF are currently included in this promulgated management method. More and more clinical evidence clarifies that the occurrence and development of T2DM can be prevented or delayed by regular intake of foods that are believed to be functional and affect glycemic control, antioxidant enzymes activity and intestinal flora, while also inhibiting the excessive production of pro-inflammatory cytokines during diabetes [13].

Therefore, in this review, we searched various online databases (PubMed, ScienceDirect, CNKI) and scientific publications from the library using qualitative systematic reviews. The review was based on MHF and FF application for possessing medicinal value against T2DM by modulating the gut microbiota (Figure 1A).

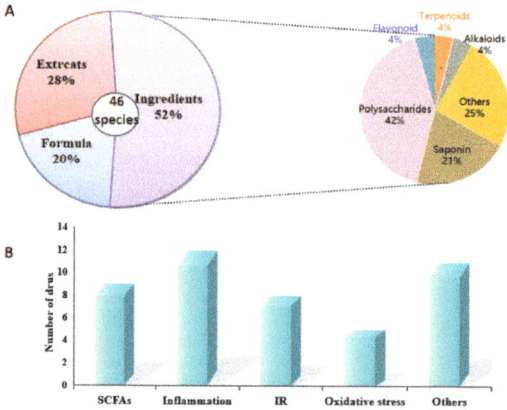

Figure 1. Analysis of MFH and FF showing anti-diabetic effects by modulating gut microbiota in this review. (**A**) Classification about the active MFH and FF species. (**B**) the relational mechanism of MFH and FF on T2DM associated with gut micorobiota.

2. Association between Gut Microbiota and T2DM

2.1. Alteration of Gut Microbiota Composition with T2DM

Although T2DM is caused due to various factors, the human gut microbiota plays a vital role in the progression of T2DM [4]. The impact of gut microbiota on T2DM has attracted widespread attention; studies have been done over the past few years to research the relationship between the two [12]. 'Human microbiome' was firstly defined by Joshua Lederberg in 2001 as an ecological community of symbiotic and pathogenic microorganisms that share our body space. An adult is colonized by almost 100 trillion microbes, which mainly exist in the gastrointestinal tract, with the largest group living in the colon. Human health is strongly affected by the microbiota that coexist with our body [14]. The diversity of the intestinal flora of T2DM patients is significantly decreased compared to that of healthy controls [15,16]. As Larson et al. reported, the abundance of Firmicutes phylum in diabetic patients was reduced when compared to non-diabetic patients, and the ratio of Bacteroides to Firmicutes was positively correlated with blood glucose levels [17].

2.2. Mechanism of Gut Microbiota Alteration Causing T2DM

T2DM, characterized by "leaky gut" syndrome, is known to have markedly enhanced intestinal permeability, allowing bacteria to translocate across the intestinal epithelium, resulting in host metabolic endotoxemia and triggering low-grade inflammation. In T2DM, the abundance and diversity of the gut microbiota both decreased, accompanied by an increase in the abundance of pathogenic microorganisms and a decrease in the abundance of symbiotic microorganisms [18]. For example, the generas *Faecalibacterium*, *Roseburia* and *Bifdobacterium*, with noticeable abilities to reduce intestinal permeability, have been shown to be exhausted in T2DM [19]. The changes in the above-mentioned microbiota would lead to low-grade inflammation, resulting in a decrease in mucus layer and disintegration of the epithelial membrane. This is followed by an increase in intestinal permeability, allowing lipopolysaccharides (LPS) to enter the blood circulation. Bacterial fragments and LPS can be recognized by innate toll-like receptors (TLRs), particularly TLR-4, which subsequently stimulates the activation of transcription factor κB (NF-κB) and the release of pro-inflammatory mediators in intracellular signaling pathways [20]. The release of pro-inflammatory cytokines would further result in the destruction of glucose metabolism and insulin signaling pathways [21]. Metabolic endotoxemia and low-grade inflammation occurs, subsequently. The systemic low-grade inflammation affects all vital organs or tissues, such as the pancreas, liver, and kidney [22]. For example, the level of TNF-α in T2DM is significantly increased, which is closely related to islet dysfunction [16,23]. Under this circumstance, the homeostasis of glucose metabolism no longer exists and thus results in type 2 diabetes. In this condition, the steady state of glucose metabolism collapses and T2DM is developed [24].

3. Bioactive Ingredients of MFH and FF Target for Microbiota in T2DM

The diet and its metabolites have a major physiological impact on the composition of gut microbiota and the health of the host [22]. In China, MFH and FF refers to a group of foods that can also be used as medicines, many of which possessed anti-hyperglycemic activities. Regular consumption of MFH, which is considered to affect glycemic control, activation of antioxidant enzymes and gut microbiota, and to inhibit the excessive production of pro-inflammatory cytokines, to prevent or treat T2DM [25]. MFH and FF have been widely sought recently, and research into their use for T2DM has evoked considerable interest. Herein, the bioactive ingredients of MFH and MHF were divided into: saponins, polysaccharides, flavonoids, terpenoids, alkaloids, and others, and their anti-diabetic effects via gut miocrobiota regulation were listed in Table 1, and the chemical structures of the representative compounds are shown in Figure 2.

Table 1. Effects of ingredients from MFH and FF on T2DM via gut microbiota.

	Ingredients	Source	Microbiota Findings	Mechanism	Study Types and Sequencing Method	Animals	Dose and Duration	Refs.
Saponins	Ginsenoside Rk3	Panax notoginseng	↑ Lactobacillaceae, Helicobacteraceae, Neococcaceae, Bifidobacteriaceae; ↓ Ratio of Firmicute to Bacteroidet;	Inhibit the inflammatory cascade by suppressing the TLR4/NF-κB pathway	In vivo; 16S rRNA Sequencing Analysis	C57BL/6 Mice	60 mg/kg/day; 8 weeks	[26]
	20(S)-ginsenoside Rg3	Panax ginseng C. A. Meyer	↑ Bacterial diversity	Improve bacterial diversity	In vivo; principal component analysis	Male Wistar rats	20 mg/kg/day; 2 weeks	[27]
	Ginsenoside Rb1	Panax ginseng C. A. Meyer	Unclear	Inhibit deglycosylation in the diabetic rats	In vivo; 16S rRNA Sequencing Analysis	Male Sprague-Dawley rats	100 mg/kg/day; 72 h	[28]
	Saponin-containing Korean red ginseng extracts	Korean red ginseng (Panax ginseng Meyer)	↑ Parabacteroides, Allistipes, Lactobacillus; ↓ Barnesiella, Mucispirillum, Lactococcus, Oscillibacter, Helicobacter	Improve IR and glucose intolerance	In vivo; 16S rRNA Sequencing Analysis	C57BL/6	235 mg/kg/day; 4 weeks	[29]
	Saponin extract of Polygonatum sibiricum	Polygonatum sibiricum (Liliaceae)	↑ Bifidobacteria, Lactobacillus; ↓ Enterobacteriaceae, Enterococcus, C. perfringens	Improve IR	In vivo; Bacteria plate count	ICR male mice	1.0, 1.5, or 2.0 g/kg/day; 5 weeks	[30]
	Polysaccharides (MDG-1) from Ophiopogonis Radix	Ophiopogon japonicus (Thunb.) Ker-Gawl. (Liliaceae)	↑ Lactobacillus, Bifidobacterium; ↓ Escherichia coli, Streptococcus	Improve SCFAs metabolism	In vivo; 16S rRNA Sequencing Analysis	KKay mice	300 mg/kg/day; 8 weeks	[31,32]
	Homogeneous polysaccharides from crude Lycium barbarum polysaccharides	Lycium barbarum L.	↑ Firmicutes/Bacteroides, SCFAs	Regulate SCFAs levels	In vitro; 16S rRNA Sequencing Analysis	C57BL/6	50 mg/kg/day; 12 weeks	[33]
	Polygonatum sibiricum polysaccharide	Polygonatum sibiricum (Liliaceae)	↑ Firmicutes, Veillomella, Escherichia-Shigella, Klebsiella; ↓ Proteobacteria, Bacteroides	Regulate bacterial diversity	In vivo; 16S rRNA Sequencing Analysis	/	/	[34]
	polysaccharide-rich extracts of A. venetum	Apocynum venetum	↑ Odoribacter, Anaeroplasma, Parasutterella, Muribaculum; ↓ Enterococcus, Klebsiella, Aerococcus.	Attenuate oxidative stress and SCFAs levels	In vivo; 16S rRNA Sequencing Analysis	Male C57BL/6 J mice	400 mg/kg/day; 4 weeks	[35]
Polysaccharides	Maydis stigma polysaccharides	Zea mays subsp. mays	↑ Lactobacillus and Bacteroides	Restore the intestinal microflora balance	In vivo; 16S rRNA Sequencing Analysis	Male KM mice	400, 600, 800 mg/kg/day; 5 weeks	[36]
	Plantago asiatica L. polysaccharides	Plantago asiatica L.	↑ Colon bacterial diversity, Bacteroides vulgatus, Lactobacillus fermentum, Prevotella loescheii, Bacteroides vulgates	Increase the levels of SCFAs	In vivo; 16S rRNA Sequencing Analysis	Wistar rats	100, 200 or 400 mg/kg/day; 5 weeks	[37]
	Pseudostellariae Radix	Pseudostellaria heterophylla (Miq.) Pax ex Paxet Hoffm.	↑ Lactobacillus, Bifidobacterium	Attenuate oxidative stress; suppress inflammatory response	In vivo; 16S rRNA Sequencing Analysis	Male C57BL/6 J	500 mg/kg/day; 4 weeks	[38]
	Polysaccharides of Lactobacillus plantarum-fermented Momordica charantia	Momordica charantia L.	↑ Lactococcus laudensis, Prevotella loescheii, diversity of gut microbiota, SCFAs ↓ pH value	Attenuate oxidative stress	In vivo; 16S rRNA Sequencing Analysis	Male Wistar rats	50, 100 mg/kg/day; 4 weeks	[39]
	mulberry fruit polysaccharide	Morus alba L.	↑ Lactobacillus, Allobaculum, Bacteroides, Akkermansia, SCFA (butyrate, propionate). ↓ Firmicutes, Bacillus, Lactobacillus	Attenuate oxidative stress	In vivo; 16S rRNA Sequencing Analysis	Male db/db mice	500, 800 mg/kg/day; 8 weeks	[40]

Table 1. Cont.

	Ingredients	Source	Microbiota Findings	Mechanism	Study Types and Sequencing Method	Animals	Dose and Duration	Refs.
	Pumpkin polysaccharide	Cucurbita moschata (Duch. ex Lam.)	↑ Bacteroidetes, Prevotella, Deltaproteobacteria, Oscillospira, Veillonellaceae, Phascolarctobacterium, Sutterella, Bilophila	Increase SCFAs production	In vivo; 16S rRNA Sequencing Analysis	Male Wistar rats	1000 mg/kg/day; 4 weeks	[41]
Flavonoids	Baicalein	Oroxylum indicum, Scutellaria baicalensis	↑ Bacteroides, Bacteroidales S24-7	Alleviate inflammation and IR	In vivo; 16S rRNA Sequencing Analysis	Male Wistar rats	50, 150 mg/kg/day; 4 weeks	[42]
Terpenoids	2β-hydroxybetulinic acid 3β-oleate	Euryale ferox salisb.	Unclear	Reduce blood glucose, regulate dyslipidemia and antioxidant enzymes, protect pancreatic β-cell	In vivo	Male Wistar rats	60 mg/kg/day; 45 days	[43]
Alkaloids	Berberine	Coptidis rhizoma and Berberis vulgaris	↑ Bacteroidetes, Lactobacillaceae; diversity of the gut microbiota ↓ Proteobacteria, Verrucomicrobia	Alleviate inflammation via NF-κB signaling pathways	In vivo; Real-Time PCR Assay	Male Sprague-Dawley rats	200 mg/kg/day; 6 weeks	[44,45]
	total glycoside from R. glutinosa leaves	Rehmannia glutinosa	↑ Firmicutes, norank_f_Bacteroidales_S24-7_group	Regulate glycolipid, inhibit the expression of α-SMA, TGF-β1, Smad3 and Smad4 in the kidney tissues	In vivo; 16S rRNA Sequencing Analysis	db/db mice	520 mg/kg/day; 6 weeks	[46]
	low-polar S. grosvenorii glycosides	Siraitia grosvenorii (Swingle) C.	↑ Elusimicrobium, Lachnospiraceae_UCG-004	Increase SCFAs production (acetate, butyrate, and 1β-hydroxycholic acid)	In vivo; 16S rRNA Sequencing Analysis	Sprague-Dawley rats	20 mg/kg/day; 14 days	[47]
Others	sea buckthorn protein	Hippophae rhamnoides L.	↑ Bifidobacterium, Lactobacillus, Bacteroides ↓ Clostridium coccoides, PH value;	Increase intestinal microorganism diversity and SCFAs levels	In vivo; 16S rRNA Sequencing Analysis	ICR mice	50, 100 and 200 mg/kg/day; 30 days	[48]
	Long chain of inulin-type fructans	inulin	↑ Firmicutes/Bacteroidetes ratio; Ruminococcaceae, Lactobacilli	Regulate SCFAs levels	In vivo; 16S rRNA Sequencing Analysis	Female NOD/LtJ mice	5% diet; 24 weeks	[49]
	cinnamon oil	Cortex Cinnamomi	↑ Bacteroides ↓ Clostridia flora IV	Improve IR	In vivo; 16S rRNA Sequencing Analysis	Sprague-Dawley rats	0.384 g/kg/day; 30 days	[50,51]

Abbreviations: SCFAs, short-chain fatty acid. IR, insulin resistance. ↑, Increase. ↓, Decrease.

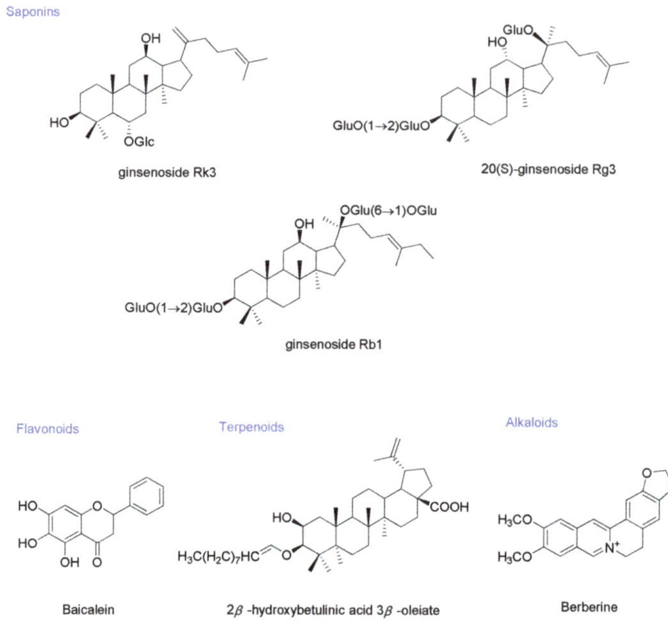

Figure 2. Chemical structures of the representative hypoglycemic compounds from MFH and FF that can modulate gut microbiota in T2DM.

3.1. Saponins

Saponins are a class of glycosides composed of triterpenes or spirostanes, which are widely present in nature [52]. Saponins have been reported to have a wide range of hypoglycemic targets and pathways, which can directly repair damaged islet cells and increase insulin levels to maintain normal blood sugar. Saponins can also regulate blood lipids and improve glucose tolerance. This suggests that they have broad research and development prospects as anti-diabetic drugs [53]. In this review, saponins from *Panax ginseng*, Panax notoginseng, Korean red ginseng and Polygonatum sibiricum were researched. It was observed that these saponins can intervene on T2DM and are associated with their modulating the imbalance of gut microbiota and inhibiting the low-grade inflammation and insulin resistance.

Ginseng, a perennial herb of the genus Panax, has been used widely as a TCM herbs in China and Asia for thousands of years. About 4000 years ago, "Shen Nong Ben Cao Jing" is the earliest surviving TCM monograph in China. It records the use of ginseng as a health medicine to delay aging and nourish the body without side effects [54]. According to Zhang Zhongjing's Shang Han Za Bing Lun in the Han Dynasty, ginseng was used to cure thirst, which is the main symptom of "Xiaoke" (diabetes). Additionally, the "Tai Ping Hui Min He Ji Ju Fang", an official traditional Chinese medicine book in Song Dynasty, recorded the use of ginseng to treat "Xiaoke disease". Many of the Chinese patent medicines approved by the government for the treatment of diabetes contain ginsenosides, such as Tianqi capsules [55], Jinlida Granule [56], and ShenMai Injection [28,57]. Ginseng has several therapeutic functions, such as anti-stress, maintaining and strengthening the central and immune system, preventing certain chronic diseases, and delaying aging. While American ginseng is more effective in treating cardiovascular disease [58]. Ginsenosides are extracted from the roots and rhizomes of *Panax ginseng* C. A. Meyer. Research has shown that ginsenosides show noticeable anti-diabetic activities and have been used as adjuvants for diabetes treatment in China. It was reported that saponins isolated from ginseng, such as

Ginsenoside Rk3, and 20(S)-ginsenoside Rg3 showed potential anti-diabetic activities by regulation of gut microbiota.

It was observed that Ginsenoside Rk3 at the dose of 30 and 60 mg/kg/day could alleviate the abundance imbalance of gut microbiota and inhibit the expression of pro-inflammatory cytokines by reducing intestinal permeability and LPS levels, thereby preventing low-grade colon inflammation caused by a high-fat diet in mice. An 8-week intervention of Rk3 could significantly decrease the ratio of Firmicute to Bacteroidete, and restore the abundance of Lactobacillaceae, Helicobacteraceae, Neococcaceae, and Bifidobacteriaceae at the dose of 60 mg/kg/day. Ginsenoside Rk3 can effectively improve the C57BL/6 Mice metabolic disorder of gut microbiota by decreasing the ratio of Firmicute/Bacteroidete, and inhibit the inflammatory cascade by suppressing the TLR4/NF-κB pathway [26]. It was found that 20(S)-ginsenoside Rg3 at a dose of 20 mg/kg can reduce the blood glucose by regulating the metabolism of gut flora in T2DM rats [27].

Polygonatum sibiricum, a perennial herb of Liliaceae family, has diverse activities, such as hypoglycemic effect, regulating blood lipids, delaying aging, and strengthening immunity. A saponin was isolated from P. sibiricum (PSS) and administered to diabetic mice at the dose of 1.0, 1.5, or 2.0 g/kg/day. It was found that PSS could alleviate the symptoms of polyphagia and polydipsia and regulate the gut microbiota in the diabetic mice. PPS increased the abundance of probiotics (including Bifidobacteria and Lactobacillus), and down-regulated the harmful bacteria (such as Enterobacteriaceae, Enterococcus, and C. perfringens) [30].

3.2. Polysaccharides

Polysaccharides are formed by the polymerization of monosaccharide molecules through glycosidic bonds, which are generally composed of hundreds or even thousands of monosaccharides molecules with a relatively high molecular weight. Polysaccharides, as a kind of abundant natural product, are found in organisms such as fungi and plant roots [59]. As prebiotics, polysaccharides have been found to affect the populations and metabolism of the gut microbiota, and attracted widespread attention in biochemical and medical research [60]. The polysaccharides from MFH have been studied to show potential impact on T2DM, which is associated with the regulation of gut microbiota.

Ophiopogonis Radixa, the Chinese name Maidong, is the tuberous roots of *Ophiopogon japonicus* (Thunb.) Ker-Gawl (Liliaceae), which is a popular TCM. Maidong is widely used as a functional food in China. Maidong has been used to relieve diabetes and cardiovascular diseases for years [31]. The polysaccharide is one of the main active ingredients of Maidong. A homogeneous polysaccharide fraction was isolated and characterized from Ophiopogonis Radix collected from Sichuan. Ophiopogonis Radix and was analyzed for anti-diabetic effects in targeting β-cell dysfunction, insulin enhancement and inhibiting α-amylase and α-glucosidase [61]. The anti-diabetic effects of polysaccharides, isolated from Maidong, have been reported [62,63]. More than 15 kinds of polysaccharides have been isolated from Maidong, which show a good anti-diabetic effect, and the main mechanism is associated with improving β-cell dysfunction, enhancing insulin and inhibiting α-glucosidase and α-amylase [64]. For example, MDG-1, a kind of polysaccharide isolated from Maidong, possessed anti-diabetic effects in diabetic mice and regulated intestinal flora in obese mice [31,64]. In KKay mice, the abundance of Escherichia coli and Streptococcus increased, while the abundance of Lactobacillus and Bifidobacterium decreased. However, oral administration of 300 mg/kg MDG-1 can reduce the number of pathogenic E. coli and Streptococcus, and increase the number of Lactobacillus ($p < 0.05$). It has been proven that oral MDG-1 can improve the glucose tolerance of diabetic mice and is related to its regulating effect on the intestinal microecological balance [32].

Lycium barbarum L. and its mature fruits have been used as a TCM and functional food in China for about 2000 years. The leaves of *L. barbarum*, also named Tianjing grass, are widely used as tea, food and medicine in China due to its activities of reinforcing deficiency and benefiting essence, as well as anti-thermic and eye-clearing effects [65,66].

An HFD/STZ-induced T2DM rat model was established to study the anti-diabetic effects of the water extract of *L. barbarum* leaf (LLB). It was found that LLB can improve T2DM, which is mainly associated with the reversal of gut microbiota imbalance, and regulation of nicotinate/nicotinamide, arachidonic acid/purine metabolism. Administration of LLB at 2.08 g/kg T2DM rats significantly reduced excessive abundance of Parasutterella, Marvinbryantia, Blautia, Ruminococcus_1, and Prevotellaceae_NK3B31_group, and reversed the ratio of Firmicutes to Bacteroidetes in the gut microbiota of diabetic rats [66]. The homogeneous polysaccharide (LBP-W) was purified from crude *Lycium barbarum* polysaccharides (LBPs), and administration of 50 mg/kg LBP-W could improve obesity by modulating the composition of gut microbiota and the metabolism of SCFAs in C57BL/6 mice on a high fat diet. LBP-W intervention reversed the HFD-induced changes in Firmicutes and Bacteroides, and the ratio of Firmicutes/Bacteroides was noticeably reduced ($p < 0.01$) [33].

Plantago asiatica L. is a kind of TCM and has been used as a folk medicine worldwide [67,68]. A high-fat diet and STZ induced T2DM rat model has been established, and the anti-diabetic effect of *Plantago asiatica* L. polysaccharide (PLP) was studied. It was observed that administration of PLP (at dose of 100, 200 or 400 mg/kg) significantly decreased the level of blood glucose, insulin, serum lipids, non-esterifified fatty acid and maleic dialdehyde, and noticeably increased the activities of antioxidant enzymes in T2DM rats after 4 weeks of PLP intervention. The concentrations of SCFA were noticeably higher in the feces of diabetic rats after treating with PLP. Moreover, colon bacterial diversity and abundance of bacteria, including Bacteroides vulgatus, Lactobacillus fermentum, Prevotella loescheii and Bacteroides vulgates were markedly increased by PLP intervention. It indicated that the anti-diabetic effect of PLP inT2DM rats was related to the regulation of gut microbiota and increased levels of SCFAs production [37].

Apocynum venetum is a perennial herbaceous or half-shrub plant, and its leaves have been traditionally consumed as a tea beverage in China. *A. venetum* is widely distributed in saline-alkali land, riverbanks, fluvial plains and sandy soils of Asia and North America [69]. Hypoglycemic and hypolipidemic effects of polysaccharide-rich extracts from *A. venetum* leaves on T2DM mice has been studied. Treatment of alkaline extracted polysaccharide-rich products markedly decreased the levels of fasting blood glucose, serum insulin, and serum lipids. Meanwhile, the reduced glycogen contents in liver were prominently improved, and the oxidative damage was markedly ameliorated by alkaline extracted polysaccharide products in diabetic mice. Furthermore, the polysaccharide-rich extracts could reverse the gut microbiota dysbiosis in T2DM mice by increasing the abundance of genera Odoribacter, Anaeroplasma, Parasutterella, and Muribaculum, while decreasing the abundance of genera Enterococcus, Klebsiella, and Aerococcus. Thus, polysaccharide-rich extracts of *A. venetum* showed good anti-diabetic effects for treating T2DM, which was associated with the intervention of gut microbiota [35].

In this review, polysaccharides from MFH and FF were summarized and their impacts on T2DM by regulating gut microbiota were listed in Table 1. It was found that the polysaccharides play an important role in maintaining intestinal flora steady state, which was associated with the promotion of short-chain fatty acids (SCFAs). SCFA mainly include acetate, butyrate and propionate at the ratio of 3:1:1 in human gut microbiota, which are usually present in the human intestine at a ratio of 3:1:1 and are in a steady state [70]. Butyrate possesses anti-inflammatory effects and can reduce intestinal permeability, and propionate also maintains gluconeogenesis in the intestines, thereby making better use of energy [24]. Individuals with T2DM have reduced butyrate-producing gut microbiota, which promotes low-grade inflammation [70].

3.3. Flavonoids

Flavonoids are meaningful natural compounds that exist widely in the plant kingdom and have a basic 2-phenyl-chromone structure. They are a class of secondary plant compound with noticeable physiological effects and various health benefits [9]. Flavonoids possess extensive pharmacological effects, among which are antioxidant and free radical scavenging activities, which are of particular interest to the pharmaceutical industry [71]. Flavonoids are widely reported to prevent and treat T2DM by affecting the function of islet β-cells and anti-lipid peroxidation [72]. However, not so many flavonoids from natural herbs were found to intervene T2DM by the regulation of gut microbiota.

Baicalein is a dietary flavonoid and is a main component of Oroxylum indicum and Scutellaria baicalensis. It is used as a dietary supplement or as tea in Asia, Europe and the Americas. Based on Zhang's study in 2018, four weeks intervention of baicalein (50, 150 mg/kg·d) significantly decreased the blood glucose and LPS and improved insulin resistance, inflammation, and lipid profile in T2DM rat dose-developmentally. These anti-diabetic effects are owing to the increase in SCFAs content and the thickness of the intestinal mucus layer, which is closely related to the regulation of the intestinal microbiota, especially the abundance of Bacteroides and Bacteroides S24-7. They had the highest relative abundance in rats receiving 150 mg/kg baicalein, and they were positively correlated with improving T2DM-related phenotypes [42]. As reported, Bacteroidales S24-7, Prevotella, Blautia, and Butyricoccus are the key SCFA-producing bacteria, which may relieve inflammation and insulin resistance, by reducing the intestinal endotoxins entering the circulation, thereby alleviating T2DM [73,74].

Plumula nelumbinis, also named "Lian-Zi-Xin" in Chinese, is the dried embryo of the ripe seeds of Nelumbo nucifera Gaertn (Nelumbonaceae). It is a traditional Chinese medicine (TCM), and also an ordinary health food. It is commonly used in several counties around the world. In TCM, Lian-Zi-Xin has been used to clear heart heat, calm the mind, and treat high fever, promote astringent essence and hemostasis [75,76]. As Qiuzhe Li reported in 2015, the total flavonoids from Lotus plumule showed noticeable anti-diabetic effects by reducing the blood glucose level, regulating blood lipid levels and improving the glucose tolerance in the T2DM mice.

3.4. Terpenoids

Terpenes are natural hydrocarbons and can be linked in diverse ways through isoprene or isopentane. It mainly includes monoterpenes, sesquiterpenes, diterpenes and triterpenes, which play a vital role in organisms. Studies have shown that some terpenoids possess a preventive effect on T2DM; the mechanism may be mediated by protecting islet β-cells and increasing glucose tolerance and hepatic glycogen synthesis [71]. However, there are few studies on the effects of terpenoids treating T2DM by regulating gut microbiota.

A pentacyclic triterpene, 2β-hydroxybetulinic acid 3β-oleiate (HBAO), was isolated from the seeds of Euryale ferox salisb. Oral administration of 60 mg/kg/d HBAO could ameliorate glycemic homeostasis and alleviate oxidative stress in the streptozocin (STZ)-induced diabetic rats. It was observed that HBAO normalized the blood glucose, glycosylated hemoglobin (HbA1c), hepatic hexokinase and plasma insulin, improved damaged pancreatic β-cell, regulated dyslipidemia and antioxidant enzymes (such as superoxide dismutase, catalase and glutathione peroxidase) in the diabetic rats ($p < 0.05$) [43]. STZ-induced diabetic mice were administrated by the triterpenoid-rich extracts of Euryale ferox shell (ES) orally at doses of 200, 300, 400, 500 ± 2 mg/L for 4 weeks. It was found that the triterpenoid-rich extracts of ES could regulate glucose metabolism ($p < 0.01$), normalize the body weight of the diabetic mice ($p < 0.01$), reduce the expression of the negative regulation protein PTP1B gene and increase insulin receptor IRS-1 protein expression ($p < 0.05$) [77].

3.5. Alkaloids

Alkaloids are a class of nitrogen-containing organic compounds derived in nature, mainly in the plant kingdom. Most alkaloids are alkaline and have significant biological activity and are a kind of important bioactive ingredient in MFH and FF [71]. It has been found that the hypoglycemic activities of alkaloids are mainly mediated by inhibition of gluconeogenesis, regulation of gut microbiota structure, promotion of glycolysis and anti-glucagon activities, promotion of the secretion of pancreatic β-cells, and scavenging of oxygen free radicals [78]. For example, neferine could reduce the levels of blood glucose, improve insulin resistance and regulate the disorder of lipid metabolism in T2DM rats [75]. Isoliensinine was found to attenuate T2DM with hyperlipidemia in a KK-Ay mouse model by regulating GLUT4, SREBP-1c, PPARγ, AMPK and ACC phosphorylation [76]. However, there are few studies on the effects of alkaloids treating T2DM through gut microbiota regulation.

Berberine is an isoquinoline quaternary alkaloid that is widely found in Coptidis rhizoma and Berberis vulgaris [79]. Berberine has a long history in Chinese and Western medicine treatment [80]. In China, Berberine has been used to treat diarrhea caused by bacteria as an over-the-counter drug for years [45,81]. Berberine was administrated to T2DM rats, and it was found that the anti-diabetic effects of Berberine is related to its regulation of gut microbiota. The community richness and diversity of the gut microbiota were noticeably increased by Berberine, and the abundance of Bacteroidetes was increased, while the number of Proteobacteria and Verrucomicrobia were decreased. At the family level, a probiotic Lactobacillaceae was markedly increased after Berberine intervention, which was negatively related to the risk of T2DM [44]. It suggested that Berberine can alleviate T2DM in rats by modulating gut microbiota composition.

3.6. Others

Some other kinds of compounds in medical herbs, such as proteins, fibers, essential oil and glycosides, also show significant hypoglycemic activities. We also researched and summarized those kinds of ingredients from MFH and FF to find the potential antidiabetic compounds.

Rehmannia glutinosa is a kind of perennial herbaceous plant of the *Scrophulariaceae* family. The *R. glutinosa* leaves' total glycoside (DHY) is mainly composed of iridoid glycosides and phenylethanoid glycosides extracted from *R. glutinosa* leaves. Studies have shown that DHY has been used in the clinical treatment of various kidney diseases, due to its protection on kidneys by improving glomerular permeability and reducing proteinuria. DHY was also found to improve STZ-induced gut microbiota imbalance in diabetic nephropathy rats [46]. DHY was observed to significantly decrease the levels of blood glucose, serum lipid (such as total cholesterol and triglyceride) and improve kidney damage, and inhibit the expression of α-SMA, TGF- β1, Smad3 and Smad4 in the kidney tissues of *db/db* mice. DHY had noticeable up-regulation effect on *Firmicutes* in *db/db* mice. At the genus level, DHY were dominant for the recovery of *norank_f_Bacteroidales_S24_7_group* in *db/db* mice. Therefore, DHY may restore the dysfunctional intestinal flora to normal and regulate glycolipid level of *db/db* mice [46].

Salvia miltiorrhiza Bge., a TCM for promoting blood circulation and removing blood stasis, has been used as a health-care food recently. The aerial parts of *S. miltiorrhiza* Bge. (DJ) are rich in phenolic acids similar to the rhizome [82]. The 60% ethanol extracts of DJ were found to strengthen the intestinal barrier of diabetic mice by up-regulating the tight junction proteins expressions in ileum and colon, but not in duodenum. DJ could modulate the diabetes-induced gut microbiota imbalance. At phylum level, that the number of *Proteobacteria* was significantly increased while *Tenericutes* was significantly decreased in DJ group compared to the control group [82].

Dietary fibers can modify the gut barrier and microbiota homeostasis, thereby impacting the progression of diabetes. Inulin-type fructans (ITFs) are natural soluble dietary fibers with different fermentation degrees in chicory root, which can regulate the occurrence and development of diabetes. Female nonobese diabetic mice were weaned to long-and short-chain ITFs, ITF(l) and ITF(s) supplemented diet up to 24 weeks. Expression of barrier reinforcing tight junction proteins occludin and claudin-2, antimicrobial peptides-defensin-1, and cathelicidin-related antimicrobial peptide as well as short-chain fatty acid production were enhanced by ITF(l). It was found that ITF(l) enhanced *Firmicutes/Bacteroidetes* ratio to an antidiabetogenic balance and enriched modulatory *Ruminococcaceae* and *Lactobacilli* [49]. The inulin was found to alleviate different stages of T2DM in diabetic mice by modulating gut microbiota. It increased the relative abundance of *Cyanobacteria* and *Bacteroides*, and reduced the relative abundance of *Deferribacteres* and *Tenericutes*. Dietary inulin can ameliorate diverse stages of T2DM by suppressing inflammation and modulating gut microbiota, especially in pre-diabetic and early diabetic stages, thus it potentially serves as an inexpensive intervention for the prevention and treatment of T2DM patients [15].

4. Herb Extracts of MFH and FF Target for Microbiota in T2DM

4.1. Single Herb Extracts of MFH and FF Target for Microbiota in T2DM

Generally, MFH and FF are usually taken in the form of decoction or direct consumption. Therefore, the anti-diabetic effect of the water extracts or total extracts is worthy of attention. We investigated the anti-diabetic effects of the extracts of MFH and FF by regulating the imbalance of the intestinal microbiota, such as *Fructus Aurantii Immaturus*, *Atractylodis macrocephalae Rhizoma*, Radix *Puerariae*, sea buckthorn, *Anemarrhena asphodeloides*, *Dendrobium officinale*, listed in Table 2.

Table 2. The role and mechanism of extracts in MFH and FF on T2DM through modulating gut microbiota.

MFH/FF	Source	Microbiota Findings	Mechanism	Test Sections	Study Type and Sequencing Method	Animals	Dose and Duration	Refs.
Fructus Aurantii Immaturus	Citrus aurantium L.	↓ Lachnospiraceae NK4A136, Prevotellaceae UCG-003, Prevotellaceae NK3B31, Lachnospiraceae UCG-008, Ruminiclostridium 9, Ruminococcaceae UCG-014; ↑ Lactobacillus, Alloprevotella, Treponema 2	Restore the intestinal microflora balance	Water extracts of fried Fructus Aurantii Immaturus with wheat bran decoction	In vivo; 16S rRNA Sequencing Analysis	Male Sprague-Dawley rats	9 g/kg/day; 14 d	[83]
Atractylodes macrocephala Koidz	Atractylodes macrocephala Koidz (Compositae)	↑ Bacteroides thetaiotaomicron, Methanobrevibacter smithii	Upregulate GLP-1R, PI3K, PDX-1 expressions, and suppress inflammation (decrease FOXO1, NF-κB p65)	Water extracts of Atractylodis macrocephaliae Rhizoma (AMK)	In vivo; 16S rRNA Sequencing Analysis	db/db mice	100 mg/kg/day; 3 weeks	[84]
Anemarrhena asphodeloides	Anemarrhena asphodeloides Bge.	Blautia coccoides (in vitro) ↓ Proteobacteria, Facklamia, Oligella, and Klebsiella	Suppress the increased oxidative stress and inflammatory activation.	Water extract of A. asphodeloides	In vivo; 16S rRNA Sequencing Analysis	Male SPF Wistar rats	20, 60, 180 mg/kg/day; 4 weeks.	[85]
Lycium barbarum	Lycium barbarum L.	↑ the ratio of Firmicutes to Bacteroidetes; ↓ Parasutterella, Marvinbryantia, Blautia, Ruminococcus_1, Prevotellaceae_NK3B31_group	Improve liver, kidney, and pancreas injury and regulate metabolic profiles	Water extract of L. barbarum leaf	In vivo; 16S rRNA Sequencing Analysis	(SPF)-grade rat	1.04, 2.08 g/kg/day; 4 weeks	[66]
Alpinia oxyphylla Miq.	Alpinia oxyphylla Miq. (Zingiberaceae)	↑ Akkermansia; ↓ Helicobacter	Modulate gut microbiota composition	Water extract of Alpinia oxyphylla Miq.	In vivo; 16S rRNA Sequencing Analysis	db/db mice	100, 300, 500 mg/kg/day; 8 weeks	[86]
Chinese propolis	Chinese propolis	↑ Roseburia, Intestinimonus, Parabacteroides goldsteinii, Parabacteroides distasonis; ↓ Faecalibacterium, Prevotella, Bacteroides vulgatus	Reduce inflammation	Ethanol extract of propolis	In vivo; 16S rRNA Sequencing Analysis	C57BL/6	200, 300 mg/kg/day; 12 weeks	[87,88]
Puerariae Radix	Pueraria lobata	↑ Lactococcus, Ruminococcus	Inhibit obesity and inflammatory-related parameters	30% ethanol extracts of dried root of P. lobata	In vivo; 16S rRNA Sequencing Analysis	Female C57BL/6 J mice	400 mg/kg/day; 10 weeks	[89]
Mulberry leaf	Morus alba L.	↑ Bacteroidetes, Proteobacteria; Clostridia	Improve IR	mulberry leaf powder	In vivo; 16S rRNA Sequencing Analysis	Sprague-Dawley male rats	20% (w/w) in diet; 13 weeks	[90]
Coicis Semen	Coix lacryma-jobi L. var. ma-yuen (Roman.) Stapf	↑ Lactobacillus, Coprococcus, Akkermansia, Akkermansia muciniphila, Lactobacillus agilis	Improve glucose homeostasis	Coicis Semen power included in diet	In vivo; 16S rRNA Sequencing Analysis	C57BL/6 mice	0.5 g/100 g; 5 weeks	[91]
Astragali Radix	Astragalus membranaceus (Fisch.) Bge. var. mongholicus (Bge.)	↑ ratio of Firmicutes/Bacteroidota; Lactobacillales	Regulate gut microbiota	Astragali Radix decoction vesicle-like nanoparticles extracted by ltracentrifugation;	In vivo; 16S rRNA Sequencing Analysis	db/db mice	5.3, 10.6, 21.1 g/kg/day; 3 weeks	[92]
Dendrobium candidum	Dendrobium candidum Wall Ex Lindl	↑ Akkermansia, Parabacteroides	Improve glucose intolerance and IR	Dendrobium officinale extract	In vivo; 16S rRNA Sequencing Analysis	T2D mice	1.0 g/kg/day; 30 days	[93]

Table 2. *Cont.*

MFH/FF	Source	Microbiota Findings	Mechanism	Test Sections	Study Type and Sequencing Method	Animals	Dose and Duration	Refs.
hemp seed	*Cannabis sativa* L.	↑ *Bacteroidetes*; ↓ *Firmicutes*	Modulate gut microbiota	hemp seed oil-water mixture	In vivo; 16S rRNA Sequencing Analysis	Female KM mice	0.2, 0.4 mL; 10 days	[94]
Dioscoreae Rhizoma	*Dioscorea opposita* Thunb.	↑ *Bifidobacterium, Adolescentis, Bifidobacterium infantis*	Modulate gut microbiota	yam gruel	In vivo; 16S rRNA Sequencing Analysis	Human patients	150 g/day; 3 months	[95]

Abbreviations: IR, insulin resistance. ↑, Increase. ↓, Decrease.

Atractylodis macrocephalae Rhizoma is widely used as a functional food in Asia. The water extracts of *A. macrocephalae* (AMK) at a dose of 100 mg/kg noticeably increased the relative abundance of *Bacteroides thetaiotaomicron* and *Methanobrevibacter smithii* in gut microbiota of the diabetic mice. It was found that AMK could significantly decrease the blood glucose and serum lipids, and improve the insulin resistance, which was associated with its inhibitory effects on inflammation and its regulation of gut miocrobiota imbalance.

Chinese propolis, is a resinous substance collected by bees from plants exudates that is mixed with wax and mandibular gland secretions [96]. Propolis has long been recognized as a natural nutraceutical has shown a beneficial effect on alleviating by exerting good anti-inflammatory, anti-oxidant effects [96]. Studies have reported that propolis extract could boost lipid metabolism, alleviate insulin resistance, and delay obesity in high-fat diet-fed mice and rats with T2DM [87]. Propolis were abserved to reverse the elevation of *Firmicutes* and inflammatory biomarkers expression induced by HFD in the obese mice [88]. Propolis intervention can regulate gut microbiota by decreasing *Alistipes*, and increasing *Lactobacillus* in male mice, which are playing an important role in the preventive effect on obesity and T2DM.

4.2. Herb Formula Consisted of MFH for T2DM by Regulating Microbiota

Chinese herbal formulas with anti-diabetic effects have been well studied, and many of them have commonly been used in "Xiaoke" patients since ancient times. In the traditional Chinese medicine system, the relationship between the gut microbiota and disease is actually the relationship between the intestine and disease, which was early mentioned in the *"Huang Di Nei Jing"*. Therefore, we summarized the herb formulas consisted of MFH, which act anti-diabetic effects by regulating the imbalance of gut microbiota, and listed in Table 3.

Wumei Wan was first recorded in Zhang Zhongjing's *"Shanghan lun"*, and is the main prescription for the treatment of Jueyin disease. "Xiaoke" disease was considered to be one of Jueyin diseases as recorded in ancient China. It was found that Wumei Wan (at the dose of 20, 10, 5 g/kg/d) could significantly enrich the functional bacteria, such as *Firmicutes, DeltaProteobacteria*, and *Lactobacillus*, and decrease the abundance of *Bacteroidetes, Actinobacteria, Bacteroides, Clostridium* in the T2DM rats [97]. It has been proven that Wumei Pill can regulate the balance of intestinal flora in T2DM model rats, increase the content of short-chain fatty acids (including acetic acid, propionic acid, butyric acid), thereby lowering blood glucose and ameliorating T2DM. Daesiho-Tang is another important formulation in TCM, known for its anti-diabetic and anti-hepatotoxic effects. It has been found that Daesiho-Tang treatment noticeably increased the relative abundance of *Bacteroidetes, Bacteroidetes/Firmicutes* ratio, *Akkermansia Bifidobacterium, Lactobacillus*, and decreased the level of *Firmicutes* [98].

Table 3. The role and mechanism of formula extracts in MFH and FF on T2DM through modulating gut microbiota.

MFH and FF	Microbiota Findings	Mechanism	Test Sections	Study Type and Sequencing Method	Animals	Dose and Duration	Ref.
Wumeiwan	↓ *Bacteroidetes, Actinobacteria, Bacteroides, Clostridium*; ↑ *Firmicutes, DeltaProteobacteria, Lactobacillus*	Improve SCFA, inhibit inflammatory mediums (TNF-α, IL-10)	Decoction concentrate	In vivo; 16S rRNA Sequencing Analysis	Sprague-Dawley rats	5, 10, 20 g/kg/day; 4 weeks	[97]
Daesiho-Tang	↑ *Bacteroidetes, Bacteroidetes/Firmicutes ratio, Akkermansia Bifidobacterium, Lactobacillus*; ↓ *Firmicutes*	Modulate intestinal microbiota	Water extracts	In vivo; 16S rRNA Sequencing Analysis	Male C57BL/6 mice	700 mg/kg/day; 12 weeks	[98]
Gegen Qinlian Decoction	↑ *Lactobacillus johnsonii, Stomatobaculum longum* strain ACC2, *Bacteroides vulgatus*	Suppress inflammation: reduce the levels of LPS; TNF-α, IL-6	Crude drugs	In vivo; 16S rRNA Sequencing Analysis	KK-Ay mice	4.44, 13.30, 40.00 g/kg/day; 4 weeks	[99]
A mixture of *D. officinale* and American ginseng	↑ ratio of *Bacteroidetes* to *Firmicutes, Prevotella, Akkermansia*; and SCFA-producing bacteria; ↓ S24-7/*Rikenella/Escherichia coli*.	Decrease inflammation (IL-6 and TNF-α) and oxidative stress; improve intestinal flora balance	Mixture of *D. officinale* and American ginseng	In vivo; 16S rRNA Sequencing Analysis	Dogs	160 mg/kg/day; 60 days	[100]
Chinese Herbal Formula Shenzhu Tiaopi Granule	↑ *Lactobacillus*; ↓ *Firmicutes/Bacteroidetes* ratio, *Bacteroides, Allobaculum, Desulfovibrionaceae*	Inhibit inflammation, ameliorate IR	Shenzhu Tiaopi Granule	In vivo; 16S rRNA Sequencing Analysis	Male Goto-Kakizaki (GK)	1000 mg/kg/day; 8 weeks	[101]
Qijian Mixture	↑ *Bacteroidetes*	Inhibit inflammation and oxidative stress	Qijian Mixture	In vivo; 16S rRNA Sequencing Analysis	Male KKay mice	1.795, 5.385 g/kg/day; 5 weeks	[102]
Anemarrhena asphodeloides Bge. and *Phellodendron chinense* Schneid	↓ *Bacteroidetes; Bacilli, Lactobacillus*; ↑ *Firmicutes, Proteobacteria; Clostridia, Romboutsia, Bacteroides*	Improve intestinal microbiota	Decoction concentrate	In vivo; 16S rRNA Sequencing Analysis	Sprague-Dawley rats	6.48 g/kg/day; 30 days	[103]
Combination of Aronia, Red Ginseng, Shiitake Mushroom and Nattokinase	↓ *Clostridiales*; ↑ *Bacteroidales*	Improve IR	Water extracts of the combination	In vivo; 16S rRNA Sequencing Analysis	Sprague Dawley rats	0.5, 1.0 g/kg/day; 12 weeks	[104]
Scutellaria baicalensis Georgi. SR and *Coptis chinensis* Franch, CR	↑ SCFAs-producing bacteria: *Bacteroidales* S24-7 group_norank, *Eubacterium nodatum* group, *Parasutterella, Prevotellaceae* UCG-001, *Ruminiclostridium, Ruminiclostridium*; ↓ Secondary bile acid-producing bacteria *Escherichia Shigella*;	Increase microbially derived SCFAs	Water extracts	In vivo; 16S rRNA Sequencing Analysis	Male Sprague-Dawley rats	6.3 g/kg/day; 1 month	[105]

Abbreviations: IR, insulin resistance. ↑, Increase. ↓, Decrease.

5. Conclusions and Perspective

T2DM, as one of the major public health problems worldwide, is currently prevailing and seems likely to continue for some time. Therefore, there is an urgent need for new methods to prevent and treat this disease. However, most of the treatments currently in use, especially drugs with proven effects, generally focus on agents designed to directly affect signaling pathways that directly modulate the blood glucose, which usually show some side effects. However, better underlying causes of T2DM indicates that regulating the gut microbiota may be a potential way to treat this disorder.

Natural plants, especially medicine food homology and functional foods, are considered to be an ideal candidate for oral treatment because of their effective, non-toxic, few side effects, and have received widespread attention in the of management of T2DM. As described in this review, research, especially in animal models, supports this view. Additionally, studies on MFH and FF suggests that their beneficial effects on T2DM may be partly mediated by their influences on gut microbiota. In fact, approaches such as inhibiting low-grade inflammation to prevent T2DM through regulating gut microbiota have existed, but recent studies on impacts of gut microbiota suggest it may be a possible medium for preventing this disorder. In this regard, further studies on the impacts of MFH and FF on the gut microbiota are worthy of in-depth attention, in humans, paving the way for better treatment and prevention of T2DM.

Author Contributions: X.X. and J.X. designed and revised the manuscript; J.X. analyzed the data. X.X. wrote the paper, and both authors critically reviewed and approved the final form of the manuscript. All data were generated in-house, and no paper mill was used. All authors have read and agreed to the published version of the manuscript.

Funding: This work was financially supported by National Natural Science Foundation of China (Grant No. 82104061); LiaoNing Revitalization Talents Program (XLYC1802037).

Conflicts of Interest: The authors declare no conflict of interest.

References

1. Choi, J.H.; Jin, S.W.; Choi, C.Y.; Kim, H.G.; Lee, G.H.; Kim, Y.A.; Chung, Y.C.; Jeong, H.G. Capsaicin Inhibits Dimethylnitrosamine-Induced Hepatic Fibrosis by Inhibiting the TGF-beta1/Smad Pathway via Peroxisome Proliferator-Activated Receptor Gamma Activation. *J. Agric. Food Chem.* **2017**, *65*, 317–326. [CrossRef]
2. Da Rocha Fernandes, J.; Ogurtsova, K.; Linnenkamp, U.; Guariguata, L.; Seuring, T.; Zhang, P.; Cavan, D.; Makaroff, L.E. IDF Diabetes Atlas estimates of 2014 global health expenditures on diabetes. *Diabetes Res. Clin. Pract.* **2016**, *117*, 48–54. [CrossRef]
3. Danda, R.S.; Habiba, N.M.; Rincon-Choles, H.; Bhandari, B.K.; Barnes, J.L.; Abboud, H.E.; Pergola, P.E. Kidney involvement in a nongenetic rat model of type 2 diabetes. *Kidney Int.* **2005**, *68*, 2562–2571. [CrossRef]
4. Al-Jameel, S.S. Association of diabetes and microbiota: An update. *Saudi J. Biol. Sci.* **2021**, *28*, 4446–4454. [CrossRef] [PubMed]
5. Needell, J.C.; Zipris, D. The Role of the Intestinal Microbiome in Type 1 Diabetes Pathogenesis. *Curr. Diabetes Rep.* **2016**, *16*, 89. [CrossRef] [PubMed]
6. Koh, A.; De Vadder, F.; Kovatcheva-Datchary, P.; Backhed, F. From Dietary Fiber to Host Physiology: Short-Chain Fatty Acids as Key Bacterial Metabolites. *Cell* **2016**, *165*, 1332–1345. [CrossRef]
7. Qin, J.; Li, Y.; Cai, Z.; Li, S.; Zhu, J.; Zhang, F.; Liang, S.; Zhang, W.; Guan, Y.; Shen, D.; et al. A metagenome-wide association study of gut microbiota in type 2 diabetes. *Nature* **2012**, *490*, 55–60. [CrossRef]
8. Zhang, F.; Wang, M.; Yang, J.; Xu, Q.; Liang, C.; Chen, B.; Zhang, J.; Yang, Y.; Wang, H.; Shang, Y.; et al. Response of gut microbiota in type 2 diabetes to hypoglycemic agents. *Endocrine* **2019**, *66*, 485–493. [CrossRef] [PubMed]
9. Gong, X.; Ji, M.; Xu, J.; Zhang, C.; Li, M. Hypoglycemic effects of bioactive ingredients from medicine food homology and medicinal health food species used in China. *Crit. Rev. Food Sci. Nutr.* **2020**, *60*, 2303–2326. [CrossRef]
10. Kankanala, J.; Kirby, K.A.; Huber, A.D.; Casey, M.C.; Wilson, D.J.; Sarafianos, S.G.; Wang, Z. Design, synthesis and biological evaluations of N-Hydroxy thienopyrimidine-2,4-diones as inhibitors of HIV reverse transcriptase-associated RNase H. *Eur. J. Med. Chem.* **2017**, *141*, 149–161. [CrossRef]
11. Chen, Y.; Zhao, Z.; Fan, H.; Li, Z.; He, Y.; Liu, C. Safety and therapeutic effects of anti-fibrotic Traditional Chinese Medicine Fuzheng Huayu on persistent advanced stage fibrosis following 2 years entecavir treatment: Study protocol for a single arm clinical objective performance criteria trial. *Contemp. Clin. Trials Commun.* **2020**, *19*, 100601. [CrossRef] [PubMed]
12. Zhou, M.; Hong, Y.; Lin, X.; Shen, L.; Feng, Y. Recent pharmaceutical evidence on the compatibility rationality of traditional Chinese medicine. *J. Ethnopharmacol.* **2017**, *206*, 363–375. [CrossRef] [PubMed]

13. Alkhatib, A.; Tsang, C.; Tiss, A.; Bahorun, T.; Arefanian, H.; Barake, R.; Khadir, A.; Tuomilehto, J. Functional Foods and Lifestyle Approaches for Diabetes Prevention and Management. *Nutrients* **2017**, *9*, 1310. [CrossRef] [PubMed]
14. Relman, D.A.; Falkow, S. The meaning and impact of the human genome sequence for microbiology. *Trends Microbiol.* **2001**, *9*, 206–214. [CrossRef]
15. Li, B.Y.; Xu, X.Y.; Gan, R.Y.; Sun, Q.C.; Meng, J.M.; Shang, A.; Mao, Q.Q.; Li, H.B. Targeting Gut Microbiota for the Prevention and Management of Diabetes Mellitus by Dietary Natural Products. *Foods* **2019**, *8*, 440. [CrossRef]
16. Cunningham, A.L.; Stephens, J.W.; Harris, D.A. Gut microbiota influence in type 2 diabetes mellitus (T2DM). *Gut Pathog.* **2021**, *13*, 50. [CrossRef]
17. Larsen, N.; Vogensen, F.K.; van den Berg, F.W.; Nielsen, D.S.; Andreasen, A.S.; Pedersen, B.K.; Al-Soud, W.A.; Sorensen, S.J.; Hansen, L.H.; Jakobsen, M. Gut microbiota in human adults with type 2 diabetes differs from non-diabetic adults. *PLoS ONE* **2010**, *5*, e9085. [CrossRef]
18. Tilg, H.; Moschen, A.R. Microbiota and diabetes: An evolving relationship. *Gut* **2014**, *63*, 1513–1521. [CrossRef]
19. Cani, P.D.; Possemiers, S.; Van de Wiele, T.; Guiot, Y.; Everard, A.; Rottier, O.; Geurts, L.; Naslain, D.; Neyrinck, A.; Lambert, D.M.; et al. Changes in gut microbiota control inflammation in obese mice through a mechanism involving GLP-2-driven improvement of gut permeability. *Gut* **2009**, *58*, 1091–1103. [CrossRef]
20. Cani, P.D.; Bibiloni, R.; Knauf, C.; Waget, A.; Neyrinck, A.M.; Delzenne, N.M.; Burcelin, R. Changes in gut microbiota control metabolic endotoxemia-induced inflammation in high-fat diet-induced obesity and diabetes in mice. *Diabetes* **2008**, *57*, 1470–1481. [CrossRef]
21. Sedighi, M.; Razavi, S.; Navab-Moghadam, F.; Khamseh, M.E.; Alaei-Shahmiri, F.; Mehrtash, A.; Amirmozafari, N. Comparison of gut microbiota in adult patients with type 2 diabetes and healthy individuals. *Microb. Pathog.* **2017**, *111*, 362–369. [CrossRef]
22. Dabke, K.; Hendrick, G.; Devkota, S. The gut microbiome and metabolic syndrome. *J. Clin. Investig.* **2019**, *129*, 4050–4057. [CrossRef]
23. Li, W.; Yuan, G.; Pan, Y.; Wang, C.; Chen, H. Network Pharmacology Studies on the Bioactive Compounds and Action Mechanisms of Natural Products for the Treatment of Diabetes Mellitus: A Review. *Front. Pharmacol.* **2017**, *8*, 74–84. [CrossRef] [PubMed]
24. Hung, W.-W.; Hung, W.-C. How gut microbiota relate to the oral antidiabetic treatment of type 2 diabetes. *Med. Microecol.* **2020**, *3*, 100007. [CrossRef]
25. Li, L.J.; Wu, Z.W.; Xiao, D.S.; Sheng, J.F. Changes of gut flora and endotoxin in rats with D-galactosamine-induced acute liver failure. *World J. Gastroenterol.* **2004**, *10*, 2087–2090. [CrossRef]
26. Chen, Y.; Yang, H.; Deng, J.; Fan, D. Ginsenoside Rk3 Ameliorates Obesity-Induced Colitis by Regulating of Intestinal Flora and the TLR4/NF-kappaB Signaling Pathway in C57BL/6 Mice. *J. Agric. Food Chem.* **2021**, *69*, 3082–3093. [CrossRef] [PubMed]
27. Niu, J.; Pi, Z.F.; Yue, H.; Yang, H.; Wang, Y.; Yu, Q.; Liu, S.Y. Effect of 20(S)-ginsenoside Rg3 on streptozotocin-induced experimental type 2 diabetic rats: A urinary metabonomics study by rapid-resolution liquid chromatography/mass spectrometry. *Rapid Commun. Mass Spectrom.* **2012**, *26*, 2683–2689. [CrossRef] [PubMed]
28. Bai, L.; Gao, J.; Wei, F.; Zhao, J.; Wang, D.; Wei, J. Therapeutic Potential of Ginsenosides as an Adjuvant Treatment for Diabetes. *Front. Pharmacol.* **2018**, *9*, 423. [CrossRef]
29. Lee, S.Y.; Yuk, H.G.; Ko, S.G.; Cho, S.G.; Moon, G.S. Gut Microbiome Prolongs an Inhibitory Effect of Korean Red Ginseng on High-Fat-Diet-Induced Mouse Obesity. *Nutrients* **2021**, *13*, 926. [CrossRef]
30. Luo, J.; Chai, Y.; Zhao, M.; Guo, Q.; Bao, Y. Hypoglycemic effects and modulation of gut microbiota of diabetic mice by saponin from Polygonatum sibiricum. *Food Funct.* **2020**, *11*, 4327–4338. [CrossRef]
31. Wang, H.-Y.; Guo, L.-X.; Hu, W.-H.; Peng, Z.-T.; Wang, C.; Chen, Z.-C.; Liu, E.Y.L.; Dong, T.T.X.; Wang, T.-J.; Tsim, K.W.K. Polysaccharide from tuberous roots of Ophiopogon japonicus regulates gut microbiota and its metabolites during alleviation of high-fat-induced type-2 diabetes in mice. *J. Funct. Foods* **2019**, *63*, 103593–103603. [CrossRef]
32. Wang, L.; Wang, S.; Wang, Y.; Ruan, K.F.; Feng, Y. Effect of MDG-1 on oral glucose tolerance and intestinal microecological balance in diabetic mice. *World Chin. J. Dig.* **2011**, *19*, 2058–2062. [CrossRef]
33. Yang, Y.; Chang, Y.; Wu, Y.; Liu, H.; Liu, Q.; Kang, Z.; Wu, M.; Yin, H.; Duan, J. A homogeneous polysaccharide from Lycium barbarum: Structural characterizations, anti-obesity effects and impacts on gut microbiota. *Int. J. Biol. Macromol.* **2021**, *183*, 2074–2087. [CrossRef] [PubMed]
34. Yang, M.C.; Yuan, M.X.; Lu, W.; Bao, Y.H.; Chai, Y.Y. In Vitro Digestion Properties of Polygonatum sibiricum Polysaccharide and Its Regulatory Action on the Gut Microbiota in T2DM Mice. *Mod. Food Sci. Technol.* **2021**, *37*, 8–22.
35. Yuan, Y.; Zhou, J.; Zheng, Y.; Xu, Z.; Li, Y.; Zhou, S.; Zhang, C. Beneficial effects of polysaccharide-rich extracts from Apocynum venetum leaves on hypoglycemic and gut microbiota in type 2 diabetic mice. *Biomed. Pharmacother.* **2020**, *127*, 110182. [CrossRef]
36. Wang, C.; Yin, Y.; Cao, X.; Li, X. Effects of Maydis stigma polysaccharide on the intestinal microflora in type-2 diabetes. *Pharm. Biol.* **2016**, *54*, 3086–3092. [CrossRef]
37. Nie, Q.; Hu, J.; Gao, H.; Fan, L.; Chen, H.; Nie, S. Polysaccharide from *Plantago asiatica* L. attenuates hyperglycemia, hyperlipidemia and affects colon microbiota in type 2 diabetic rats. *Food Hydrocol.* **2019**, *86*, 34–42. [CrossRef]
38. Wang, Q.; Chai, D.D.; Wu, X.H.; Ren, L.W.; Liu, Y.N.; Yu, Z.W. Radix Pseudostellariae polysaccharide attenuates high fat diet induced hepatic insulin resistance in mice. *Chin. J. Pathophysiol.* **2015**, *31*, 5–10.
39. Gao, H.; Wen, J.J.; Hu, J.L.; Nie, Q.X.; Chen, H.H.; Xiong, T.; Nie, S.P.; Xie, M.Y. Polysaccharide from fermented *Momordica charantia* L. with *Lactobacillus plantarum* NCU116 ameliorates type 2 diabetes in rats. *Carbohydr. Polym.* **2018**, *201*, 624–633. [CrossRef]

40. Chen, C.; You, L.J.; Huang, Q.; Fu, X.; Zhang, B.; Liu, R.H.; Li, C. Modulation of gut microbiota by mulberry fruit polysaccharide treatment of obese diabetic db/db mice. *Food Funct.* **2018**, *9*, 3732–3742. [CrossRef]
41. Liu, G.; Liang, L.; Yu, G.; Li, Q. Pumpkin polysaccharide modifies the gut microbiota during alleviation of type 2 diabetes in rats. *Int. J. Biol. Macromol.* **2018**, *115*, 711–717. [CrossRef]
42. Zhang, B.; Sun, W.; Yu, N.; Sun, J.; Yu, X.; Li, X.; Xing, Y.; Yan, D.; Ding, Q.; Xiu, Z.; et al. Anti-diabetic effect of baicalein is associated with the modulation of gut microbiota in streptozotocin and high-fat-diet induced diabetic rats. *J. Funct. Foods* **2018**, *46*, 256–267. [CrossRef]
43. Ahmed, D.; Khan, M.I.; Sharma, M.; Khan, M.F. Novel pentacyclic triterpene isolated from seeds of Euryale Ferox Salisb. ameliorates diabetes in streptozotocin induced diabetic rats. *Interdiscip. Toxicol.* **2018**, *11*, 275–288. [CrossRef]
44. Gong, J.; Hu, M.; Huang, Z.; Fang, K.; Wang, D.; Chen, Q.; Li, J.; Yang, D.; Zou, X.; Xu, L.; et al. Berberine Attenuates Intestinal Mucosal Barrier Dysfunction in Type 2 Diabetic Rats. *Front. Pharmacol.* **2017**, *8*, 42–54. [CrossRef] [PubMed]
45. Liu, D.; Zhang, Y.; Liu, Y.; Hou, L.; Li, S.; Tian, H.; Zhao, T. Berberine Modulates Gut Microbiota and Reduces Insulin Resistance via the TLR4 Signaling Pathway. *Exp. Clin. Endocrinol. Diabetes* **2018**, *126*, 513–520. [CrossRef]
46. Xu, Z.; Dai, X.X.; Zhang, Q.Y.; Su, S.L.; Yan, H.; Zhu, Y.; Shang, E.X.; Qian, D.W.; Duan, J.A. Protective effects and mechanisms of Rehmannia glutinosa leaves total glycoside on early kidney injury in db/db mice. *Biomed. Pharmacother.* **2020**, *125*, 109926. [CrossRef] [PubMed]
47. Zhang, Y.; Peng, Y.; Zhao, L.; Zhou, G.; Li, X. Regulating the gut microbiota and SCFAs in the faeces of T2DM rats should be one of antidiabetic mechanisms of mogrosides in the fruits of Siraitia grosvenorii. *J. Ethnopharmacol.* **2021**, *274*, 114033–114044. [CrossRef]
48. Yuan, H.; Shi, F.; Meng, L.; Wang, W. Effect of sea buckthorn protein on the intestinal microbial community in streptozotocin-induced diabetic mice. *Int. J. Biol. Macromol.* **2018**, *107*, 1168–1174. [CrossRef] [PubMed]
49. Chen, K.; Chen, H.; Faas, M.M.; de Haan, B.J.; Li, J.; Xiao, P.; Zhang, H.; Diana, J.; de Vos, P.; Sun, J. Specific inulin-type fructan fibers protect against autoimmune diabetes by modulating gut immunity, barrier function, and microbiota homeostasis. *Mol. Nutr. Food Res.* **2017**, *61*, 1601006. [CrossRef]
50. Lira Neto, J.C.G.; Damasceno, M.M.C.; Ciol, M.A.; de Freitas, R.; de Araujo, M.F.M.; Teixeira, C.R.S.; Carvalho, G.C.N.; Lisboa, K.; Marques, R.L.L.; Alencar, A.; et al. Efficacy of Cinnamon as an Adjuvant in Reducing the Glycemic Biomarkers of Type 2 Diabetes Mellitus: A Three-Month, Randomized, Triple-Blind, Placebo-Controlled Clinical Trial. *J. Am. Coll. Nutr.* **2021**, 1–9, (online ahead of print). [CrossRef]
51. Peng, X.C.; Huang, L.Z.; Zhan, H.L.; Wang, C.; Zhang, N.; Liu, L. Effects of essential oil from Cinnamomum Cassia on Clostridia flora IV and Bacteroides in gut of rats. *Chin. Tradit. Herb. Drugs* **2013**, *44*, 437–443.
52. Liu, J.; Henkel, T. Traditional Chinese medicine (TCM): Are polyphenols and saponins the key ingredients triggering biological activities? *Curr. Med. Chem.* **2002**, *9*, 1483–1488. [CrossRef]
53. Adeshirlarijaney, A.; Gewirtz, A.T. Considering gut microbiota in treatment of type 2 diabetes mellitus. *Gut Microbes* **2020**, *11*, 253–264. [CrossRef] [PubMed]
54. Sun, Y.; Guo, M.; Feng, Y.; Zheng, H.; Lei, P.; Ma, X.; Han, X.; Guan, H.; Hou, D. Effect of ginseng polysaccharides on NK cell cytotoxicity in immunosuppressed mice. *Exp. Ther. Med.* **2016**, *12*, 3773–3777. [CrossRef] [PubMed]
55. Pang, B.; Zhang, Y.; Liu, J.; He, L.S.; Zheng, Y.J.; Lian, F.M. Correction to: Prevention of Type 2 diabetes with the Chinese herbal medicine tianqi capsule: A systematic review and meta-analysis. *Diabetes Ther.* **2017**, *8*, 1243–1245. [CrossRef] [PubMed]
56. Tian, J.; Lian, F.; Yang, L.; Tong, X. Evaluation of the Chinese Herbal medicine jinlida in Type 2 diabetes patients based on stratification: Results of subgroup analysis from a 12-week trial. *J. Diabetes* **2018**, *10*, 112–120. [CrossRef]
57. Zhang, Y.C.; Lu, B.J.; Zhao, M.H.; Rong, Y.Z.; Chen, R.M. Effect of shengmai injection on vascular endothelial and heart functions in patients with coronary heart disease complicated with diabetes mellitus. *Chin. J. Integr. Med.* **2008**, *14*, 281–286. [CrossRef]
58. Wang, Y.; Choi, H.K.; Brinckmann, J.A.; Jiang, X.; Huang, L. Chemical analysis of Panax quinquefolius (North American ginseng): A review. *J. Chromatogr. A* **2015**, *14*, 1426. [CrossRef]
59. Gan, L.; Zhang, S.H.; Yang, X.L.; Xu, H.B. Immunomodulation and antitumor activity by a polysaccharide protein complex from Lycium barbarum. *Int. Immunopharmacol.* **2004**, *4*, 563–569. [CrossRef]
60. Parnell, J.A.; Reimer, R.A. Prebiotic fiber modulation of the gut microbiota improves risk factors for obesity and the metabolic syndrome. *Gut Microbes* **2012**, *3*, 29–34. [CrossRef]
61. He, J.; Ye, L.; Fang, C.; Li, J.; Liu, J.; Zhang, W. Identification of changes in volatile organic compounds in Ophiopogonis Radix containing spoiled products in different proportions by headspace-gas chromatography-ion mobility spectrometry. *J. Food Biochem.* **2021**, e13802. [CrossRef] [PubMed]
62. Yang, Y.; Zhou, Y. Shashen-Maidong Decoction-Mediated IFN-gamma and IL-4 on the Regulation of Th1/Th2 Imbalance in RP Rats. *BioMed Res. Int.* **2019**, *2019*, 6012473. [PubMed]
63. He, Q.; Zhang, T.; Jin, B.; Wu, Y.; Wu, J.; Gao, P.; Wu, S. Exploring the Regulatory Mechanism of Modified Huanglian Maidong Decoction on Type 2 Diabetes Mellitus Biological Network Based on Systematic Pharmacology. *Evid. Based Complement. Altern. Med.* **2021**, *2021*, 1768720. [CrossRef]
64. Mao, D.; Tian, X.Y.; Mao, D.; Hung, S.W.; Wang, C.C.; Lau, C.B.S.; Lee, H.M.; Wong, C.K.; Chow, E.; Ming, X.; et al. A polysaccharide extract from the medicinal plant Maidong inhibits the IKK-NF-kappaB pathway and IL-1beta-induced islet inflammation and increases insulin secretion. *J. Biol. Chem.* **2020**, *295*, 12573–12587. [CrossRef] [PubMed]

65. Liu, L.; Lao, W.; Ji, Q.S.; Yang, Z.H.; Yu, G.C.; Zhong, J.X. Lycium barbarum polysaccharides protected human retinal pigment epithelial cells against oxidative stress-induced apoptosis. *Int. J. Ophthalmol.* **2015**, *8*, 11–16. [PubMed]
66. Zhao, X.Q.; Guo, S.; Lu, Y.Y.; Hua, Y.; Zhang, F.; Yan, H.; Shang, E.X.; Wang, H.Q.; Zhang, W.H.; Duan, J.A. Lycium barbarum L. leaves ameliorate type 2 diabetes in rats by modulating metabolic profiles and gut microbiota composition. *Biomed. Pharmacother.* **2020**, *121*, 109559. [CrossRef]
67. Samuelsen, A.B. The traditional uses, chemical constituents and biological activities of Plantago major L. A review. *J. Ethnopharmacol.* **2000**, *71*, 1–21. [CrossRef]
68. Michaelsen, T.E.; Gilje, A.; Samuelsen, A.B.; Hogasen, K.; Paulsen, B.S. Interaction between human complement and a pectin type polysaccharide fraction, PMII, from the leaves of Plantago major L. *Scand. J. Immunol.* **2000**, *52*, 483–490. [CrossRef]
69. Ren, H.; Cao, J.; Chen, Y.; Li, G. Current research state and exploitation of Apocynum venetum L. *North. Hortic.* **2008**, *7*, 4.
70. Everard, A.; Cani, P.D. Diabetes, obesity and gut microbiota. *Best Pract. Res. Clin. Gastroenterol.* **2013**, *27*, 73–83. [CrossRef]
71. Jin, D.L.; Chen, X.B. Progress in research on hypoglycemic effect of traditional Chinese medicine. *Zhejiang J. Integr. Tradit. Chin. West. Med.* **2015**, *25*, 1–3.
72. Chen, F.; Liu, D.B. Advances in anti-diabetes mechanism of active components in Traditional Chinese Medicine. *Acta Chin. Med. Pharmacol.* **2012**, *40*, 1–5.
73. Zhang, B.; Yue, R.; Chen, Y.; Yang, M.; Huang, X.; Shui, J.; Peng, Y.; Chin, J. Gut Microbiota, a Potential New Target for Chinese Herbal Medicines in Treating Diabetes Mellitus. *Evid. Based Complement. Altern. Med.* **2019**, *2019*, 2634898. [CrossRef] [PubMed]
74. Zhou, S.S.; Xu, J.; Zhu, H.; Wu, J.; Xu, J.D.; Yan, R.; Li, X.Y.; Liu, H.H.; Duan, S.M.; Wang, Z.; et al. Gut microbiota-involved mechanisms in enhancing systemic exposure of ginsenosides by coexisting polysaccharides in ginseng decoction. *Sci. Rep.* **2016**, *6*, 22474. [CrossRef] [PubMed]
75. Zheng, J.; Tian, W.; Yang, C.; Shi, W.; Cao, P.; Long, J.; Xiao, L.; Wu, Y.; Liang, J.; Li, X.; et al. Identification of flavonoids in Plumula nelumbinis and evaluation of their antioxidant properties from different habitats. *Ind. Crop. Prod.* **2019**, *127*, 36–45. [CrossRef]
76. Chen, S.; Li, X.; Wu, J.; Li, J.; Xiao, M.; Yang, Y.; Liu, Z.; Cheng, Y. Plumula Nelumbinis: A review of traditional uses, phytochemistry, pharmacology, pharmacokinetics and safety. *J. Ethnopharmacol.* **2021**, *266*, 113429. [CrossRef]
77. Yuan, H.; Meng, S.; Wang, G.; Gong, Z.; Sun, W.; He, G. Hypoglycemic effect of triterpenoid-rich extracts from Euryale ferox shell on normal and streptozotocin-diabetic mice. *Pak. J. Pharm. Sci.* **2014**, *27*, 859–864.
78. Zhang, T.T.; Jiang, J.G. Active ingredients of traditional Chinese medicine in the treatment of diabetes and diabetic complications. *Expert Opin. Investig. Drugs* **2012**, *21*, 1625–1642. [CrossRef]
79. Wang, N.; Tan, H.Y.; Li, L.; Yuen, M.F.; Feng, Y. Berberine and Coptidis Rhizoma as potential anticancer agents: Recent updates and future perspectives. *J. Ethnopharmacol.* **2015**, *176*, 35–48. [CrossRef]
80. Schiffelers, M. Liposome encapsulated berberine treatment attenuates cardiac dysfunction after myocardial infarction. *J. Control. Release* **2017**, *247*, 7.
81. Lan, J.; Zhao, Y.; Dong, F.; Yan, Z.; Zheng, W.; Fan, J.; Sun, G. Meta-analysis of the effect and safety of berberine in the treatment of type 2 diabetes mellitus, hyperlipemia and hypertension. *J. Ethnopharmacol.* **2015**, *161*, 69–81. [CrossRef]
82. Gu, J.-F.; Su, S.-L.; Guo, J.-M.; Zhu, Y.; Zhao, M.; Duan, J.-A. The aerial parts of Salvia miltiorrhiza Bge. strengthen intestinal barrier and modulate gut microbiota imbalance in streptozocin-induced diabetic mice. *J. Funct. Foods* **2017**, *36*, 362–374. [CrossRef]
83. Wang, T.; Sun, J.; Liu, C.; He, Q.; Zhou, X.; Wan, J. Effects of Fried Fructus Aurantii Immaturus with Wheat Bran Decoction on Intestinal Flora in rats with Functional Dyspepsia. *Chin. Pharm. J.* **2021**, *56*, 1068–1075.
84. Zhang, W.-Y.; Zhang, H.-H.; Yu, C.-H.; Fang, J.; Ying, H.-Z. Ethanol extract of Atractylodis macrocephalae Rhizoma ameliorates insulin resistance and gut microbiota in type 2 diabetic db/db mice. *J. Funct. Foods* **2017**, *39*, 139–151. [CrossRef]
85. Yan, H.; Lu, J.; Wang, Y.; Gu, W.; Yang, X.; Yu, J. Intake of total saponins and polysaccharides from Polygonatum kingianum affects the gut microbiota in diabetic rats. *Phytomedicine* **2017**, *26*, 45–54. [CrossRef] [PubMed]
86. Xie, Y.; Xiao, M.; Ni, Y.; Jiang, S.; Feng, G.; Sang, S.; Du, G. Alpinia oxyphylla Miq. Extract Prevents Diabetes in Mice by Modulating Gut Microbiota. *J. Diabetes Res.* **2018**, *2018*, 4230590. [CrossRef] [PubMed]
87. Xue, M.; Liu, Y.; Xu, H.; Zhou, Z.; Ma, Y.; Sun, T.; Liu, M.; Zhang, H.; Liang, H. Propolis modulates the gut microbiota and improves the intestinal mucosal barrier function in diabetic rats. *Biomed. Pharmacother.* **2019**, *118*, 109393. [CrossRef]
88. Zheng, Y.; Wu, Y.; Tao, L.; Chen, X.; Jones, T.J.; Wang, K.; Hu, F. Chinese Propolis Prevents Obesity and Metabolism Syndromes Induced by a High Fat Diet and Accompanied by an Altered Gut Microbiota Structure in Mice. *Nutrients* **2020**, *12*, 959. [CrossRef]
89. Choi, Y.; Bose, S.; Shin, N.R.; Song, E.J.; Nam, Y.D.; Kim, H. Lactate-Fortified Puerariae Radix Fermented by Bifidobacterium breve Improved Diet-Induced Metabolic Dysregulation via Alteration of Gut Microbial Communities. *Nutrients* **2020**, *12*, 276. [CrossRef]
90. Sheng, Y.; Zheng, S.; Ma, T.; Zhang, C.; Ou, X.; He, X.; Xu, W.; Huang, K. Mulberry leaf alleviates streptozotocin-induced diabetic rats by attenuating NEFA signaling and modulating intestinal microflora. *Sci. Rep.* **2017**, *7*, 12041. [CrossRef]
91. Liu, S.; Li, F.; Zhang, X. Structural modulation of gut microbiota reveals Coix seed contributes to weight loss in mice. *Appl. Microbiol. Biotechnol.* **2019**, *103*, 5311–5321. [CrossRef] [PubMed]
92. Gao, W.; Hou, M.; Chen, X.; Wang, P.; Ren, J.; Liu, J. Mechanism of Astragali Radix Vesicle-like Nanoparticles for Reducing Blood Glucose in db/db Diabetic Mice by Regulating Gut Microbiota. *Chin. J. Exp. Tradit. Med. Formulae* **2021**, *27*, 111–118.
93. Wang, S.; Li, X.Y.; Shen, L. Modulation effects of Dendrobium officinale on gut microbiota of type 2 diabetes model mice. *FEMS Microbiol. Lett.* **2021**, *368*, 1–5. [CrossRef]

94. Wang, H. Effects of Hemp Seed Oil-Water Mixture on Intestinal Microbial and Intestinal Immunity in Mice. Master's Thesis, Guangdong Pharmaceutical University, Guangzhou, China, 2016.
95. Xin, H. Effect Study of Yam Gruel on Bifidobacterium in the Gut with Diabetic Patients of Type 2. Master's Thesis, Fujian University of Traditional Chinese Medicine, Fuzhou, China, 2016.
96. Sforcin, J.M.; Bankova, V. Propolis: Is there a potential for the development of new drugs? *J. Ethnopharmacol.* **2011**, *133*, 253–260. [CrossRef] [PubMed]
97. Zhou, G.; Wu, F.; Zhu, J.; Gao, Y.; Wan, H. Effect of Wumeiwan on Intestinal Microflora, Inflammatory Factor and Short Chain Fatty Acids in Type 2 Diabetic Rat. *Chin. J. Exp. Tradit. Med. Formulae* **2020**, *26*, 8–15.
98. Hussain, A.; Yadav, M.K.; Bose, S.; Wang, J.H.; Lim, D.; Song, Y.K.; Ko, S.G.; Kim, H. Daesiho-Tang Is an Effective Herbal Formulation in Attenuation of Obesity in Mice through Alteration of Gene Expression and Modulation of Intestinal Microbiota. *PLoS ONE* **2016**, *11*, e0165483. [CrossRef]
99. Zhang, C.; Ma, G.; Deng, Y.; Wang, X.; Chen, Y.C.; Tu, X.Y.; Yu, M.; Sheng, J. Effect of Gegen Qinlian Decoction on LPS, TNF-α, IL-6, and intestinal flora in diabetic KK-Ay mice. *Chin. Tradit. Herb. Drugs* **2017**, *48*, 1611–1616.
100. Liu, C.-Z.; Chen, W.; Wang, M.-X.; Wang, Y.; Chen, L.-Q.; Zhao, F.; Shi, Y.; Liu, H.-J.; Dou, X.-B.; Liu, C.; et al. Dendrobium officinale Kimura et Migo and American ginseng mixture: A Chinese herbal formulation for gut microbiota modulation. *Chin. J. Nat. Med.* **2020**, *18*, 446–459. [CrossRef]
101. Zhao, J.; Li, Y.; Sun, M.; Xin, L.; Wang, T.; Wei, L.; Yu, C.; Liu, M.; Ni, Y.; Lu, R.; et al. The Chinese Herbal Formula Shenzhu Tiaopi Granule Results in Metabolic Improvement in Type 2 Diabetic Rats by Modulating the Gut Microbiota. *Evid. Based Complement. Altern. Med.* **2019**, *2019*, 6976394. [CrossRef]
102. Gao, K.; Yang, R.; Zhang, J.; Wang, Z.; Jia, C.; Zhang, F.; Li, S.; Wang, J.; Murtaza, G.; Xie, H.; et al. Effects of Qijian mixture on type 2 diabetes assessed by metabonomics, gut microbiota and network pharmacology. *Pharmacol. Res.* **2018**, *130*, 93–109. [CrossRef] [PubMed]
103. Fan, S.; Zhang, C.; Li, X.; Ao, M.; Yu, L. Effect of Raw and Salt-processed Herb Pair Anemarrhenae Rhizoma-Phellodendri Chinensis Cortex on Gut Microbiota of Type 2 Diabetic Rats Based on 16S T Sequencing Technique. *Pharmacol. Clin. Chin. Med.* **2020**, *36*, 150–156.
104. Yang, H.J.; Kim, M.J.; Kwon, D.Y.; Kim, D.S.; Zhang, T.; Ha, C.; Park, S. Combination of Aronia, Red Ginseng, Shiitake Mushroom and Nattokinase Potentiated Insulin Secretion and Reduced Insulin Resistance with Improving Gut Microbiome Dysbiosis in Insulin Deficient Type 2 Diabetic Rats. *Nutrients* **2018**, *10*, 948. [CrossRef] [PubMed]
105. Xiao, S.; Liu, C.; Chen, M.; Zou, J.; Zhang, Z.; Cui, X.; Jiang, S.; Shang, E.; Qian, D.; Duan, J. Scutellariae radix and coptidis rhizoma ameliorate glycolipid metabolism of type 2 diabetic rats by modulating gut microbiota and its metabolites. *Appl. Microbiol. Biotechnol.* **2020**, *104*, 303–317. [CrossRef] [PubMed]

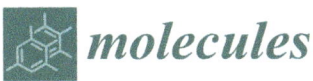

Review

Phytotherapeutic Approaches to the Prevention of Age-Related Changes and the Extension of Active Longevity

Olga Babich [1], Viktoria Larina [1], Svetlana Ivanova [2,3,*], Andrei Tarasov [4], Maria Povydysh [5,6], Anastasiya Orlova [6,7], Jovana Strugar [6] and Stanislav Sukhikh [1]

1. Institute of Living Systems, Immanuel Kant Baltic Federal University, A. Nevskogo Street 14, Kaliningrad 236016, Russia; olich.43@mail.ru (O.B.); surinac@mail.ru (V.L.); SSukhikh@kantiana.ru (S.S.)
2. Natural Nutraceutical Biotesting Laboratory, Kemerovo State University, Krasnaya Street 6, Kemerovo 650043, Russia
3. Department of General Mathematics and Informatics, Kemerovo State University, Krasnaya Street 6, Kemerovo 650043, Russia
4. Department of Pediatrics and Preventive Medicine, Medical Institute, Immanuel Kant Baltic Federal University, 14 A. Nevskogo ul., Kaliningrad 236016, Russia; drup1@yandex.ru
5. Department of Biochemistry, Saint Petersburg State Chemical Pharmaceutical University, Professora Popova 14A, Saint Petersburg 197376, Russia; maria.povydysh@pharminnotech.com
6. Department of Pharmacognosy, Saint Petersburg State Chemical Pharmaceutical University, Professora Popova 14A, Saint Petersburg 197376, Russia; lanas_95@mail.ru (A.O.); jovana.strugar12@gmail.com (J.S.)
7. Department of Science and Training of Scientific and Pedagogical Personnel, Saint Petersburg State Chemical Pharmaceutical University, Professora Popova 14A, Saint Petersburg 197376, Russia
* Correspondence: pavvm2000@mail.ru; Tel.: +7-384-239-6832

Citation: Babich, O.; Larina, V.; Ivanova, S.; Tarasov, A.; Povydysh, M.; Orlova, A.; Strugar, J.; Sukhikh, S. Phytotherapeutic Approaches to the Prevention of Age-Related Changes and the Extension of Active Longevity. *Molecules* **2022**, *27*, 2276. https://doi.org/10.3390/molecules27072276

Academic Editors: Toshio Morikawa and Ricardo Calhelha

Received: 9 February 2022
Accepted: 30 March 2022
Published: 31 March 2022

Publisher's Note: MDPI stays neutral with regard to jurisdictional claims in published maps and institutional affiliations.

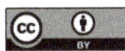

Copyright: © 2022 by the authors. Licensee MDPI, Basel, Switzerland. This article is an open access article distributed under the terms and conditions of the Creative Commons Attribution (CC BY) license (https://creativecommons.org/licenses/by/4.0/).

Abstract: Maintaining quality of life with an increase in life expectancy is considered one of the global problems of our time. This review explores the possibility of using natural plant compounds with antioxidant, anti-inflammatory, anti-glycation, and anti-neurodegenerative properties to slow down the onset of age-related changes. Age-related changes such as a decrease in mental abilities, the development of inflammatory processes, and increased risk of developing type 2 diabetes have a significant impact on maintaining quality of life. Herbal preparations can play an essential role in preventing and treating neurodegenerative diseases that accompany age-related changes, including Alzheimer's and Parkinson's diseases. Medicinal plants have known sedative, muscle relaxant, neuroprotective, nootropic, and antiparkinsonian properties. The secondary metabolites, mainly polyphenolic compounds, are valuable substances for the development of new anti-inflammatory and hypoglycemic agents. Understanding how mixtures of plants and their biologically active substances work together to achieve a specific biological effect can help develop targeted drugs to prevent diseases associated with aging and age-related changes. Understanding the mechanisms of the biological activity of plant complexes and mixtures determines the prospects for using metabolomic and biochemical methods to prolong active longevity.

Keywords: aging of the human body; medicinal plants; antioxidant; anti-inflammatory; anti-glycation; anti-neurodegenerative properties

1. Introduction

One of humanity's global problems is the preservation of quality of life as the average age of the population rises. According to the 2019 Revision of World Population Prospects, by 2050, 1 in 6 people in the world will be over 65 (16% of the population), compared to 1 in 11 in 2019 (9% of the population) [1]. By 2050, one in four people in Europe and North America will be 65 years of age or older. In 2018, for the first time in history, the number of people aged 65 and over exceeded the number of children under the age of five worldwide. The number of people aged 80 and over is projected to triple, from 143 million in 2019 to 426 million in 2050 [1].

Chronic diseases were responsible for more than two-thirds of deaths worldwide (38 million) in 2014, according to the World Health Organization [2]. Most deaths from chronic diseases were associated with cancer, cardiovascular disease, chronic respiratory disease, or diabetes. Although chronic diseases have a major cumulative impact on human health and aging, epidemiology has historically studied chronic diseases separately [3]. Understanding the epidemiology of particular diseases requires a clinical assessment of each chronic disease that contributes to aging. Accounting for multiple chronic diseases at the same time, on the other hand, more accurately reflects the experience of patients who accumulate conditions associated with aging and better reflects overall health. Well-established data show that the incidence of cancer, cardiovascular disease, chronic respiratory disease, and diabetes is associated with common modifiable risk factors such as alcohol use, body mass index (BMI), smoking, unhealthy diet, and physical inactivity, which account for more than two-thirds of the diseases that cause human aging [4].

A significant increase in the proportion of the elderly in populations of developed countries has resulted in an increase in mortality from major diseases of old age (cardiovascular diseases, malignant neoplasms, neurodegenerative processes, decreased resistance to infection, diabetes mellitus) [5]. As a result, it is no coincidence that the concept of healthy aging is listed as one of the top priorities in the UN Program on Aging's project "Programs for Scientific Research on Aging in the Twenty-First Century" [5].

Human aging is accompanied by the accumulation of unhealthy changes in the structure of cell biopolymers and the intercellular matrix. The age-related increase in the level of oxidative processes in cells and tissues is one of the most important factors influencing these changes [6]. With aging, assimilation processes in organs and tissues weaken, and the system of neurohumoral regulation of metabolism and body functions undergoes restructuring. Moreover, one of the leading reasons for this is systemic inflammation and the development of atherosclerotic processes. Oxidative stress associated with inflammation leads to significant changes in the structure of biomolecules. The rate of nonenzymatic protein modifications—oxidation, glycation, and lipooxidation, as well as amyloidogenesis—increases dramatically with age [7]. As a result, aging is often accompanied by the development of metabolic disorders (the most common of which is type 2 diabetes) as well as neurodegenerative diseases. In the process of aging, numerous changes of various natures accumulate in the human body. Therefore, it appears obvious that in order to effectively prolong active longevity, a coordinated effect on all of these factors associated with body aging is required. At the same time, we must not forget that neurodegenerative changes and diabetes mellitus complications are irreversible. Therefore, it is preferable to prevent them, for example, by using substances that prevent the development of these diseases with age—geroprotectors [8]. Clearly, a pharmaceutical strategy that aims to simultaneously prevent the full range of age-related molecular changes such as inflammation, oxidative stress, oxidative and glycoxidative protein modifications, and amyloidogenesis would be more effective than current approaches.

Over the past decades, natural compounds of plant origin have been intensively studied as potential antioxidants, antiglycators, and neuroprotective agents. However, their combined application remains largely intuitive [9]. One of the promising objects for preventing oxidative, inflammatory, neurodegenerative and glycating aging processes are the components of medicinal plants [9]. It has been shown that many secondary plant metabolites can effectively control the aging process and delay the development of age-related diseases [9].

Therefore, the goal of this research was to study the concept of using medicinal plants and their highly purified complexes, which have the optimal combination of antioxidant, anti-inflammatory, anti-glycating, and anti-neurodegenerative properties, to slow down the onset of age-related changes and prolong active longevity.

The scientific publications and patents of Russian and foreign authors on the effect of medicinal plants and herbal preparations on antioxidant activity, the ability to reduce the harmful effects of free radicals and, as a result, oxidative and aging processes in the human body, were the subjects of this study. Several keyword combinations were used to search PubMed for studies published between 1999 and 2022, including natural compounds, flavonoids, bioflavonoids, aging; medicinal plants; antioxidant, anti-inflammatory, antiglycation, and anti-neurodegenerative properties. Abstracts, bibliographies, editorials, and pieces written in languages other than English and Russian were excluded. Generalization was the primary method [10]. The results of practical studies and original studies of the composition and antioxidant properties of medicinal ingredients, as well as statistical and clinical data on the antioxidant activity of plant ingredients (for example, plant extracts), scientific principles for the use of plant ingredients in the production of medicines, and the results of practical and original studies of the composition and antioxidant properties of medicinal ingredients were analyzed.

2. Antioxidant Properties of Medicinal Plants and Their Complexes

There is no doubt about the importance of disturbances in the regulation of free-radical processes that occur in the body during aging, which is one of the causes of severe pathologies such as atherosclerosis, myocardial infarction, diabetes, cancer, and a number of other diseases, the emergence and progression of which depend on the effect of unfavorable environmental factors, and in some cases, genetic anomalies. In living cells, there is a perfect system of antioxidant protection that regulates the formation of free radicals (FRs) and limits the accumulation in cells of both the FRs themselves and the toxic products of their activity. Accumulation of FRs in the body with aging increases due to a decrease in the effectiveness of the natural antioxidant system caused by exposure to radiation, UV radiation, smoking, alcohol, constant stress, and poor nutrition. Cells use a variety of body defense mechanisms against the toxic effects of free radicals. As a result, therapy with antioxidants (AO) is increasingly being used in the treatment of a variety of diseases. At the same time, the production of branded antioxidant preparations, which include various components of natural or synthetic origin, is expanding [11].

As previously stated [12], free radicals are atoms, molecules, or ions that have unpaired electrons and are extremely active in chemical reactions with other molecules. In a biological system, free radicals are often formed from oxygen, nitrogen, and sulfur molecules. These free radicals are members of the reactive oxygen species (ROS), reactive nitrogen species (RNS), and reactive sulfur species (RSS) groups of molecules. For example, ROS include free radicals such as superoxide anion, perhydroxyl radical, hydroxyl radical, nitric oxide, and other compounds such as hydrogen peroxide, singlet oxygen, hypochlorous acid, and peroxynitrite [13]. ROS are produced during cellular metabolism and functional activity and play an important role in cell signaling, apoptosis, gene expression, and ion transport [14]. However, excessive amounts of ROS can have harmful effects on many molecules, including proteins, lipids, RNA, and DNA, because they are very small and highly reactive. ROS can attack bases in nucleic acids, amino acid side chains in proteins, and double bonds in unsaturated fatty acids, in which the hydroxyl radical is the strongest oxidizing agent. ROS attacking macromolecules are often referred to as oxidative stress. Cells can usually protect themselves from ROS damage by using intracellular enzymes to maintain low ROS homeostasis. ROS levels can grow rapidly during periods of environmental stress and cellular malfunction, causing considerable cell damage in the body. Thus, oxidative stress makes a significant contribution to the pathogenesis of inflammatory diseases, cardiovascular diseases, cancer, diabetes, Alzheimer's disease, and, in general, aging of the body [15]. The human body and other species have developed an antioxidant defense mechanism that comprises enzymatic, metal chelating, and scavenging activities to neutralize free radicals once they have been created in order to avoid or mitigate ROS-induced oxidative damage. Furthermore, plant antioxidants can aid in maintaining a healthy antioxidant level in the body [16].

The last twenty years have been marked by increased attention, both in medicine and the chemical industry, to the products of processing of medicinal plant raw materials (MPRM), which contain a rich complex of biologically active substances (BAS), many of which exhibit antioxidant activity [16,17]. The search, methods for isolation and study of promising natural sources of substances with antiradical activity (ARA) and antioxidant activity (AOA), along with the development of accessible and rapid methods for determining AOA, is currently one of the urgent tasks in preventing aging of the human body for modern medicine, pharmacy, cosmetology, and food industry.

The group of substances that prevent the formation of strong oxidizing agents in vivo during the aging of the human body is diverse. These include the SH-containing amino acid cysteine, some peptides, and proteins (glutathione, albumin), ubiquinone, ascorbic and uric acids, tocopherols, carotenoids, flavonoids, etc. (Figures 1 and 2). The detection of AOA makes it possible to judge the possible physiological value of the studied plant objects. Determining the content of individual AOs is, as a rule, insufficient since, in this case, the processes of mutual oxidation/reduction and the influence of the analyte matrix are not taken into account [18,19].

A significant amount of natural AO of the phenolic class present in MPRM determines their antioxidant effect. The content of flavonoids, along with ascorbic acid and provitamin A, is the most important indicator of the biological value of MPRM. The synergism of the action of ascorbic acid with flavonoids in the regulation of redox processes is significant [20]. The biological activity of natural AO is based on the processes of inhibition of the developing radical oxidation of tissue lipids through the interaction of active radicals with bioantioxidants [21]. It is noteworthy that the AOA value of flavonoids significantly decreases as the number of free phenolic hydroxyl groups in the molecules decreases: quercetin > rutin > luteolin-7-glucoside > apigenin > naringenin > 7-hydroxy-flavone [22]. For example, an assessment of the AOA of various natural flavonoids showed that quercetin and cyanidin have the highest AOA after theaflavin. Quercetin glycosides, such as rutin, have a lower AOA; flavones and flavone glycosides are characterized by the smallest AOA among this group of substances. Therefore, the antioxidant properties of plant raw materials can be judged based on the quantitative content of phenolic substances [20].

It has been established that polyphenols, tocopherols, and flavonoids exhibit AOA. The theory of radical oxidation distinguishes between the mechanisms of linear termination of radical chains on an inhibitor and the mechanism of inhibition, which is realized through the formation of complexes of active radicals with systems with conjugated π-bonds. For example, spatially shielded phenols, tocopherols, interact according to the first mechanism; these inhibitors have a distinct induction period. The second mechanism is realized more often for natural mixtures, including essential oils. Chamazulene and neryl methyl butanoates, two of the compounds found in them, may act as second-type inhibitors [23]. Antioxidants are widely used as the main means of therapy or as additional means of correction in the treatment of atherosclerosis, coronary heart disease, acute cerebrovascular accident, inflammatory processes, diabetes mellitus, a wide range of eye diseases, etc. [24].

Natural antioxidants used in pharmacy easily and organically enter into metabolic processes in the body during aging and practically do not have side effects common in synthetic drugs [25]. However, Henkel et al. [26] found that increased attention is paid to antioxidant therapy to prevent the rapid aging of the population. These substances are appealing because they are considered natural and are associated with a healthy diet. The hypothesis is that reducing oxidative stress can prevent disease processes such as cancer or coronary heart disease. Because the majority of the general population is comprised of reasonably healthy individuals, it is critical that these supplements be free of toxicity and side effects. While early research on antioxidant supplements suggested they could help prevent disease, more recent clinical trials and meta-analyses have cast doubt on their effectiveness. Several studies have shown that overconsumption of supplements can actually be harmful [27–30]. These studies have shown that excessive antioxidant levels can be teratogenic for embryos [31]. As a result, recent attention has been focused on adjusting the use of antioxidants for the treatment of male infertility, with particular emphasis on the potentially dangerous consequences of antioxidant therapy [26].

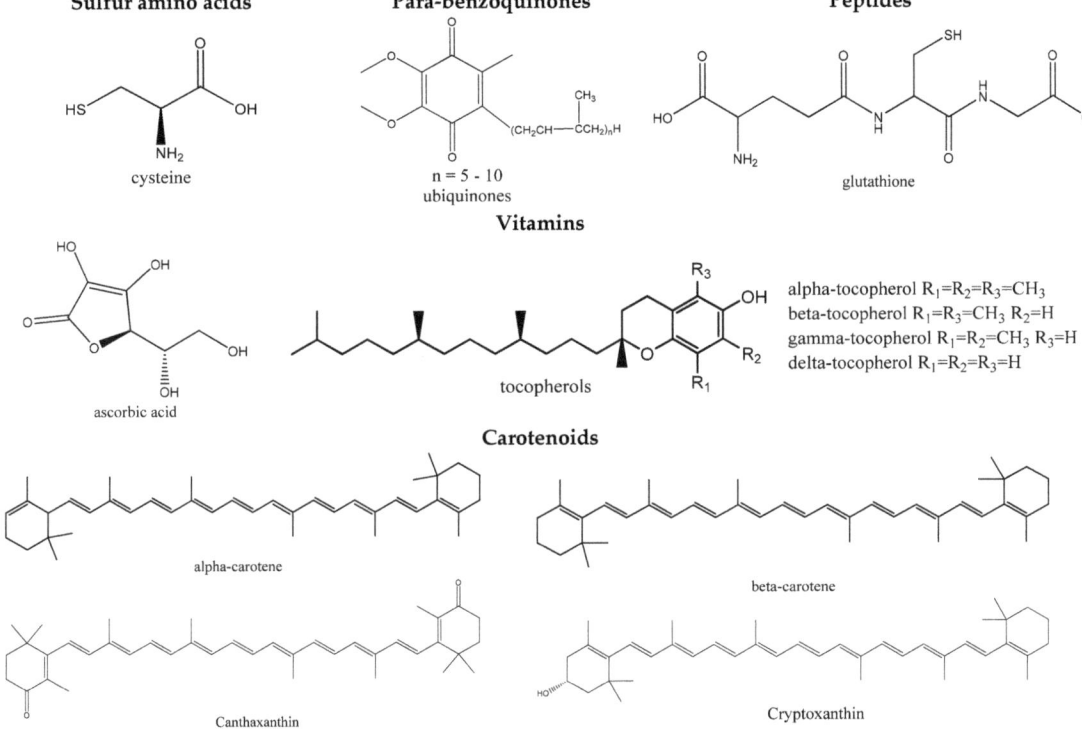

Figure 1. Structural formulas of some antioxidants.

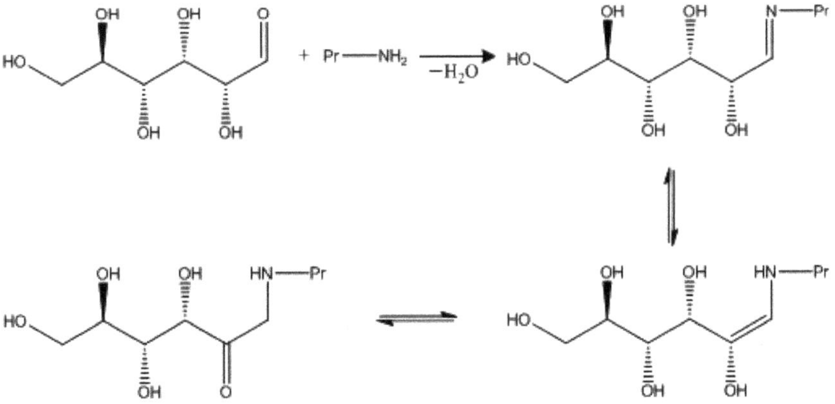

Figure 2. Maillard reaction scheme.

However, their composition is difficult to control [31]. The synergy of the action of complexes of plant and synthetic drugs may be the solution to this problem. Synergy is a process in which certain substances interact with each other to achieve a combined effect that is greater than the sum of their individual effects [32]. It can be considered as a natural direct strategy for increasing the efficacy of drugs with antioxidant activity. Hence, synergistic effects can be observed when plant preparations interact with conventional drugs or biochemical compounds. It is essential to identify and utilize these interactions because any advancement made as a result of such a process could be used to successfully treat human diseases. Even in diseases as complex as cancer or aging, favorable synergistic interactions between plants and medications must be investigated in order to get the optimum results, such as increased patient benefit or the avoidance of negative side effects. Multi-drug therapy is an effective strategy for directly blocking or destroying harmful agents (such as cancer cells, free radicals, or pathogens) while also activating the human body's defense or repair mechanisms. This is because the previously accepted dogma of monodrug therapy has gradually been abandoned; for decades, pharmacological research has been based on the identification of a single active principle [33]. In terms of herbal medicine research, traditional Chinese medicine, Ayurveda, and traditional Western herbal medicine have only recently been scientifically validated and appreciated. Furthermore, over the last two decades, there has been an increase in the use of traditional medicines in combination with complementary and alternative medicine (CAM), which includes not only homeopathy, naturopathy, chiropractic, and energy medicine, but also ethnopharmacology and herbal medicine [34]. It is becoming clear that many diseases have a diverse etiology and can be treated more effectively with a combination drug strategy than with a single therapy. In Western countries, effective combination drug therapy is typically used for multifactorial or complex disease treatment (for example, cancer, hypertension, metabolic and inflammatory diseases, acquired immunodeficiency syndrome (AIDS), aging, oxidative and infectious processes) [35]. Herbal medicine and ethnopharmacology play an important role in the prevention of body aging in this context, as they are based on herbs or plants, which are secundum naturam, a complex pool of millions of molecules. It should be noted that human pharmacotherapy began with the use of plants in ancient times, probably mimicking the self-medication of animals.

Due to the huge popularity of CAM (including ethnopharmacology and herbal medicine), there is a need to focus on the risk/benefit ratio of herbal medicines and updated information. As a result, new information on synergistic anticancer and antioxidant effects of herbal medications and standard synthetic treatments is needed to explore the interaction of plants and drugs. In this regard, research into the complex of medicinal preparations with antioxidant properties is an urgent task.

The group of antioxidant protection of the human body from aging includes fat-soluble plant antioxidants: vitamins of group E (tocopherols), ubiquinone, vitamins of group A (retinols) and provitamins of group A (α-, β-, γ-carotenes), vitamins of group D (calciferols), K (phylloquinone and menaquinone), lipoic acid, etc. [36].

The mechanism of the antioxidant action of these compounds is due to their high donor properties (decrease in the amount of free oxygen in the cell, for example, by activating its utilization, increasing the activity of oxidation and phosphorylation processes), and the ability to restore lipid radicals. All of these compounds are classified as antiradical protection substances or direct antioxidants. Endogenous direct antioxidants are antioxidants that form less reactive radicals and have a more pronounced antioxidant activity. Thus, tocopherols are of the greatest importance among all known endogenous antioxidants [37]. However, the total antioxidant activity of these substances (the ability to inhibit peroxide free radical reactions at all stages of oxidative stress) is determined not only by their antiradical activity but also by the ability of the formed radical of the antioxidant itself, in parallel with recombination reactions with the formation of stable molecules, to initiate new chains of free radical oxidation upon interaction with each new molecule of an oxidized compound [38].

Endogenous direct plant antioxidants, which form less reactive radicals, have a more pronounced antioxidant activity. Thus, tocopherols are of the greatest importance among all known endogenous antioxidants. To date, seven different compounds that exhibit E-vitamin activity have been isolated from natural plant sources and studied. Phospholipids of mitochondria and endoplasmic reticulum of membranes have a specific affinity for α-tocopherols. The presence of a side isoprene chain in tocopherols, corresponding in length to the fatty acid residues of phospholipids, provides them with the ability to integrate into the membrane with subsequent formation of complexes between the methyl groups of the side chain and double bonds of fatty acids [39].

Plant α- and γ-tocopherols (vitamin E) have a pronounced antioxidant activity; the antiradical activity is higher for α-tocopherol and the antioxidant activity is higher for γ-tocopherol. α-Tocopherol provides 60% of the anti-radical action of all fat-soluble plant antioxidants. In addition to the antiradical action, α-tocopherol has the greatest ability to stabilize membranes and form complexes with fatty acids, leading to an increase in membrane resistance to free radicals [40]. Fat-soluble plant antioxidants are retinols and their precursors, mainly β-carotene [41].

The study of the pharmacological activity of *Calluna vulgaris* (L.) Hull., including as an antioxidant agent, is of undoubted interest. Since ancient times, this plant has been used in folk medicine for the treatment of various diseases: atherosclerosis, coronary heart disease, diabetes mellitus, and diseases of the musculoskeletal system. The chemical composition of the plant is quite diverse and includes the following groups of compounds: flavonoids (from 0.5% to 5.5%), catechins, proanthocyanidins (up to 7–8%), phenolic acids (from 5% to 9%), organic acids, amino acids (up to 17%), polysaccharides (about 5%), etc. [42]. It is known that the flavonoids of *Calluna vulgaris* have a pronounced antioxidant activity [43]. Inflammation in damaged tissues intensifies the formation of free radicals, the excess of which can adversely affect healthy cells and tissues. In this case, the use of antioxidants can reduce the risk of oxidative damage.

The selection of dosage form, including the justification of the extractant, plays an important role in the development of a drug. It is critical that the active substances be extracted as much as possible when preparing a dosage form such as an extract. During the extraction of *Calluna vulgaris* shoots with ethyl alcohol, mainly quercetin and its glycosides pass into the extraction. Chepel V. et al. [44] associated the antioxidant properties of *Calluna vulgaris* shoots with kaempferol-3-β-D-galactoside. This compound predominated in the ethyl acetate fraction of the ethanol extract from the aerial part of the plant. Previously, the *Calluna vulgaris* shoot extract was found to be safe for long-term use in an experiment on rats [45]. *Calluna vulgaris* was studied as a plant antioxidant in order to establish the nature of the dose–effect relationship for *Calluna vulgaris* shoot extract in an in vivo model, as well as to evaluate the antioxidant activity of its main component, quercetin-3-β-D-glucoside [42]. *Comarum palustre* L. has a wide spectrum of biological activity, including wound healing, analgesic, anti-inflammatory, immunostimulating, antirheumatic, and antioxidant actions [44]. *Comarum palustre* L. is widely used in traditional and folk medicine. The chemical composition of *Comarum palustre* L. is characterized by great diversity; it includes a polyphenolic complex, essential oils, resins, organic, hydroxycinnamic acids, and their derivatives [43], including chlorogenic acid.

Chlorogenic acid (CA)-3-O-caffeoylquinic acid and its isomers are powerful antioxidants. The properties of CA have been intensively studied over the past few years due to the discovery of a wide range of biological activities. CA exhibits the ability to inhibit tumor growth (in vitro), has an inhibitory effect on colorectal cancer, liver cancer, and laryngeal cancer, helps prevent type 2 diabetes mellitus, and has antihypertensive, antiviral, antibacterial, and antifungal effects [46]. At the same time, CA has relatively low toxicity and no side effects. Because of these properties, CA is used in food supplements and cosmetics with antioxidant properties. It has also been established that one of the molecular-cellular mechanisms of action of the *Comarum palustre* L. extract is its ability to inhibit the processes of free radical oxidation of biomacromolecules, probably due to the high content of substances of a phenolic nature. It has been shown that the mechanism of the antioxidant activity of this phytoextract is associated with its ability to increase the potential of the endogenous defense system of the body [47].

Artemisia vulgáris L. has been used as a medicinal plant since ancient times. It is also used in modern scientific medicine. In modern folk medicine of the countries of Central Asia, the herb *Artemísia vulgáris* L. in the form of a decoction is used as a laxative, diaphoretic, diuretic, and anthelmintic, is used as a sedative and anticonvulsant in Chinese medicine, and in Russian folk medicine in the treatment of bronchial asthma, bleeding, pyoderma, and as an antitoxic, antioxidant, and tonic. Extracts of *Artemisia vulgaris* L. have a cytotoxic effect on leukemia cells. Their choleretic, hypoglycemic, antioxidant, and hypolipidemic properties have also been determined [48]. *Artemisia vulgaris* herb contains essential oils (0.07–0.20%), which contains: limonene, terpinolene, fenchone, aromadendrene, thayyl alcohol, thujone (alpha and betta), alpha-pinene, beta-pinene, camphor, and others [49]; triterpenoids: alpha-amyrin, fernenol; steroids: beta-sitosterol, stigmasterol; amino acids: arginine, histidine, asparagine, proline, lysine, alanine, valine, glycine, isoleucine, aspartic acid, methionine; phenolcarboxylic acids (not less than 0.5% in terms of chlorogenic acid); coumarins (1.2%): scopoletin, umbelliferone, imperatorin, esculetin, xanthotoxol, coumarin [48]; flavonoids (not less than 0.5% in terms of rutin): quercetin, kaempferol, isorhamnetin, apigenin; carbohydrates: polysaccharides, inulin, starch [49]; and artemisinin, a substance with antioxidant properties, was also discovered in the herb [50].

One study [51] investigated the effect of various factors on the yield, antioxidant activity (AA), and total phenol content (TPC) of plant extracts (guava leaves). The effect of leaf sample pretreatment before extraction, extraction method, and leaf age were studied. The results showed that sonication is the most suitable method for plant extraction as it produces an extract with a significantly higher AA. Blanching followed by cooling with ice water was proposed for the leaf pretreatment process. The study of leaf maturity showed that young leaves show the greatest activity. Hot water was the best solvent for extracting the active ingredients. An aqueous extract of young leaves pre-treated by blanching and cooling showed the highest AA values. These values are 1.88-times higher than those of the synthetic antioxidant butylated hydroxytoluene. It was concluded that the extraction of plant extract bioactive components and their antioxidant capacity is influenced by pre-treatment and drying processes, extraction method, and leaf maturity [51].

3. Anti-Neurodegenerative Properties of Medicinal Plants and Their Complexes

Millions of patients in the world suffer from chronic neurodegenerative diseases (Parkinson's and Alzheimer's diseases, Huntington's chorea, hyperprolactinemia, etc.). The key link in the pathogenesis of neurodegenerative diseases is the degeneration of specific neurons, which over time leads to dysfunction in the regulation of which they are involved—cognitive functions in Alzheimer's disease, motor behavior in Parkinson's disease, etc. [52].

Alzheimer's disease (AD) has a special place among neurodegenerative diseases (ND) in terms of its negative significance for society [52]. According to the World Health Organization experts, AD is the most common cause of dementia in the elderly. The global prevalence of dementia in the world will practically double every 20 years to 65.7 million in 2030 and 115.4 million in 2050. A particularly sharp increase in patients will occur in middle- and low-income countries. The prevalence of the disease increases as the age category increases. In people older than 65 years, the number of patients doubles every five years. The available statistical data give grounds to consider AD, along with cardiovascular and oncological diseases, as one of the most serious medical problems in developed countries [53]. The risk of developing Alzheimer's disease is significantly higher in women than in men, mainly due to the higher life expectancy of women compared to men [53].

The etiology of Alzheimer's disease is still an open question. Currently, factors and diseases have been identified that increase the risk of AD developing. Risk factors are advanced age, obesity, insulin resistance, vascular factors, dyslipidemia, hypertension, CNS traumatic injury, and depression. The anatomical pathology of AD at the microscopic level includes neurofibrillary tangles (NFT), senile plaques (SP), and cerebrocortical atrophy, which mainly develops in the association regions and medial areas of the temporal lobe. Alzheimer's disease is accompanied by proteinopathy—the accumulation in the brain tissues of abnormally folded proteins—of amyloid-beta and tau protein. Plaques are formed from small peptides 39–43 amino acids long called amyloid-beta (A-beta, Aβ). Amyloid beta is a fragment of a larger precursor protein, APP. This transmembrane protein plays an important role in neuron growth, survival, and recovery from damage. In Alzheimer's disease, for unknown reasons, APP undergoes proteolysis—it is divided into peptides under the influence of enzymes. Aβ strains formed by one of the peptides stick together in the intercellular space into dense formations known as senile plaques [54]. In Alzheimer's disease, changes in the structure of the tau protein lead to the disintegration of microtubules in brain cells. More specifically, Alzheimer's disease is also referred to as tauopathies, diseases associated with abnormal aggregation of the tau protein. Each neuron contains a cytoskeleton made up of microtubules that carry nutrients and other molecules from the center to the periphery of the cell, to the end of the axon, and back. Microtubules are made up of the tau protein, which stabilizes them along with several other proteins once they are phosphorylated. In Alzheimer's disease, tau protein is over-phosphorylated.

Herbal preparations can play an important role in the prevention and treatment of neurodegenerative diseases, including Alzheimer's and Parkinson's diseases. This review summarizes research by scientists worldwide on these diseases. Many studies by international and Russian scientists have relied on preliminary and clinical studies [55–57]. Alzheimer's and Parkinson's diseases are among the major neurodegenerative disorders (NDDs) that impose a significant socioeconomic burden. People have been searching for a cure for NDDs using natural herbs for centuries. It is reported that many medicinal plants and their secondary metabolites are able to alleviate the symptoms of NDDs [58,59]. The major identified mechanisms by which phytochemicals exert their neuroprotective effects and potential neurological health support during aging include antioxidant, anti-inflammatory, antithrombotic, antiapoptotic, acetylcholinesterase and monoamine oxidase inhibition, and neurotrophic activity [60,61]. Studies [62,63] reviewed clinical trials and provided statistical data on the mechanisms of action of some major herbal products with potential in the treatment of NDD, according to their molecular targets, as well as their regional sources. A number of studies have demonstrated the beneficial properties of plant extracts or their bioactive compounds against NDDs [64,65]. Plant products potentially offer new treatment options for patients with NDD that are a cheaper and culturally acceptable alternative to traditional therapies for millions of people around the world with age-related NDDs [66,67].

The mechanisms of this effect are not always known. Perhaps antioxidant, adaptogenic mechanisms play a role here. Due to the content of carotenoids, some medicinal plants and their complexes prevent the occurrence of Alzheimer's disease. This fact was evaluated in a number of studies [68–72]. Alzheimer's disease is the most devastating neurodegenerative disease affecting the aging population worldwide. Endogenous and exogenous factors are involved in the triggering of this complex and multifactorial disease, the hallmark of which is amyloid-β (Aβ), formed as a result of the breakdown of the amyloid precursor protein under the action of β- and γ-secretase. Although there is no cure for Alzheimer's disease at this time, many neuroprotective natural products, such as polyphenol and carotenoid compounds, have shown promising preventive activity as well as helping to slow the disease's progression [68]. Studies [68,70] have focused on the chemistry as well as the structure of carotenoid compounds and their neuroprotective activity against Aβ aggregation using molecular docking assays. Besides the most common anti-amyloidogenic carotenoid, lutein, cryptocapsin, astaxanthin, fucoxanthin, and the apocarotenoid bixin have all been studied [70]. Structure-based computer analysis of drug design and molecular docking simulations have revealed important interactions between carotenoids and Aβ through hydrogen bonding and van der Waals interactions and have shown that carotenoids are potent anti-amyloidogenic molecules with a potential role in preventing Alzheimer's disease, especially since most of them can cross the blood–brain barrier and are considered nutraceuticals [71]. As a result of these findings, we now have a better understanding of how carotenoids inhibit Aβ aggregation. The potential role of carotenoids as new therapeutic molecules in the treatment of Alzheimer's disease and other neurodegenerative diseases has been discussed [72].

Nobiletin and tangeretin, flavonoids isolated from the peel and other parts of citrus fruits, have a neuroprotective effect in experiments in vitro and in vivo and are promising in the prevention and treatment of Alzheimer's and Parkinson's diseases [73]. Citrus naringenin prevents dopamine synthesis disorders in the brain which prevents the development of Parkinson's disease. Sedative, muscle relaxant, anti-hallucinogenic, neuroprotective, memory-enhancing, and anti-Parkinsonian properties of medicinal plants have been noted.

Polyphenols, due to the antioxidant, anti-inflammatory properties of medicinal plants and their extracts, have a neuroprotective effect in epilepsy and other neurodegenerative diseases; resveratrol and flavonoids prevent the occurrence and development of neurodegenerative diseases and have a neuroprotective effect. Due to its antioxidant, anti-inflammatory properties, methanol extract of ginger root can serve as an additional tool in the treatment and prevention of Alzheimer's disease [74]. Experimental studies have shown that taking cinnamon powder (*Cinnamonum cassia*, *Cinnamonum verum*) prevents T-cell dysfunction, thereby providing a therapeutic and prophylactic effect in autoimmune diseases, including multiple sclerosis [75]. Lemon oil reduces lipid peroxidation in the hippocampus, thereby preventing the development of neurodegenerative diseases [76]. Experimental studies have shown the presence of neuroprotective properties in *Terminalia chebula* Retz. seed extracts [77]. Chebulic acid has pronounced neuroprotective properties [78]. Ellagic acid has the same properties [78]. *Silibum marianum* Gaerth silubin has immunosuppressive properties, and this makes it possible to use it in multiple sclerosis [79]. Silubin prevents memory impairment and destruction of nerve cells caused by oxidation, which opens up prospects for its use in the treatment of Alzheimer's disease [80]. Ferulic acid (*Ferula assa foetida* L.), due to its antioxidant properties, has a therapeutic effect in neurodegenerative diseases such as Alzheimer's and Parkinson's diseases [81].

Experimental studies have shown that alcoholic extracts of date fruits (*Phoenix dactylifera* L.) have a neuroprotective effect in ischemic damage to the nervous tissue [82]. Experimental studies have shown that the date diet, due to its antioxidant properties, can serve as a prophylactic for Alzheimer's disease [83]. As we have already noted, acetyl and butyrylcholinesterase enzymes play an important role in the pathogenesis of the development of complications from the nervous system in Alzheimer's disease. In the plant world, biologically active substances that inhibit these enzymes are common. The hot infusion of orange (*Citrus sinensis* (L.) Osbeck.) peel has been found to inhibit MAO and butyrylcholinesterase, which opens up great prospects for its use in the treatment of neurodegenerative diseases [84]. It has also been determined that aqueous extracts of oranges inhibit acetylcholinesterase, and they can serve as a therapeutic agent in the treatment of Alzheimer's disease [85]. Anticholinesterase activity has been shown for a number of natural compounds, due to which they can be used for the prevention and treatment of Alzheimer's disease: essential oil of leaves and flowers of *Polygonum hydropiper* L., phenolics and flavonoids in *Inula britannica* L. [86,87], rosmarinic acid from extracts of *Hypericum perforatum* L. [88], phenolics from extracts of *Terminalia chebula* Retz [89], alkaloids of *Fumaria vailantii* Loisl. [90], extracts *Coriandrum sativum* L. [91], a mixture of chokeberry and lemon juices [92], ursolic acid and oil of *Origanum majorana* L. [93], extracts of *Myristica fragrans* Houtt. [94], alcohol *Foeniculum vulgare* Mill. fruit extracts and its oil [95], extracts of *Thymus serpyllum* L. [96], extracts of *Rumex confertus* Willd. leaves [97], mulberry root bark extracts [98], *Pleurotus ostreatus* (Fr.) [99], castor bean leaf extracts [100].

The stems and fruits of black pepper (*Piper nigrum* L.) have shown the ability to inhibit acetylcholinesterase, and butyrylcholinesterase. Cucumber fruit extracts have anticholinesterase and antimonoamine oxidase activity, which opens up prospects for their use in the treatment of neurodegenerative diseases [101]. Substances that prevent the formation of amyloid fibrils have been identified among the biologically active substances of plants. Grape seed gallic acid prevents the formation and accumulation of amyloid fibrils, which play the main pathogenetic role in Alzheimer's and Parkinson's diseases [102]. Experimental studies have revealed the properties of alcoholic extracts of buckwheat (*Fagopyrum esculentum* Moench.) to inhibit the production of β-amyloid and prevent memory impairment [103]. In the pathogenesis of Alzheimer's disease, deficiency of P-glycoprotein with adenosine transferase protein (ABCB1), which is involved in the transport of β-amyloid from the brain tissue into the blood, plays an important role. Experimental studies have shown that *Hypericum perforatum* L. extracts increase the rate of transport of β-amyloid into the blood, thereby providing a preventive and therapeutic effect in Alzheimer's disease [104]. Similar properties have been found in curcumin.

Quinolinic acid is formed due to the degradation of tryptophan. The accumulation of this substance stimulates the processes of neuroinflammation and demyelination, and the development of degenerative diseases such as multiple sclerosis. Experimental studies have shown that alcohol *Terminalia chebula* Retz. extracts inhibit the accumulation of this substance and the development of oxidative stress in the nervous tissue under the influence of quinolinic acid [105]. Calamus (*Acorus calamus* L.) root preparations [106] and asparagus (*Asparagus officinalis* L.) extracts [107] reduce damage to the nervous tissue by β-amyloid, thereby preventing the development of Alzheimer's disease. Experimental studies have shown that curcumin (*Curcuma longa* L.) prevents degradation caused by toxic factors of nigral dopaminergic neurons and prevents the development of Parkinson's disease [108]. Methanol extracts of black pepper (*Piper nigrum* L.) reduce oxidative stress in the hippocampus under the influence of β-amyloid [109]. In addition, pepper fruits improve memory by stimulating the trophism of the nervous tissue, especially in the hippocampus. *Acorus calamus* L. β-azarone is considered a potentially effective agent in the treatment of neurodegenerative diseases, including Alzheimer's disease [110]. Ginseng preparations have been shown to be effective in the treatment of Parkinson's disease due to their neuroprotective properties of ginseng [111].

Experimental studies have shown that taking extracts of *Hypericum perforatum* L. has a therapeutic effect in Parkinson's disease [112]. Plant extracts are also promising as a therapeutic agent for multiple sclerosis [113]. A similar effect was shown for cinnamon (*Cinnamomum Blume* L.) extract [114]. A number of medicinal plants and their metabolites have a therapeutic effect in Alzheimer's disease: nobiletin and narirutin, flavanoids from lemon fruits [115,116]; tangeretin has therapeutic potential in inflammatory and degenerative processes in the nervous tissue accompanied by microglial activation [117]; seeds and roots of *Peganum harmala* L. [118], *Crocus sativus* L. stigmas [119], *Trigonella foenum-graecum* L. seeds [120,121]. Experimental studies have shown that fenugreek seed extracts have a therapeutic effect on motor disorders in animal models of Parkinson's disease. Randomized, placebo-controlled clinical trials have shown that IBHB (fenugreek seed extract) is a safe, effective adjuvant treatment for patients with L-DOPA-dependent Parkinson's disease.

Filipendula ulmaria L. Maxim, due to the presence of flavonoids such as kaempferol, luteolin, and apigenin, has a therapeutic effect in neurodegenerative diseases such as Alzheimer's disease, Parkinson's disease, epilepsy, multiple sclerosis, and stroke [122]. Animal experiments have shown that meadowsweet has a therapeutic effect and prevents the processes of demyelinization in encephalomyelitis [123]. Glabridin, extracted from mistletoe (*Víscum álbum* L.), protects against the deterioration of cognitive processes and memory caused by exposure to chemical agents. This opens up prospects for the use of glabridin in the treatment of Alzheimer's disease. Neuroprotective properties of rosehip extracts (*Rosa cinnamonea* L.) have been noted. Experimental studies have shown that a herbal preparation of rose hips, tansy herb, and nettle prevents memory impairment in Alzheimer's disease [124]. *Valeriana officinalis* L. extract improves cognitive functions caused by exposure to amyloid β in models of Alzheimer's disease [125]. The anti-neurodegenerative effects of various plant components are summarized in Table 1. The table demonstrates a fairly wide range of plants of various species that exhibit significant antioxidant activity. Many plant species considered include neurodegenerative and antioxidant components.

Table 1. Anti-neurodegenerative action of various plant components.

Plant	Active Components	Activity	Sources
Citrus limon	Nobiletin, flavonoids	Neuroprotective action	[76]
	Tangeretin	Neuroprotective action	[76]
	Essential oil Glycosides Phytoncides Macro-, microelements Organic acids Vitamins Pectin substances	Therapeutic potential in inflammatory and degenerative processes in the nervous tissue accompanied by microglia activation	[115]
	Narirutin	Therapeutic effect in Alzheimer's disease	[115]
	Naringenin	Prevention of impaired dopamine synthesis in the brain and the development of Parkinson's disease	[76]
Rauvolfia serpentina	Reserpine Macro-, microelements Organic acids Vitamins Indole flavonoids	Therapy of hypertension and psychotic disorders (schizophrenia, anxiety, insomnia); reduces Aβ toxicity in an Alzheimer's disease model	[126]
	Punicalagin Macro-, microelements Organic acids	Amyloid load reduction and behavior improvement in an Alzheimer's model	[127]
Punica granatum	Vitamins Flavonoids Fatty acids	β-secretase inhibition	[128]
	Ellagic acid	β-secretase inhibition	[128]
Terminalia chebula	Chebulic acid, ellagic acid Macro-, microelements Vitamins Triterpenoids Saponins Quinolinic acid	Neuroprotective action	[77]
Silybum marianum	Buformin Flavonoids	Immunosuppressive action preventing memory impairment	
	Silibin Silychristin Silydianin	Immunosuppressive action preventing the destruction of nerve cells caused by oxidation	[79]

Table 1. Cont.

Plant	Active Components	Activity	Sources
Inula britannica	Rosmarinic acid, Flavonoids, Essential oil, Carotene, Lactones, Tannins	Anticholinesterase activity	[87]
Fumaria officinalis	Alkaloids, Glycosides, Vitamins, Organic acids, Sugars Resins, Essential oil traces	Anticholinesterase activity	[90]
Vitis vinifera	Gallic acid, Organic acids	Prevention of formation and accumulation of amyloid fibrils	[129]
	Limonene, Geranyl, Phenyl acetate Squalene	Increasing the rate of transport of β-amyloid into the blood	[130]
Curcuma longa	Curcumin, Carbohydrates, Essential oils, Fatty acids Curcuminoids	Prevention of toxic-induced degradation of black dopaminergic neurons and impeding the development of Parkinson's disease	[131]
Acorus calamus	β-azarone, Essential oils, Polysaccharides phenolic compounds	Inhibition of the release of pro-inflammatory mediators and cytokines; decreased JNK phosphorylation, inhibition of NF-κB nuclear translocation	[106]
	Kaempferol, luteolin, apigenin	Therapeutic effect in neurodegenerative diseases	[122]
Filipendula ulmaria	Nitrogen compounds, Higher fatty acids, Ethers	Prevention of demyelination processes in encephalomyelitis	[123]
Viscum album	Glabridin, Flavonoids, Terpenoids, Hormones	Protection against deterioration of cognitive processes and memory caused by exposure to chemical agents	[132]

Table 1 demonstrates only the main components of the presented plants that affect the antioxidant activity. It should be noted that these plants also contain other components (for example, ellagitannins in *Filipendula ulmaria* or procyanidins in *Vitis vinifera* and wine), which have a beneficial effect on the oxidation of free radicals, antioxidant activity, and the aging process of the human body [122,123].

Essential oil is one of the key components of *Citrus limon*. Lemon essential oil is extracted by cold pressing the fruit's peel. The oil is fractionated by vacuum distillation, and essential oils with varying concentrations of the main components (limonene, other monoterpene hydrocarbons, citral, geranyl acetate, and sesquiterpenes) are produced. The three primary components responsible for the aroma of lemon are limonene (1-methyl-4-(1-methylethenyl)cyclohexene) and citral (a combination of two geometric isomers of 3,7-dimethyl-2,6-octadienal, neral and geranial). It was demonstrated that citral is unstable; it is easily oxidized in the presence of light or oxygen [133]. In addition to these components, lemon essential oil contains α-pinene, sabinene, β-pinene, β-myrcene, p-cymene, α-terpinene, limonene, γ-terpinene, linalool, neral, geranial, neryl acetate, and geranyl acetate. Lemon essential oils are powerful antioxidants. The inhibitory effect of essential oil components on model aldehyde oxidation is based on competitive reactions between these components and the aldehyde with an oxidizing agent, in this case air oxygen. The components of essential oils oxidize and transform, resulting in a change in essential oil composition, the emergence of new products, and the consumption of the main components. On the other hand, comparing the rate of oxidation (decrease in concentration) of oil components allows for evaluation of their antioxidant activity.

It was found that the antioxidant activity depends on the composition of the systems and on the concentration of essential oils. Citral and limonene had the lowest antioxidant activity; a mixture of these compounds had a higher activity. The antioxidant properties of essential oils increased as their concentration or the content of monocyclic terpene hydrocarbons in the model systems increased, especially α- and γ-terpinenes. Differences in the oxidation resistance of the main components of lemon essential oils were determined, and synergistic effects in the antioxidant activity and stability of essential oil components were found [133].

Rauwolfia serpentina Benth., a tropical plant from the *Apocynaceae* family, is a source of many indole alkaloids that are widely used in medical practice as antihypertensive, antiarrhythmic, and sedative drugs. Ajmaline is a key component among the alkaloids of this plant [134]. Ajmalin is an antiarrhythmic medication that is effective in the treatment of the cardiovascular system. Due to the endemic and endangered status of *Rauwolfia serpentina*, as well as its slow growth rate and relatively low content of ajmaline alkaloids, these compounds are currently obtained from in vitro cultivated tissues of this plant. Indole alkaloids *Rauwolfia serpentina* are also represented by reserpine, serpentine, rescinnamine, or yohimbine. *Rauwolfia* alkaloids have various pharmacological properties. They mainly affect the central nervous system [134].

One of the modern directions of pharmaceutical research is the search for new types of plant materials to expand the range of fatty oils for medical use in aging. A promising source of fatty oils are the seeds and fruits of oleaginous plants. In particular, pomegranate seeds are a source of fatty oil of an atypical chemical composition, which has been found to contain the following fatty acids: palmitic (C16:0), linoleic (C18:2, cis), oleic (C18:1, cis), linolelaidic (C18:2, trans), stearic (C18:0), punicic (C18:3, 9cis, 11trans, 13cis), α-eleostearic (C18:3, 9cis, 11trans, 13trans), catalpic (C18:3, 9trans, 11trans, 13cis), β-eleostearic (C18:3, 9trans, 11trans, 13trans), eicosene (C20:1, cis), arachidonic (C20:0), lignoceric (C24:0), and conjugated linolenic acids [135]. Thus, pomegranate oil consists of triglycerides containing unsaturated fatty acids, mainly punicic acid, which has a pronounced positive biological effect on the body [135].

The study of *Terminalia chebula* revealed its antioxidant, antibacterial, antitumor, neuroprotective, anti-inflammatory, antidiabetic, hepatoprotective, antimutagenic, antiproliferative, radioprotective, cardioprotective, antiarthritic, anticaries, and wound healing properties [136]. *Terminalia chebula* fruits contain 1,2,3-tri-O-galloyl-6-O-cinnamoyl-β-d-glucose, 1,2,3,6-tetra-O-galloyl-6-O-cinnamoyl-β-d-glucose, 4-O-(2″,4″-di-O-galloyl-α-l-rhamnosyl)ellagic acid, 1′-O-methyl neochebulin, dimethyl neochebulinate, 6′-O-methyl neochebulinate, dimethyl neochebulinate, dimethyl neochebulinate, dimethyl 4′-epineochebulinate, methyl chebulate, derivatives of polyhydroxytriterpenoids-23-O-neochebuloylarjungenin 28-O-β-d-glycopyranosyl ester, 23-O-4′-epi-neochebuloylarjungenin, and 23-O-galloylpinfaenoic acid 28-O-β-d-glucopyranosyl ester. The hydrolysable tannins chebumeinin and chebumeinin B were also found [137–139]. The bark of the plant contains triterpenoids-termichebuloside, dimeric triterpenoid saponin, termichebulolide, oleanolic acid-type lactone [140]. The plant contains Cl, Co, Cr, Fe, K, Mn, Na, Se and Zn salts [141]. Plant seed extracts have been demonstrated to exhibit neuroprotective effects in experimental studies. Chebulic acid has pronounced neuroprotective properties [142]. Ellagic acid from Chebulic myrobalans has the same properties [143]. Plant extracts are promising for the treatment of Alzheimer's disease because of their antioxidant and anti-inflammatory characteristics [138]. Experiments have demonstrated that plant extracts suppress the enzyme acetylcholinesterase, which is involved in the progression of Alzheimer's disease [144,145]. Quinolinic acid is formed due to the degradation of tryptophan. The accumulation of this substance stimulates the processes of neuroinflammation and demyelination, and the development of degenerative diseases such as multiple sclerosis. Experimental studies have shown that alcoholic extracts of Chebulic myrobalans inhibit the accumulation of this substance and the development of oxidative stress in the nervous tissue under the influence of quinolinic acid [146].

The healing properties of *Sílybum mariánum* have been known since ancient times. Both the plant and the extract obtained from it are utilized in folk medicine. *Silybum marianum* has a number of protective properties against liver diseases and neurogenerative diseases [147]. It is a natural antioxidant. *Sílybum mariánum* seeds contain flavonoids from which a pharmacological agent silymarin is produced. Silymarin contains three main components: flavonoids silybin, silychristin, and silydianin. Silymarin has an antioxidant effect in Alzheimer's disease. The seeds are rich in fatty oils (20–30%), proteins (25–30%), also contain tocopherol (0.038%) and sterols (0.63%) including cholesterol, campesterol, stigmasterol, sitosterol, and others. Fatty oils are an indispensable nutritional factor that provides a person with essential fatty acids (linoleic, linolenic, and arachidic), which are not synthesized in the human body. They are also used in the production of medicines. The identified new fatty oils containing a high amount of essential fatty acids (C18:2, 18:5) belonging to the class of ω-2, ω-3 acids are of great interest [147].

Inula britannica contains flavonoids, essential oils, carotene, sesquiterpene lactones, including britanin, tannins, and other substances. The seeds contain traces of alkaloids, and the roots contain the bitter substance insulin and other compounds, which has led to their widespread use in medicine (official, folk, veterinary) and food industry [148]. Components typical of the *Asteraceae* family as a whole were detected in the glandular trichomes secretion of *I. britannica*—essential oils including sesquiterpene lactones and phenolic compounds (flavonoids). The fact that the content of trichomes stain with methylene blue, which belongs to the group of basophilic dyes, indicates the predominance of oxidized components in the composition of the essential oil (sesquiterpene lactones, flavonoids, phenolic acids). The glandular trichomes of *I. britannica* synthesize essential oils (at the initial stages of formation) and oleoresins (formed). The secret of the glandular trichomes of I. britannica is formed by a polysaccharide mucus, which includes neutral sugars (the secret is not stained with methylene blue); the content of numerous non-glandular trichomes is filled with essential oil, which is released when the terminal cell is broken off [149].

Fumaria officinalis contains about 1% of a mixture of isoquinoline (styloptin, protopin, cryptopin, synactin, biculin, adlumin, etc.) and spirobenzylisoquinoline (fumarophycin, parfumin, fumaritrin, etc.) alkaloids [150,151]. Alkaloids adlumicein methyl ester, parfumine, and N-methylhydrastine methyl ester were identified in *Fumaria officinalis* [150]. In *Fumaria officinalis*, isoquinoline alkaloids protopine, cryptopine, fumaranine, fumarostrezhdin, parfumidin, synactin, etc. were identified. These substances have a neurodegenerative effect in Alzheimer's disease and aging [151]. Glycosides, vitamins C, K, organic acids, sugars, resins, traces of essential oil were also found. Spirobenzylisoquinoline alkaloid fumariline was determined in seeds [150,152].

Vitis vinifera is a promising source of biologically active substances. Along with fruits, which are valuable medicinal plant raw materials, leaves are often used for the manufacture of a number of medicines and biologically active food supplements, which have antioxidant, cardiovascular, anti-sclerotic, capillary-strengthening, and anti-inflammatory effects [153]. Twenty compounds belonging to different chemical groups were identified in the lipophilic fraction: (a) high molecular weight fatty acids and their derivatives (myristic, palmitic, linolenic, palmitoleic acids); (b) compounds of terpene nature, which are an integral part of the essential oil fraction (d-limonene, geranyl, phenylacetate, squalene, etc.); (c) diterpene alcohol phytol; (d) fat-soluble vitamins α- and γ-tocopherols; (e) a pyrazole derivative; (f) higher aliphatic hydrocarbons and other organic substances [153].

Curcuma longa L. has a wide range of biological effects, including anti-inflammatory and antioxidant properties. Its specific effect on various organs and tissues has been revealed, i.e., on the skin, gastrointestinal tract, liver, and respiratory system. As part of the components of turmeric, carbohydrates (4.7–8.2%), essential oils (2.44%), fatty acids (1.7–3.3%), and curcuminoids (curcumin, demethoxycurcumin, and bisdemethoxycurcumin) have been isolated, the content of which is approximately 2%, although they can reach 2.5–5.0% of dry weight, as well as other polypeptides such as turmerin (0.1% dry extract) [154]. One of the main active components of Curcuma longa L. is curcumin, a polyphenol, the main representative of the curcuminoids group. The antitumor, antioxidant, and anti-inflammatory activity of curcumin has been confirmed. Curcumol, a component of turmeric essential oil, has anti-epileptic properties. Anti-epileptic properties were determined in the bisabolene terpenoids of turmeric. In experimental animals, curcumin reduced movement disorders and stiffness caused by haloperidol. Experimental studies demonstrated that curcumin prevents the degradation caused by toxic factors of nigral dopaminergic neurons and prevents the development of Parkinson's disease. Curcumin has a positive therapeutic effect in all neurodegenerative diseases [154].

Biologically active substances of Acorus calamus are represented by essential oil, polysaccharide complex, phenolic compounds [155]. The composition of the essential oil includes: d-alpha-pinene, d-camphene, d-camphor, borneol, eugenol, methyleugenone, azaron, beta-azaron, calamen, sesquiterpene ketone akorone, caryophyllene, proazulene, and other terpenoids. Acorus calamus is used for the treatment and prevention of cardiovascular diseases, neurodegenerative disorders, epilepsy, Parkinson's, and Alzheimer's diseases [155].

The medicinal plant Filipendula ulmaria is a source of highly effective preparations of various actions: anti-inflammatory, immunostimulating, antitumor, antioxidant, adaptogenic, and nootropic [156]. Filipendula ulmaria contains isobutylamine, isoamylamine, higher fatty acids (stearic and lenolenic), hexanal, 6,10,14-trimethyl-2 peptadecanone, 2 nonadecanone, 14-methyl pentadecanoic acid ester, dodecanoic, tetradecanoic, pentadecanoic and hepatodecanoic acids, 1-nonadecene, hexadecanoic acid ester, 1-octadecanol, 9,12 octadecadienoic acid [156].

The chemical composition of Viscum species, in particular Viscum album, has not been sufficiently studied, but it is known that their medicinal effectiveness is due to the content of a number of chemically complex and diverse active substances. These include polypeptides, carbohydrates, amines, organic acids (lactic, isovaleric, caproic, etc.), rubber steroids, cardenolides and triterpene glycosides (viscumneoside V, naringenin, rhamnocitrin, etc.), phenols, higher fatty acids, saponins, and many others [28]. For Viscum album, 41 components of the extract have been presented, which include 11 flavonoids, 2 hormones, 14 benzenoids, 1 inositol, 2 pyrimidines, 4 triterpenoids, 5 steroids, viscoline, and a new flavonone-(2S)-7,4'-dihydroxy-5,3'-di-methoxyflavanone [157]. White mistletoe is used as an analgesic, astringent and enveloping agent, for the treatment of hypertension, gastrointestinal, uterine and hemorrhoidal bleeding, metabolic disorders, early menopause in women, dehelmintization, as well as an anti-inflammatory, anticancer, and antioxidant agent [157].

4. Anti-Inflammatory Properties of Medicinal Plants and Their Complexes

It is estimated that more than 150,000 plant species have been studied, many of which contain valuable therapeutic agents, and the use of new compounds from plants for pharmaceutical purposes has been gradually increasing in recent years [158]. Since ancient times, plants have played an important role in protecting human health. When adapting against pathogen attack and environmental stress, plants produce several substances that exhibit biological activity. These organic molecules are secondary metabolites and also exhibit biological activity. Among the various functions, the anti-inflammatory effect of plants is distinguished. It is known that inflammation is an evolutionarily conserved defense process and a critical survival mechanism [159]. It consists of complex successive changes in tissue aimed at eliminating the original cause of damage to the cell, which could be caused by infectious agents or substances released during their metabolism (microorganisms and toxins), as well as physical factors (radiation, burns, and injuries), or chemicals (caustic substances). Signs of inflammation are local redness, swelling, pain, burning, and loss of function [160].

In general, this complex biological response leads to the restoration of homeostasis. However, in cases of sustained release of inflammatory mediators and activation of insecure signaling pathways, the inflammatory process persists, and a chronic pro-inflammatory state may occur [161]. Chronic inflammation may be associated with diseases such as obesity, diabetes, cancer, and cardiovascular disease. Medicinal plants play an important role in the development of new potent anti-inflammatory drugs [162]. Ethnobotanical research made it possible to combine a variety of plants with biological activity by methods of observation, description, and experimental studies, which greatly contributed to the discovery of natural plant products of biological action. The use of plant-based medicinal natural compounds for the treatment of many diseases has become a trend in modern clinical research. Polyphenolic compounds have attracted significant attention due to their modulating effect on inflammasomes [163]. These multiprotein complexes are associated with the onset and progression of metabolic disorders and chronic diseases caused by inflammation [163].

Over the past decades, hundreds of research and review articles have been published on the anti-inflammatory activity of plants [164]. It is important to note that the extraction of plant raw materials is an important step that makes it possible to obtain a preparation with a specialized action [164]. When a set of natural compounds is used, there is a high possibility of synergy between the active ingredients, which can be lost when each of these ingredients is isolated. This synergism has been found in several medical tests, including anti-inflammatory activity. On the other hand, a mixture of different compounds can also lead to inhibitory effects, namely that one component can reduce the biological activity of another. Medicinal plants are used instead of non-steroidal anti-inflammatory drugs, given that the use of these drugs is associated with undesirable effects on the gastrointestinal tract and kidneys. The biggest disadvantage of strong synthetic drugs is their toxicity and recurrence of symptoms after withdrawal. Thus, screening and development of herbal preparations with anti-inflammatory action are currently needed, and much effort is being made to find anti-inflammatory preparations from medicinal plants [165]. Substances of plant origin belonging to various chemical classes have demonstrated proven anti-inflammatory activity [156]. Among them are alkaloids, terpenes [157], phenolic compounds, tannins, lignans, coumarins, saponins, and especially flavonoids [152].

The *Álnus incána* flavonoids—rutin, quercetin, and hesperidin—have been found to have an anti-inflammatory effect [153]. Studies involving the *Potentilla argentea* glycosides (kaempferol, quercetin, aromatendrenene) showed anti-inflammatory activity due to the suppression of NO levels in microglial cells [154]. *Agrimónia eupatória* terpenes, which exhibit pharmacological properties such as anti-inflammatory and antinociceptive abilities, inhibit platelet aggregation and interfere at the intracellular level with the transduction mechanism [155]. These compounds also contribute to a significant reduction in edema and exhibit effects comparable to those of hydrocortisone. Some pathologies, such as inflammation, can be exacerbated by the formation of free radicals that cause tissue damage by promoting oxidation [156]. Oxidative stress is known to play an important role in endothelial dysfunction; lung disease, gastrointestinal dysfunction, atherosclerosis, and inflammatory symptoms are implicated in all these disorders [157]. Excessive pro-inflammatory cytokines and mitochondrial dysfunction cause oxidative stress, characterized by an imbalance between the effectiveness of antioxidant protection and the rate of formation of reactive oxygen species, causing an overload of oxidants [158].

Antioxidant compounds can reduce oxidative stress, minimizing the incidence of pathologies. The search for new antioxidant agents from plant sources used against inflammation and infection may lead to the discovery of natural molecules with high anti-inflammatory potential in vitro and in vivo. These substances justify the popular use of these plant species with anti-inflammatory properties [166]. Thus, arachidonic acid metabolites play a vital role in inflammation. In the inflammatory process, arachidonic acid is released from membrane phospholipids by the enzyme phospholipase and metabolized by cyclooxygenases, lipoxygenases, and cytochromes into prostaglandins/thromboxane, leukotrienes, and epoxy/hydroxy metabolites, such as epoxyeicosatrienoic acid. Cyclooxygenase (COX), the enzyme responsible for the formation of prostaglandins from arachidonic acid, is released from cell membrane phospholipids by phospholipase [167]. COX is necessary to maintain the normal physiological state of many tissues, including protecting the gastrointestinal mucosa, controlling renal blood flow, homeostasis, autoimmune and anti-inflammatory responses, and controlling the functions of the pulmonary, nervous, and cardiovascular systems, and the reproductive functions of the human body [168]. COX expression is significantly increased during inflammation, or mitogenic stimulation [167] induced by inflammation by cytokines and endotoxins, and causes a decrease in the number of prostaglandins that contribute to the development of edema, hot flashes, fever, and hyperalgesia [168]. Therefore, activation of these enzymes stimulates intracellular signals that alter the expression of pro-inflammatory cytokines such as interleukin. COX inhibition is regarded as an important target for potential drugs for the treatment of inflammatory processes in the aging human body [169]. Inhibition of COX by plant BAS is responsible for the imbalance of arachidonic acid metabolites; plant BAS increase the production of lipoxygenase products, leukotrienes, which have pro-inflammatory properties [164]. Glycation or non-enzymatic glycosylation is a reaction between reducing carbohydrates (glucose, fructose, etc.) and free amino groups of proteins, lipids, and nucleic acids of a living organism, proceeding without the participation of enzymes. Glycation is a special case of the Maillard reaction. Non-enzymatic glycosylation of proteins is a key mechanism of tissue damage in diabetes mellitus [165].

5. Antiglycating Properties of Medicinal Plants and Their Complexes

The glycation process, which is enhanced by hyperglycemia, underlies the pathogenesis of micro and macrovascular complications of diabetes mellitus (DM), which is common in the elderly [166]. Glycosylation end products (GEP) affect type IV collagen, myelin, tubulin, plasminogen activator-1, and fibrinogen. The receptor-dependent effects of GEP are mediated by their interaction with specific receptors, which leads to the activation of the nuclear factor NF-κB, which moves to the nucleus and leads to an increase in the transcription of intercellular adhesion molecules-1, E-selectin, endothelin-1, vascular endothelial growth factor, and pro-inflammatory cytokines [167]. The first and most studied substance that inhibits protein glycation is aminoguanidine, which prevents the formation of GEP [168]. However, clinical trials of this drug were stopped due to the lack of efficacy and the presence of side effects (gastrointestinal symptoms, lupus-like, flu-like syndromes, vasculitis, anemia). Antiglycation activity was found in pyridoxamine, hydrazine derivatives of thiazolidine and carboxymidamide, structurally similar to aminoguanidine, and derivatives of phenoxyisobutyric acid [169]. All of the above determines the relevance of the search for plant substances that prevent the formation of GEP in order to create drugs for the pathogenetic prevention of DM complications.

Diabetes mellitus is a metabolic disorder characterized by hyperglycemia. The prevalence of diabetes and its associated complications has increased dramatically over the past few decades, leading to increased morbidity and premature mortality, and remains a major risk factor for cardiovascular disease worldwide [170]. Chronic hyperglycemia is the main factor causing vascular and internal organ damage in diabetes [171]. An uncontrolled excess of glucose in the blood reacts with the free amino acids of proteins to form a labile Schiff base and is stabilized in a compound known as GEP. Protein glycation causes several structural modifications and alters the function of many proteins, especially albumin. This process affects the affinity of the albumin-binding activity of drugs, hormones, fatty acids, and other substances [172]. In addition, albumin-derived GEPs have been shown to trigger the generation of intracellular reactive oxygen species, which leads to inhibition of glucose uptake and oxidative changes in intracellular proteins [173,174]. Albumin has the ability to scavenge free radicals depending on its structure, and this protective function is lost in uncontrolled diabetes [175]. Numerous GEP inhibitors, including pharmacological and natural compounds, have been investigated for their ability to prevent the complications of diabetes, but medicinal plants are considered safer than others, and many of them have the ability to reduce the harmful effects of hyperglycemia [176]. Widespread in Europe, *Solidágo virgáurea* L. and *Lamium album* L. have played a traditional role in folk medicine for centuries in the treatment of skin diseases, rheumatism, hypertension, and various infections. These plants are rich in phenolic flavonoids and phenolic acids. Many compounds of these plants have antioxidant properties that act through enzymatic and non-enzymatic pathways [177]. Recent studies have demonstrated the antibacterial and antioxidant effects of *Solidágo virgáurea* L. and *Lamium album*, as well as their hypoglycemic effects in diabetes [178]. It was found that the anti-glycation properties of the extracts of *Solidágo virgáurea* L. and *Lamium album* were strongly correlated with their antioxidant capacity (trapping DPPH-radicals). Like antioxidant capacity, anti-glycation activity correlated strongly with phenol and flavonoid content.

Phenols and flavonoids are classified as antioxidants and have been reported to have protective effects in diabetes. Some studies show that a higher content of phenol and flavonoids has a greater effect on protection against hyperglycemia [179]. Albumin glycation, including the formation of fructosamine, carbonyl groups, and amyloid β-structures, is significantly attenuated in the presence of plant extracts. The initial step in the formation of GEP, also known as the Maillard reaction, begins with the nucleophilic addition of the free amino groups of proteins to the carbonyl group of reducing sugars to reversibly form a Schiff base product, which in turn is converted to a stable fructosamine residue (ketoamine) by Amadori rearrangement (Figure 2). The Schiff base and fructosamines are called early glycation products. These adducts can undergo subsequent oxidation, rearrangement, dehydration, and cyclization to form stable agents called GEP [172]. It has been demonstrated that GEP inhibitors can prevent the formation of reactive dicarbonyls and oxygen species [169]. It has been suggested that antioxidants such as phenols and flavonoids inhibit the formation of GEP and such properties have been attributed to the structure of these compounds. In fact, adjacent OH groups have been found to be responsible for their antioxidant and antiglycation activity [173]. The relationship between antioxidant and antiglycation activity was evident in that the maximum inhibition of glycation was noted for medicinal plants, which showed the highest antioxidant properties. *Solidágo virgáurea* and *Lamium album* showed a low ability to prevent the formation of amyloid β-structures. The research results show that the extracts and complexes of these plants are able to scavenge free radicals and prevent albumin glycation, and these properties are highly correlated with each other. It has been found that a higher concentration of each extract will result in greater inhibition of albumin glycation. Thus, it has been proven that the antioxidant capacity of plants and the ability to antiglycate are due to the concentration of phenols and flavonoids [172].

6. Synergism in the Action of Medicinal Plant Complexes

Plants have been used as therapeutic agents since the beginning of human history [180]. Texts from ancient Sumeria, India, Egypt, China, and other countries contain recipes using medicinal plants for the treatment of diseases [158]. Today, the use of medicinal plants is still common, with a significant portion of the world's population relying on herbal natural products and supplements as their primary source of health care [181]. Nearly 20% of adults and 5% of children in the United States use herbal supplements for disease treatment [182]. Despite being used for centuries, the effects of herbal medicines have only been partially studied, and for most natural products on the market, there is no information on which components are responsible for the alleged biological activity. The scientific study of plant-based natural products is challenging due to their enormous complexity and diversity [183]. Efforts in natural product chemistry are generally focused on reducing complexity and identifying individual active components for drug development. However, given that plant complexes, rather than single molecules, are often used for medicinal purposes, interactions between components can be of great importance.

Understanding how combinations of plants and their complexes work together to achieve a specific biological effect can aid in dealing with the ever-increasing threat of disease resistance. Indeed, many diseases are not regulated by a single molecular target but often have a multifactorial causal relationship [184]. Numerous studies have shown that disease resistance is less likely to occur with a combination of compounds than with single active ingredients [185]. Over millennia, plants have evolved to address the multifactorial nature of disease pathogenesis by targeting pathogens through the combined action of structurally and functionally diverse components [180]. Thus, complex mixtures of natural plant substances represent an important resource for drug development, for future success in natural product research, and for understanding the interactions within and between components of mixtures of natural substances. Pharmacological studies of combined effects can be studied at the level of molecular targets, disease pathways, cellular processes, and patient responses [186]. Thus, in vitro, in vivo, preclinical, and clinical studies can provide valuable information about combined effects. Despite the fact that there is a lot of research in this area, these reviews focus on the methodology for interpreting combined effects using molecular and cellular methods [187].

Plant extracts can contain hundreds or even thousands of individual components in varying amounts [188], and the identification of compounds responsible for a given biological effect is a serious problem. Too often, it is assumed that the behavior of a mixture can be described by the presence of only a few known components. However, a number of studies have shown that the overall activity of plant extracts can result from mixtures of compounds with synergistic, additive, or antagonistic activity [189], and often efforts to isolate individual compounds fail because the activity is lost upon fractionation [190]. There are many possible explanations for this problem (including the irreversible adsorption of compounds on the packing of a chromatographic column) [191]. The loss of activity in some cases is caused by the fact that several components are required to observe the biological effect. Many researchers recognize the multifactorial nature of herbal medicines. However, the research methodology applied to herbal mixtures in most cases still tends to either take a reductionist approach (focusing on only one or two "marker compounds") or completely ignores the issue of chemical composition, testing the biological effects of complex mixtures and complexes with unknown active ingredients. The problem with the latter is that the results tend to be difficult to interpret and reproduce. Many reviews describe the methodologies that currently exist for understanding combined effects in plant complexes.

To successfully generate useful data for understanding the effects of a combination in complex mixtures, one must first select an appropriate biological assay to test the combination. Since the combined effects can manifest through a myriad of mechanisms (including changes in absorption and metabolism, effects on multiple target cells, etc.), in vivo model systems provide the most complete assessment of the overall effect on a living organism [192]. The development of high-throughput in vivo testing of plant complexes and mixtures shows promising possibilities for the identification of multi-target components in mixtures [193]. Despite this, it remains a challenge to solve the complexity of the in vivo systems that require the sacrifice of experimental animals and the maintenance of animal housing. In addition, the results cannot be successfully transferred from one animal model to another. Even when evaluating drug efficacy in human patients, there is often intercellular variability and variability in drug response across patients [158]. Because of this, it is possible that patients receiving combination therapy exhibit increased treatment efficacy because their disease is sensitive to at least one of the drugs in the combination (i.e., independent drug action) rather than due to true combination effects [158].

To overcome some of these problems, a considerable number of researchers work only with in vitro systems. However, many cell-free high-throughput assays that seek molecular targets do not accurately model the biology of an intact cell, making it impossible to discover relevant combinational effects [194]. Thus, it is better to use cellular assays that strike a balance between efficiency and preservation of molecular pathway interactions [195]. Some of the useful cell systems for detecting combined effects in vitro have been discussed in a recent publication by Pemovska et al. [196]. Cellular metabolism is a dynamic network of regulated pathways that is often reprogrammed during cancer and aging, and is recognized as a new key area of study. The first observations that transformed cells exhibit a distinct metabolic program were made by Otto Warburg almost a hundred years ago. The Warburg effect describes the phenomenon of cancer cells predominantly undergoing glycolysis and the conversion of carbon to lactate even under conditions of high oxygen content [197]. In cancer and aging, genetic events activate signaling pathways that subsequently modulate cellular metabolism to meet increased bioenergetic, biosynthetic, and redox needs [198]. Moreover, it contributes to the initiation and progression of cancer and aging, and is usually accompanied by changes in the expression of metabolic enzymes and transporters, which are important for the absorption and distribution of nutrients along biomass formation pathways, which ultimately affects the response to therapy [199,200]. Therefore, the metabolic changes specific to cancer and aging provide not only a selective advantage for survival, but also introduce metabolic limitations that provide a unique opportunity for therapeutic targeting [201]. In addition to selecting appropriate cell systems for biological testing, it is important to mimic physiological conditions in the assay itself. Indeed, most of the media used to grow cells for biological testing do not mimic physiological conditions, affecting the metabolism and phenotypic response of the cells under study [202]. Similarly, the conditions of biological assays can lead to dynamic residual complexity where the sample undergoes chemical change caused by the environment, making it difficult to interpret the results [203]. In their recent publication, Vande Voorde et al. [202] illustrated that the use of a complex culture medium designed to mimic the physiological environment of cancer cells prevents the formation of undesirable phenotypic artifacts and improves the transferability between in vitro assay results and in vivo tumor models. The use of physiologically relevant media also increases the likelihood that the components that elicit a biological response during biological testing will be soluble and stable in the biological system, facilitating the identification of active components. Primary tissue assays composed of multiple cell types, such as those used to screen drug combinations for anti-inflammatory activity in mixed lymphocyte cultures, can also be used to identify combination effects that work through multitarget mechanisms [197]. However, when screening for biological activity in vitro, investigators should be aware of potential false-positive results arising from interference compounds commonly referred to as pain, which are often identified as hits in biological screenings [203]. These false-positive results can be generated due to multiple mechanisms, including fluorescence quenching, aggregation effects, chemical reactivity, oxidation/reduction, membrane disruption, and residual complexity [203]. Synergistic results are often found in aqueous media due to aggregation effects, which can be minimized by adding a detergent to the media [204].

In addition to careful selection of the biological system to study the effects of the combination, it is necessary to collect data to effectively compare the combination of drugs with extracts and individual substances [190]. Combined effects, including synergism and antagonism, can manifest themselves over a wide range of concentrations, so it is necessary to test different ratios of the studied samples [205]. A study [206] found that human serum is a vital component of the host's innate immunity that acts as the first line of defense against invading pathogens. A key player in serum-mediated innate immune defense is a system of more than 35 proteins, collectively referred to as the complement system. Upon pathogen exposure, these proteins are activated in a cascade manner, eventually forming a membrane attack complex (MAC) on the surface of the pathogen, which directly lyses the bacterial cell. MAC formation had been demonstrated in vitro using a serum bactericidal assay (SBA) that works in the absence of blood cellular components after serum has been incubated with bacteria. The age-related differences in the bactericidal activity of human blood serum against *Pseudomonas aeruginosa* have been described. It has been demonstrated that sera from young adults were highly effective in killing *Pseudomonas aeruginosa* in vitro compared to children and the elderly. The sera of the elderly were severely compromised when killing *P. aeruginosa*, while the sera of young people showed an increased level of killing. The data revealed a positive correlation between age and bacterial cell death with higher coefficients of determination of 0.34, 0.27 and 0.58 after 60, 90 and 120 min of incubation, respectively. Therefore, this study highlighted age-related differences in the bactericidal activity of human sera [207]. One of the simplest methods for identifying potential combined effects is to test samples individually and in combination, and to determine if the combined effect of the samples is greater than, equal to, or less than the expected sum of the two samples individually.

In addition to concentration-based approaches to evaluating combined effects, time-based approaches have been developed and applied to determine antimicrobial synergism and describe the relationship between bactericidal activity and sample concentration [208]. This method involves exposing a chosen pathogen to an inhibitor (or combination of inhibitors), sampling the cultures at regular intervals, serially diluting and incubating aliquots, and comparing the resulting colony-forming units. The resulting dose–response curve can be used to determine additive, synergistic, and antagonistic effects [209]. Synergism can occur through a variety of mechanisms, including pharmacodynamic synergy through multiple target effects, pharmacokinetic synergy through modulation of drug transport, penetration and bioavailability, elimination of side effects, and the manifestation of disease resistance mechanisms [209]. While the general mechanisms by which synergistic effects may occur are relatively well understood, the mechanisms by which specific herbal preparations exert synergistic effects remain largely unknown [210], hindering attempts to standardize and optimize them for therapeutic purposes. Only by understanding the nature of the synergistic activity of plant extracts is it possible to optimize safe and effective drugs for the treatment of diseases.

Cancer cells and pathogens can quickly become resistant to drugs containing a single compound, and many cancers and resistant bacterial infections are treated with complex multi-target drug combinations to overcome the development of resistance [211]. Plants have long had to defend themselves against multifactorial diseases and have evolved to produce a variety of active components that can adhere to cell membranes, intercalate into RNA or DNA, and bind to numerous proteins [212]. Pharmacodynamic synergy results from targeting multiple pathways that may include enzymes, substrates, metabolites, ion channels, ribosomes, and signaling cascades [210]. Pharmacodynamic synergism may occur through complementary actions in which synergists in a mixture interact with multiple points in the pathway, leading to up-regulation of the drug-targeting process or down-regulation of competing mechanisms. By selectively altering target activity and expression through complementary actions, pharmacodynamic synergists can both enhance the beneficial effects of treatment and reduce the side effects of the disease [211]. For example, numerous studies have shown that many plants have synergistic neuroprotective effects both in vivo and in vitro by inhibiting free radical formation, scavenging reactive oxygen species, regulating mitochondrial target gene expression, and reducing overstimulation of nerve cells by neurotransmitters [213].

7. Conclusions

A significant increase in the proportion of the elderly population in developed countries is accompanied by an increase in mortality from major diseases of old age (diseases of the cardiovascular system, malignant neoplasms, neurodegenerative processes, reduced resistance to infection, and diabetes mellitus). One of the promising objects for the prevention of antioxidant, anti-inflammatory, neuroprotective, and anti-glycation aging processes are the components of medicinal plants.

Millions of people in the world suffer from chronic neurodegenerative diseases (Parkinson's and Alzheimer's diseases, Huntington's chorea, hyperprolactinemia, etc.), which, despite therapy, end in disability and/or death. Medicinal plants, due to the presence of biologically active substances, can play an important role in the prevention of the development of neurodegenerative diseases such as Alzheimer's disease. The mechanisms of this effect are not always known. Perhaps, antioxidant and adaptogenic mechanisms play a role here.

The search, methods of isolation, and study of promising natural sources of substances with antiradical and antioxidant activity are currently one of the urgent tasks for modern medicine, pharmacy, cosmetology, and the food industry to reduce the effects of aging of the human body. Medicinal plants play an important role in the development of new potent anti-inflammatory drugs through the production of secondary metabolites with biological activity. Medicinal plants are used in place of non-steroidal anti-inflammatory drugs, given that the use of these drugs is associated with several side effects, among which are unwanted effects on the gastrointestinal tract and kidneys.

The glycation process, which is enhanced by hyperglycemia, underlies the pathogenesis of micro and macrovascular complications of diabetes mellitus (DM), which is common in the elderly. It was found that the antiglycation properties of herbal extracts and their complexes strongly correlated with their antioxidant capacity (trapping DPPH-radicals). Like antioxidant capacity, anti-glycation activity correlated strongly with phenol and flavonoid content.

In recent years, the concept of synergy in mixtures of natural plant substances has attracted attention, and the importance of multipurpose combination therapy in human aging has come to the fore. However, the classification of combined effects in complex mixtures and the identification of constituents remains a challenge, especially when most known tools have been developed to reduce the complexity of mixtures of natural substances. Furthermore, there is still disagreement in this field about which reference models are best for identifying combined effects, making it difficult to interpret studies. The metabolomic and biochemometric approaches are promising tools for studying synergy and have only just begun to be used to identify the components involved in the combined effects [197].

Author Contributions: Conceptualization, S.S. and O.B.; methodology, A.T., V.L. and J.S.; formal analysis, S.I., M.P., A.O. and S.S.; writing—original draft preparation, V.L., J.S., A.O. and S.S.; writing—review and editing, O.B., S.I. and M.P.; project administration, S.S. All authors have read and agreed to the published version of the manuscript.

Funding: This research was funded by the RUSSIAN SCIENCE FOUNDATION, grant number 21-76-10055.

Institutional Review Board Statement: Not applicable.

Informed Consent Statement: Not applicable.

Data Availability Statement: The data are included in the manuscript.

Conflicts of Interest: The authors declare no conflict of interest.

References

1. Population Division World Population Ageing 2019. Available online: https://www.un.org/en/development/desa/population/publications/pdf/ageing/WorldPopulationAgeing2019-Report.pdf (accessed on 30 March 2022).
2. World Health Organization. *Global Status Report on Noncommunicable Diseases 2014*; WHO: Geneva, Switzerland, 2014.
3. Ng, R.; Sutradhar, R.; Yao, Z.; Wodchis, W.P.; Rosella, L.C. Smoking, drinking, diet and physical activity—Modifiable lifestyle risk factors and their associations with age to first chronic disease. *Int. J. Epidemiol.* **2020**, *49*, 113–130. [CrossRef] [PubMed]
4. Kearns, K.; Dee, A.; Fitzgerald, A.P.; Doherty, E.; Perry, I.J. Chronic disease burden associated with overweight and obesity in Ireland: The effects of a small BMI reduction at population level. *BMC Public Health* **2014**, *14*, 143. [CrossRef] [PubMed]
5. Niccoli, T.; Partridge, L. Ageing as a Risk Factor for Disease. *Curr. Biol.* **2012**, *22*, R741–R752. [CrossRef]
6. Liguori, I.; Russo, G.; Curcio, F.; Bulli, G.; Aran, L.; Della-Morte, D.; Gargiulo, G.; Testa, G.; Cacciatore, F.; Bonaduce, D.; et al. Oxidative stress, aging, and diseases. *Clin. Interv. Aging* **2018**, *13*, 757–772. [CrossRef]
7. Ferrucci, L.; Fabbri, E. Inflammageing: Chronic inflammation in ageing, cardiovascular disease, and frailty. *Nat. Rev. Cardiol.* **2018**, *15*, 505–522. [CrossRef]
8. Błaszczyk, J.W. Energy Metabolism Decline in the Aging Brain-Pathogenesis of Neurodegenerative Disorders. *Metabolites* **2020**, *10*, 450. [CrossRef]
9. Babich, O.; Sukhikh, S.; Prosekov, A.; Asyakina, L.; Ivanova, S. Medicinal Plants to Strengthen Immunity during a Pandemic. *Pharmaceuticals* **2020**, *13*, 313. [CrossRef]
10. Moher, D.; Liberati, A.; Tetzlaff, J.; Altman, D.G.; Altman, D. PRISMA Group Preferred reporting items for systematic reviews and meta-analyses: The PRISMA statement. *PLoS Med.* **2009**, *6*, e1000097. [CrossRef]
11. Sharifi-Rad, M.; Anil Kumar, N.V.; Zucca, P.; Varoni, E.M.; Dini, L.; Panzarini, E.; Rajkovic, J.; Tsouh Fokou, P.V.; Azzini, E.; Peluso, I.; et al. Lifestyle, Oxidative Stress, and Antioxidants: Back and Forth in the Pathophysiology of Chronic Diseases. *Front. Physiol.* **2020**, *11*, 694. [CrossRef]
12. Vajragupta, O.; Boonchoong, P.; Berliner, L.J. Manganese complexes of curcumin analogues: Evaluation of hydroxyl radical scavenging ability, superoxide dismutase activity and stability towards hydrolysis. *Free Radic. Res.* **2004**, *38*, 303–314. [CrossRef]
13. Giles, G.I.; Jacob, C. Reactive sulfur species: An emerging concept in oxidative stress. *Biol. Chem.* **2002**, *383*, 375–388. [CrossRef] [PubMed]
14. Geier, D.A.; Kern, J.K.; Garver, C.R.; Adams, J.B.; Audhya, T.; Nataf, R.; Geier, M.R. Biomarkers of environmental toxicity and susceptibility in autism. *J. Neurol. Sci.* **2009**, *280*, 101–108. [CrossRef] [PubMed]
15. Liu, R.H.; Finley, J. Potential cell culture models for antioxidant research. *J. Agric. Food Chem.* **2005**, *53*, 4311–4314. [CrossRef] [PubMed]
16. Babich, O.; Sukhikh, S.; Pungin, A.; Ivanova, S.; Asyakina, L.; Prosekov, A. Modern trends in the in vitro production and use of callus, suspension cells and root cultures of medicinal plants. *Molecules* **2020**, *25*, 5805. [CrossRef]
17. Yang, Y.; Asyakina, L.K.; Babich, O.O.; Dyshlyuk, L.S.; Sukhikh, S.A.; Popov, A.D.; Kostyushina, N.V. Physicochemical properties and biological activity of extracts of dried biomass of callus and suspension cells and in vitro root cultures. *Food Process. Tech. Technol.* **2020**, *50*, 480–492. [CrossRef]
18. Kurutas, E.B. The importance of antioxidants which play the role in cellular response against oxidative/nitrosative stress: Current state. *Nutr. J.* **2016**, *15*, 71. [CrossRef]
19. Zehiroglu, C.; Ozturk Sarikaya, S.B. The importance of antioxidants and place in today's scientific and technological studies. *J. Food Sci. Technol.* **2019**, *56*, 4757–4774. [CrossRef]
20. Nowak, D.; Gośliński, M.; Wojtowicz, E.; Przygoński, K. Antioxidant Properties and Phenolic Compounds of Vitamin C-Rich Juices. *J. Food Sci.* **2018**, *83*, 2237–2246. [CrossRef]
21. Gonçalves, S.; Romano, A. Inhibitory Properties of Phenolic Compounds Against Enzymes Linked with Human Diseases'. In *Phenolic Compounds—Biological Activity*; Soto-Hernandez, M., Palma-Tenango, M., Garcia-Mateos, M.d.R., Eds.; IntechOpen: London, UK, 2017. [CrossRef]
22. Wang, T.Y.; Li, Q.; Bi, K.S. Bioactive flavonoids in medicinal plants: Structure, activity and biological fate. *Asian J. Pharm. Sci.* **2018**, *13*, 12–23. [CrossRef]
23. Engwa, G.A. Free Radicals and the Role of Plant Phytochemicals as Antioxidants Against Oxidative Stress-Related Diseases. In *Phytochemicals—Source of Antioxidants and Role in Disease Prevention*; Asao, T., Asaduzzaman, M., Eds.; IntechOpen: London, UK, 2018. [CrossRef]
24. Dal, S.; Sigrist, S. The Protective Effect of Antioxidants Consumption on Diabetes and Vascular Complications. *Diseases* **2016**, *4*, 24. [CrossRef]
25. Nile, S.H.; Keum, Y.S.; Nile, A.S.; Jalde, S.S.; Patel, R.V. Antioxidant, anti-inflammatory, and enzyme inhibitory activity of natural plant flavonoids and their synthesized derivatives. *J. Biochem. Mol. Toxicol.* **2018**, *32*, e22002. [CrossRef] [PubMed]
26. Henkel, R.; Agarwal, A. Harmful Effects of Antioxidant Therapy. In *Male Infertility*; Parekattil, S., Esteves, S., Agarwal, A., Eds.; Springer: Cham, Switzerland, 2020. [CrossRef]
27. Bjelakovic, G.; Nikolova, D.; Gluud, L.L.; Simonetti, R.G.; Gluud, C. Mortality in randomized trials of antioxidant supplements for primary and secondary prevention: Systematic review and meta-analysis. *JAMA* **2007**, *297*, 842–857. [CrossRef] [PubMed]

28. Ye, W.; Nanga, R.P.; Kang, C.B.; Song, J.H.; Song, S.K.; Yoon, H.S. Molecular characterization of the recombinant Achain of a type II ribosome-inactivating protein (RIP) from Viscum album coloratum and structural basis on its ribosome-inactivating activity and the sugar-binding properties of the B-chain. *J. Biochem. Mol. Biol.* **2006**, *39*, 560–570. [CrossRef]
29. Bjelakovic, G.; Nikolova, D.; Simonetti, R.G.; Gluud, C. Antioxidant supplements for prevention of gastrointestinal cancers: A systematic review and meta-analysis. *Lancet* **2004**, *364*, 1219–1228. [CrossRef]
30. Stanner, S.A.; Hughes, J.; Kelly, C.N.; Buttriss, J. A review of the epidemiological evidence for the "antioxidant hypothesis". *Public Health Nutr.* **2004**, *7*, 407–422. [CrossRef] [PubMed]
31. Wang, C.C.; Rogers, M.S. Oxidative stress and fetal hypoxia. In *Reactive Oxygen Species and Disease*; Laszlo, G., Ed.; Research Signpost: Trivandrum, India, 2007; pp. 257–282.
32. Rembold, C.M. Vitamin and antioxidant supplements do not prevent adverse cardiovascular events. *Ann. Int. Med.* **2013**, *158*, JC10. [CrossRef]
33. Pezzani, R.; Salehi, B.; Vitalini, S.; Iriti, M.; Zuñiga, F.A.; Sharifi-Rad, J.; Martorell, M.; Martins, N. Synergistic Effects of Plant Derivatives and Conventional Chemotherapeutic Agents: An Update on the Cancer Perspective. *Medicina* **2019**, *55*, 110. [CrossRef]
34. Doos, L.; Roberts, E.O.; Corp, N.; Kadam, U.T. Multi-drug therapy in chronic condition multimorbidity: A systematic review. *Fam. Pract.* **2014**, *31*, 654–663. [CrossRef]
35. Obodozie-Ofoegbu, O. *Readings in Advanced Pharmacokinetics—Theory, Methods and Applications. Pharmacokinetics and Drug Interactions of Herbal Medicines: A Missing Critical Step in the Phytomedicine/Drug Development Process*; IntechOpen: London, UK, 2012.
36. Katselou, M.G.; Matralis, A.N.; Kourounakis, A.P. Multi-target drug design approaches for multifactorial diseases: From neurodegenerative to cardiovascular applications. *Curr. Med. Chem.* **2014**, *21*, 2743–2787. [CrossRef]
37. Buompadre, M.C. Neuropatía óptica aguda: Diagnósticos diferenciales [Acute optic neuropathy: Differential diagnoses]. *Rev. Neurol.* **2013**, *57*, S139–S147.
38. Lankin, V.Z.; Postnov, A.Y.; Rodnenkov, O.V.; Rodnenkov, O.V.; Konovalova, G.G.; Doroshchuk, N.A.; Tikhaze, A.K.; Osyaeva, M.K.; Doroshchuk, A.D.; Khesuani, Y.D.; et al. Oxidative stress as a risk factor for complications of cardiovascular diseases and premature aging under the influence of adverse climatic conditions. *Cardiol. Vestn.* **2013**, *8*, 18–22. (In Russian)
39. Moussa, Z.; Judeh, Z.M.; Ahmed, S.A. Nonenzymatic Exogenous and Endogenous Antioxidants. In *Free Radical Medicine and Biology*; Das, K., Ed.; IntechOpen: London, UK, 2019. [CrossRef]
40. Szewczyk, K.; Chojnacka, A.; Górnicka, M. Tocopherols and Tocotrienols-Bioactive Dietary Compounds; What Is Certain, What Is Doubt? *Int. J. Mol. Sci.* **2021**, *22*, 6222. [CrossRef] [PubMed]
41. Allen, L.H. *Encyclopedia of Human Nutrition*; Academic Press: Cambridge, MA, USA, 2013; Volume 2013, pp. 54–59. [CrossRef]
42. Starchenko, G.; Hrytsyk, A.; Raal, A.; Koshovyi, O. Phytochemical Profile and Pharmacological Activities of Water and Hydroethanolic Dry Extracts of *Calluna vulgaris* (L.). Hull. *Herb. Plants* **2020**, *9*, 751. [CrossRef] [PubMed]
43. Zabokritskii, N.A.; Cherepanova, O.E.; Dudukina, N.N. Seasonal dynamics of the accumulation of biologically active substances in the shoots of *Calluna vulgaris* L. *Agrar. Bull. Ural* **2017**, *3*, 31–34.
44. Chepel, V.; Lisun, V.; Skrypnik, L. Changes in the Content of Some Groups of Phenolic Compounds and Biological Activity of Extracts of Various Parts of Heather (*Calluna vulgaris* (L.) Hull) at Different Growth Stages. *Plants* **2020**, *9*, 926. [CrossRef]
45. Zhao, J. The Extraction of High Value Chemicals from Heather (*Calluna vulgaris*) and Bracken (*Pteridium aquilinum*). Ph.D. Thesis, The University of York, York, UK, 2011.
46. Popov, S.V.; Ovodova, R.G.; Yu, G.; Popova, I.R.; Nikitina, Y.; Ovodov, S. Adhesion of Human Neutrophils to Fibronectin Is Inhibited by Comaruman, Pectin of Marsh Cinquefoil *Comarum palustre* L., and by Its Fragments. *Biochemistry* **2005**, *70*, 108–112. [CrossRef]
47. Kashchenko, N.I.; Chirikova, N.K.; Olennikov, D.N. Agrimoniin, an Active Ellagitannin from Comarum palustre Herb with Anti-α-Glucosidase and Antidiabetic Potential in Streptozotocin-Induced Diabetic Rats. *Molecules* **2017**, *22*, 73. [CrossRef]
48. Ekiert, H.; Pajor, J.; Klin, P.; Rzepiela, A.; Ślesak, H.; Szopa, A. Significance of *Artemisia vulgaris* L. (Common Mugwort) in the History of Medicine and Its Possible Contemporary Applications Substantiated by Phytochemical and Pharmacological Studies. *Molecules* **2020**, *25*, 4415. [CrossRef]
49. Kshirsagar, S.G.; Rao, R.V. Antiviral and Immunomodulation Effects of *Artemisia*. *Medicina* **2021**, *57*, 217. [CrossRef]
50. Abiri, R.; Silva, A.L.M.; de Mesquita, L.S.S.; de Mesquita, J.W.C.; Atabaki, N.; de Almeida, E.B.; Shaharuddin, N.A.; Malik, S. Towards a better understanding of Artemisia vulgaris: Botany, phytochemistry, pharmacological and biotechnological potential. *Food Res. Int.* **2018**, *109*, 403–415. [CrossRef]
51. Nantitanon, W.; Yotsawimonwat, S.; Okonogi, S. Factors influencing antioxidant activities and total phenolic content of guava leaf extract. *LWT—Food Sci. Technol.* **2010**, *43*, 1095–1103. [CrossRef]
52. Ben-Shushan, S.; Miller, Y. Neuropeptides: Roles and Activities as Metal Chelators in Neurodegenerative Diseases. *J. Phys. Chem. B* **2021**, *125*, 2796–2811. [CrossRef] [PubMed]
53. Kalaria, R.N.; Maestre, G.E.; Arizaga, R.; Friedland, R.P.; Galasko, D.; Hall, K.; Luchsinger, J.A.; Ogunniyi, A.; Perry, E.K.; Potocnik, F.; et al. Alzheimer's disease and vascular dementia in developing countries: Prevalence, management, and risk factors. *Lancet Neurol.* **2008**, *7*, 812–826. [CrossRef]
54. Zhang, H.; Ma, Q.; Zhang, Y.W.; Xu, H. Proteolytic processing of Alzheimer's β-amyloid precursor protein. *J. Neurochem.* **2012**, *120*, 9–21. [CrossRef]

55. Dutysheva, E.A.; Utepova, I.A.; Trestsova, M.A.; Anisimov, A.S.; Charushin, V.N.; Chupakhin, O.N.; Margulis, B.A.; Guzhova, I.V.; Lazarev, V.F. Synthesis and approbation of new neuroprotective chemicals of pyrrolyl- and indolylazine classes in a cell model of Alzheimer's disease. *Eur. J. Med. Chem.* **2021**, *222*, 113577. [CrossRef]
56. Castillo, X.; Castro-Obregón, S.; Gutiérrez-Becker, B.; Gutiérrez-Ospina, G.; Karalis, N.; Khalil Ahmed, A.; Lopez-Noguerola, J.S.; Rodríguez, L.L.; Martínez-Martínez, E.; Perez-Cruz, C.; et al. Re-thinking the Etiological Framework of Neurodegeneration. *Front. Neurosci.* **2019**, *2019*, 13. [CrossRef]
57. Li, J.; Yu, H.; Yang, C.; Tao, M.; Yuan, D. Therapeutic Potential and Molecular Mechanisms of Echinacoside in Neurodegenerative Diseases. *Front. Pharmacol.* **2022**, *2022*, 13. [CrossRef]
58. Sharifi-Rad, J.; Melgar-Lalanne, G.; Hernández-Álvarez, A.J.; Taheri, Y.; Shaheen, S.; Kregiel, D.; Antolak, H.; Pawlikowska, E.; Brdar-Jokanović, M.; Rajkovic, J.; et al. Malva species: Insights on its chemical composition towards pharmacological applications. *Phytother. Res.* **2019**, *34*, 546–567. [CrossRef]
59. Dugger, B.N.; Dickson, D.W. Pathology of neurodegenerative diseases. *Cold Spring Harb. Perspect. Biol.* **2017**, *9*, a028035. [CrossRef]
60. Sharifi-Rad, J.; Ayatollahi, S.A.; Varoni, E.M.; Salehi, B.; Kobarfard, F.; Sharifi-Rad, M.; Iriti, M.; Sharifi-Rad, M. Chemical composition and functional properties of essential oils from *Nepeta schiraziana* Boiss. *Farmacia* **2017**, *65*, 802–812.
61. Salehi, B.; Stojanović-Radić, Z.; Matejić, J.; Sharopov, F.; Antolak, H.; Kręgiel, D.; Sen, S.; Sharifi-Rad, M.; Acharya, K.; Sharifi-Rad, R.; et al. Plants of genus Mentha: From farm to food factory. *Plants* **2018**, *7*, 70. [CrossRef] [PubMed]
62. Wink, M. Introduction: Biochemistry, Physiology and Ecological Functions of Secondary Metabolites. In *Annual Plant Reviews*; Wink, M., Ed.; Wiley-Blackwell: Oxford, UK, 2010.
63. Croteau, R.; Kutchan, T.M.; Lewis, N.G. Natural Products (Secondary Metabolites). In *Biochemistry & Molecular Biology of Plants*; Buchanan, B.B., Gruissem, W., Jones, R.L., Eds.; American Society of Plant Physiologists: Rockville, MD, USA, 2000.
64. Salehi, B.; Albayrak, S.; Antolak, H.; Kręgiel, D.; Pawlikowska, E.; Sharifi-Rad, M.; Uprety, Y.; Fokou, P.V.T.; Yousef, Z.; Zakaria, Z.A.; et al. Aloe genus plants: From farm to food applications and phytopharmacotherapy. *Int. J. Mol. Sci.* **2018**, *19*, 2843. [CrossRef] [PubMed]
65. Salehi, B.; Zucca, P.; Orhan, I.E.; Azzini, E.; Adetunji, C.O.; Mohammed, S.A.; Banerjee, S.K.; Sharopov, F.; Rigano, D.; Sharifi-Rad, J.; et al. Allicin and health: A comprehensive review. *Trends Food Sci. Technol.* **2019**, *86*, 502–516. [CrossRef]
66. Kumar, G.P.; Khanum, F. Neuroprotective potential of phytochemicals. *Pharmacogn. Rev.* **2012**, *6*, 81–90. [CrossRef] [PubMed]
67. Fujiwara, H.; Tabuchi, M.; Yamaguchi, T.; Iwasaki, K.; Furukawa, K.; Sekiguchi, K.; Ikarashi, Y.; Kudo, Y.; Higuchi, M.; Saido, T.; et al. A traditional medicinal herb *Paeonia suffruticosa* and its active constituent 1,2,3,4,6-penta-O-galloyl-beta-D-glucopyranose have potent anti-aggregation effects on Alzheimer's amyloid beta proteins in vitro and in vivo. *J. Neurochem.* **2009**, *169*, 1648–1657. [CrossRef]
68. Ramesh, B.N.; Indi, S.S.; Rao, K.S. Anti-amyloidogenic property of leaf aqueous extract of *Caesalpinia crista*. *Neurosci. Lett.* **2010**, *475*, 110–114. [CrossRef]
69. Murillo, E.; Britton, G.B.; Durant, A.A. Antioxidant activity and polyphenol content in cultivated and wild edible fruits grown in Panama. *J. Pharm. Bioallied Sci.* **2012**, *4*, 313–317.
70. Obulesu, M.; Dowlathabad, M.R.; Bramhachari, P.V. Carotenoids and Alzheimer's disease: An insight into therapeutic role of retinoids in animal models. *Neurochem. Int.* **2011**, *59*, 535–541. [CrossRef]
71. Sharifi-Rad, M.; Lankatillake, C.; Dias, D.A.; Docea, A.O.; Mahomoodally, M.F.; Lobine, D.; Chazot, P.L.; Kurt, B.; Tumer, T.B.; Moreira, A.C.; et al. Impact of Natural Compounds on Neurodegenerative Disorders: From Preclinical to Pharmacotherapeutics. *J. Clin. Med.* **2020**, *9*, 1061. [CrossRef]
72. Lakey-Beitia, J.; Kumar, D.J.; Hegde, M.L.; Rao, K.S. Carotenoids as Novel Therapeutic Molecules Against Neurodegenerative Disorders: Chemistry and Molecular Docking Analysis. *Int. J. Mol. Sci.* **2019**, *20*, 5553. [CrossRef]
73. Braidy, N.; Behzad, S.; Habtemariam, S.; Ahmed, T.; Daglia, M.; Nabavi, S.M.; Sobarzo-Sanchez, E.; Nabavi, S.F. Neuroprotective Effects of Citrus Fruit-Derived Flavonoids, Nobiletin and Tangeretin in Alzheimer's and Parkinson's disease—CNS. *Neurol. Disord. Drug Targets.* **2017**, *16*, 387–397. [CrossRef]
74. Zeng, G.-F.; Zhang, Z.-Y.; Lu, L.; Xiao, D.-Q.; Zong, S.-H.; He, J.-M. Protective Effects of Ginger Root Extract on Alzheimer Disease-Induced Behavioral Dysfunction in Rats. *Rejuvenation Res.* **2013**, *16*, 124–133. [CrossRef] [PubMed]
75. Pahan, S.; Pahan, K. Can cinnamon spice down autoimmune diseases? *J. Clin. Exp. Immunol.* **2020**, *5*, 252–258. [CrossRef] [PubMed]
76. Oboh, G.; Olasehinde, T.A.; Ademosun, A.O. Essential oil from lemon peels inhibit key enzymes linked to neurodegenerative conditions and pro-oxidant induced lipid peroxidation. *J. Oleo Sci.* **2014**, *63*, 373–381. [CrossRef]
77. Park, J.H.; Joo, H.S.; Yoo, K.Y.; Shin, B.N.; Kim, I.H.; Lee, C.H.; Choi, J.H.; Byun, K.; Lee, B.; Lim, S.S.; et al. Extract from Terminalia chebula seeds protect against experimental ischemic neuronal damage via maintaining SODs and BDNF levels. *Neurochem. Res.* **2011**, *36*, 2043–2050. [CrossRef]
78. Kim, H.J.; Kim, J.; Kang, K.S.; Lee, K.T.; Yang, H.O. Neuroprotective Effect of Chebulagic Acid via Autophagy Induction in SH-SY5Y Cells. *Biomol. Ther.* **2014**, *22*, 275–281. [CrossRef]
79. Bijak, M. Silybin, a Major Bioactive Component of Milk Thistle (Silybum marianum L. Gaernt.)—Chemistry, Bioavailability, and Metabolism. *Molecules* **2017**, *22*, 1942. [CrossRef]

80. Min, K.; Yoon, W.K.; Kim, S.K.; Kim, B.H. Immunosuppressive effect of silibinin in experimental autoimmune encephalomyelitis. *Arch. Pharm. Res.* **2007**, *30*, 265–1272. [CrossRef]
81. Nabavi, S.F.; Devi, K.P.; Malar, D.S.; Sureda, A.; Daglia, M.; Nabavi, S.M. Ferulic acid and Alzheimer's disease: Promises and pitfalls. *Mini Rev. Med. Chem.* **2015**, *15*, 776–788. [CrossRef]
82. Agbon, A.N.; Ingbian, S.D.; Dahiru, A.U. Preliminary histological and histochemical studies on the neuroprotective effect of aqueous fruit extract of *Phoenix dactylifera* L. (Date Palm) on atesunate—Induced cerebellar damage in wistar rats. *Sub-Saharan Afr. J. Med.* **2014**, *1*, 204–209. [CrossRef]
83. Ademosun, A.O.; Oboh, G. Anticholinesterase and antioxidative properties of water-extractable phytochemicals from some citrus peels. *J. Basic Clin. Physiol. Pharmacol.* **2014**, *25*, 199–204. [CrossRef] [PubMed]
84. Ademosun, A.O.; Oboh, G. Comparison of the inhibition of monoamine oxidase and butyrylcholin-esterase activities by infusions from green tea and some citrus peels. *Int. J. Alzheimers Dis.* **2014**, *2014*, 586407. [CrossRef] [PubMed]
85. Jabir, N.R.; Khan, F.R.; Tabrez, S. Cholinesterase targeting by polyphenols: A therapeutic approach for the treatment of Alzheimer's disease. *CNS Neurosci. Ther.* **2018**, *24*, 753–762. [CrossRef]
86. Ayaz, M.; Junaid, M.; Ullah, F.; Sadiq, A.; Khan, M.A.; Ahmad, W.; Shah, M.R.; Imran, M.; Ahmad, S. Comparative chemical profiling, cholinesterase inhibitions and anti-radicals properties of essential oils from *Polygonum hydropiper* L: A Preliminary anti-Alzheimer's study. *Lipids Health Dis.* **2015**, *14*, 141. [CrossRef]
87. Bae, W.Y.; Kim, H.Y.; Choi, K.S.; Chang, K.H.; Hong, Y.H.; Eun, J.; Lee, N.K.; Paik, H.D. Investigation of Brassica juncea, Forsythia suspensa, and *Inula britannica*: Phytochemical properties, antiviral effects, and safety. *BMC Complement. Altern. Med.* **2019**, *19*, 253. [CrossRef] [PubMed]
88. Nicolai, M.; Pereira, P.; Vitor, R.F.; Pinto Reis, C.; Roberto, A.; Rijo, P. Antioxidant activity and rosmarinic acid content of ultrasound-assisted ethanolic extracts of medicinal plants. *Measurement* **2016**, *89*, 328–332. [CrossRef]
89. Tubtimdee, C.; Shotipruk, A. Extraction of phenolics from *Terminalia chebula* Retz with water–ethanol and water–propylene glycol and sugaring-out concentration of extracts, eparation and Purification. *Technology* **2011**, *77*, 339–346. [CrossRef]
90. Păltinean, R.; Mocan, A.; Vlase, L.; Gheldiu, A.M.; Crișan, G.; Ielciu, I.; Voștinaru, O.; Crișan, O. Evaluation of Polyphenolic Content, Antioxidant and Diuretic Activities of Six Fumaria Species. *Molecules* **2017**, *22*, 639. [CrossRef]
91. Msaada, K.; Ben Jemia, M.; Salem, N.; Bachrouch, O.; Sriti, J.; Tammar, S.; Bettaieb, I.; Jabri, I.; Kefi, S.; Limam, F.; et al. Antioxidant activity of methanolic extracts from three coriander (*Coriandrum sativum* L.) fruit varieties. *Arab. J. Chem.* **2017**, *10*, S3176–S3183. [CrossRef]
92. Gironés-Vilaplana, A.; Valentão, P.; Andrade, P.B.; Ferreres, F.; Moreno, D.A.; García-Viguera, C. Phytochemical profile of a blend of black chokeberry and lemon juice with cholinesterase inhibitory effect and antioxidant potential. *Food Chem.* **2012**, *134*, 2090–2096. [CrossRef]
93. Chung, Y.K.; Heo, H.J.; Kim, E.; Kim, H.K.; Huh, T.L.; Lim, Y.; Kim, S.K.; Shin, D.H. Inhibitory Effect of Ursolic Acid Purified from Origanum majorana L. on the Acetylcholinesterase. *Mol. Cells* **2001**, *11*, 137–143.
94. Akinboro, A.; Mohamed, K.B.; Asmawi, M.Z.; Sulaiman, S.F.; Sofiman, O.A. Antioxidants in aqueous extract of *Myristica fragrans* (Houtt.) suppress mitosis and cyclophosphamide-induced chromosomal aberrations in Allium cepa L. cells. *J. Zhejiang Univ. Sci. B* **2011**, *12*, 915–922. [CrossRef] [PubMed]
95. Manzoor, A.; Rather, B.A.D.; Shahnawaz, N.S.; Qurishi, M.A. *Foeniculum vulgare*: A comprehensive review of its traditional use, phytochemistry, pharmacology, and safety. *Arab. J. Chem.* **2016**, *9*, 13–16. [CrossRef]
96. Šojić, B.; Tomović, V.; Kocić-Tanackov, S.; Bursać Kovačević, D.; Putnik, P.; Mrkonjić, Ž.; Đurović, S.; Jokanović, M.; Ivić, M.; Škaljac, S.; et al. Supercritical extracts of wild thyme (*Thymus serpyllum* L.) by-product as natural antioxidants in ground pork patties. *LWT* **2020**, *130*, 109661. [CrossRef]
97. Berillo, D.; Kozhahmetova, M.; Lebedeva, L. Overview of the Biological Activity of Anthraquinons and Flavanoids of the Plant Rumex Species. *Molecules* **2022**, *27*, 1204. [CrossRef]
98. Lee, S.; Kim, S.H.; Jo, Y.-Y.; Kim, S.-W.; Kim, H.-B.; Kweon, H. Characterization of Mulberry Root Bark Extracts (*Morus alba* L.) Based on the Extraction Temperature and Solvent. *Int. J. Ind. Entomol.* **2020**, *41*, 36–44. [CrossRef]
99. Ianni, F.; Blasi, F.; Angelini, P.; Simone, S.C.D.; Angeles Flores, G.; Cossignani, L.; Venanzoni, R. Extraction Optimization by Experimental Design of Bioactives from Pleurotus ostreatus and Evaluation of Antioxidant and Antimicrobial Activities. *Processes* **2021**, *9*, 743. [CrossRef]
100. Rossi, G.D.; Santos, C.D.; Carvalho, G.A.; Alves, D.S.; Pereira, L.L.; Carvalho, G.A. Biochemical analysis of a castor bean leaf extract and its insecticidal effects against *Spodoptera frugiperda* (Smith) (*Lepidoptera: Noctuidae*). *Neotrop. Entomol.* **2012**, *41*, 503–509. [CrossRef]
101. Lomarat, P.; Sripha, K.; Phanthong, P.; Kitphati, W.; Thirapanmethee, K.; Bunyapraphatsara, N. In vitro biological activities of black pepper essential oil and its major components relevant to the prevention of Alzheimer's disease. *TJPS* **2015**, *39*, 94–101.
102. Pasinetti, G.M.; Ho, L. Role of grape seed polyphenols in Alzheimer's disease neuropathology. *Nutr. Diet. Suppl.* **2010**, *2010*, 97–103. [CrossRef]
103. Enogieru, A.B.; Haylett, W.; Hiss, D.C.; Bardien, S.; Ekpo, O.E. Rutin as a Potent Antioxidant: Implications for Neurodegenerative Disorders. *Oxid. Med. Cell. Longev.* **2018**, *2018*, 6241017. [CrossRef] [PubMed]

104. Brenn, A.; Grube, M.; Jedlitschky, G.; Fischer, A.; Strohmeier, B.; Eiden, M.; Keller, M.; Groschup, M.; Vogelgesang, S. St. John's Wort Reduces Beta-Amyloid Accumulation in a Double Transgenic Alzheimer's Disease Mouse Model-Role of P-Glycoprotein. *Brain Pathol.* **2013**, *24*, 15–30. [CrossRef] [PubMed]
105. Sadeghnia, H.R.; Jamshidi, R.; Afshari, A.R.; Mollazadeh, H.; Forouzanfar, F.; Rakhshandeh, H. *Terminalia chebula* attenuates quinolinate-induced oxidative PC12 and OLN-93 cell death. *Mult. Scler. Relat. Disord.* **2017**, *14*, 60–67. [CrossRef] [PubMed]
106. Raina, V.; Srivastava, S.; Kv, S. Essential oil composition of Acorus calamus L. from the lower region of the Himalaya. *Flavour Fragr. J.* **2003**, *18*, 18–20. [CrossRef]
107. Fan, R.; Yuan, F.; Wang, N.; Gao, Y.; Huang, Y. Extraction and analysis of antioxidant compounds from the residues of *Asparagus officinalis* L. *J. Food Sci. Technol.* **2015**, *52*, 2690–2700. [CrossRef]
108. Nebrisi, E.E. Neuroprotective Activities of Curcumin in Parkinson's Disease: A Review of the Literature. *Int. J. Mol. Sci.* **2021**, *22*, 11248. [CrossRef]
109. Hritcu, L.; Noumedem, J.A.; Cioanca, O.; Hancianu, M.; Kuete, V.; Mihasan, M. Methanolic extract of *Piper nigrum* fruits improves memory impairment by decreasing brain oxidative stress in amyloid beta(1-42) rat model of Alzheimer's disease. *Cell Mol. Neurobiol.* **2014**, *34*, 437–449. [CrossRef]
110. Esfandiari, E.; Ghanadian, M.; Rashidi, B.; Mokhtarian, A.; Vatankhah, A.M. The Effects of *Acorus calamus* L. in Preventing Memory Loss, Anxiety, and Oxidative Stress on Lipopolysaccharide-induced Neuroinflammation Rat Models. *Int. J. Prev. Med.* **2018**, *9*, 85. [CrossRef]
111. Huang, X.; Li, N.; Pu, Y.; Zhang, T.; Wang, B. Neuroprotective Effects of Ginseng Phytochemicals: Recent Perspectives. *Molecules* **2019**, *24*, 2939. [CrossRef]
112. Oliveira, A.I.; Pinho, C.; Sarmento, B.; Dias, A.C. Neuroprotective Activity of *Hypericum perforatum* and Its Major Components. *Front. Plant. Sci.* **2016**, *7*, 1004. [CrossRef]
113. Mojaverrostami, S.; Bojnordi, M.N.; Ghasemi-Kasman, M.; Ebrahimzadeh, M.A.; Hamidabadi, H.G. A Review of Herbal Therapy in Multiple Sclerosis. *Adv. Pharm. Bull.* **2018**, *8*, 575–590. [CrossRef] [PubMed]
114. Sandamali, J.A.N.; Hewawasam, R.P.; Perera, K.A.; Jayatilaka, W.; Kumari, L.; Mudduwa, B. Cinnamomum zeylanicum Blume (*Ceylon cinnamon*) bark extract attenuates doxorubicin induced cardiotoxicity in Wistar rats. *Saudi Pharm. J.* **2021**, *29*, 820–832. [CrossRef] [PubMed]
115. Kimura, J.; Nemoto, K.; Yokosuka, A.; Mimaki, Y.; Degawa, M.; Ohizumi, Y. 6-demethoxynobiletin, a nobiletin-analog citrus flavonoid, enhances extracellular signal-regulated kinase phosphorylation in PC12D cells. *Biol. Pharm. Bull.* **2013**, *36*, 1646–1649. [CrossRef] [PubMed]
116. Carmona, L.; Sulli, M.; Diretto, G.; Alquézar, B.; Alves, M.; Peña, L. Improvement of Antioxidant Properties in Fruit from Two Blood and Blond Orange Cultivars by Postharvest Storage at Low Temperature. *Antioxidants* **2022**, *11*, 547. [CrossRef] [PubMed]
117. Matsuzaki, K.; Ohizumi, Y. Beneficial Effects of Citrus-Derived Polymethoxylated Flavones for Central Nervous System Disorders. *Nutrients* **2021**, *13*, 145. [CrossRef]
118. Moloudizargari, M.; Mikaili, P.; Aghajanshakeri, S.; Asghari, M.H.; Shayegh, J. Pharmacological and therapeutic effects of Peganum harmala and its main alkaloids. *Pharmacogn. Rev.* **2013**, *7*, 199–212. [CrossRef]
119. Menghini, L.; Leporini, L.; Vecchiotti, G.; Locatelli, M.; Carradori, S.; Ferrante, C.; Zengin, G.; Recinella, L.; Chiavaroli, A.; Leone, S.; et al. *Crocus sativus* L. stigmas and byproducts: Qualitative fingerprint, antioxidant potentials and enzyme inhibitory activities. *Food Res. Int.* **2018**, *109*, 91–98. [CrossRef]
120. Srinivasa, U.M.; Naidu, M.M. Chapter 6—Fenugreek (*Trigonella foenum-graecum* L.) Seed: Promising Source of Nutraceutical. In *Studies in Natural Products Chemistry*; Atta-ur-Rahman, Ed.; Elsevier: Amsterdam, The Netherlands, 2021; Volume 71, pp. 141–184. [CrossRef]
121. Gang, L.; Guangxiang, L.; Yanfeng, H.; Fangfang, T.; Zhenhua, W.; Yourui, S.; Chengjun, M.; Honglun, W. Polyphenol Stilbenes from Fenugreek (*Trigonella foenum-graecum* L.) Seeds Improve Insulin Sensitivity and Mitochondrial Function in 3T3-L1 Adipocytes. *Oxid. Med. Cell. Longev.* **2018**, *2018*, 7634362. [CrossRef]
122. Vysochina, G.I.; Kukushkina, T.A.; Vasfilov, E.S. Biologically Active Substances in *Filipendula ulmaria* (L.) Maxim. Growing in the Middle Urals. *Chem. Sustain. Dev.* **2013**, *21*, 369374.
123. Katanić, J.; Boroja, T.; Mihailović, V.; Nikles, S.; Pan, S.P.; Rosić, G.; Selaković, D.; Joksimović, J.; Mitrović, S.; Bauer, R. In vitro and in vivo assessment of meadowsweet (*Filipendula ulmaria*) as anti-inflammatory agent. *J. Ethnopharmacol.* **2016**, *193*, 627–636. [CrossRef]
124. Winther, K.; Vinther Hansen, A.S.; Campbell-Tofte, J. Bioactive ingredients of rose hips (*Rosa canina* L) with special reference to antioxidative and anti-inflammatory properties: In vitro studies. *Bot. Targets Ther.* **2016**, *6*, 11–23. [CrossRef]
125. Wang, Q.; Wang, C.; Shu, Z.; Chan, K.; Huang, S.; Li, Y.; Xiao, Y.; Wu, L.; Kuang, H.; Sun, X. Valeriana amurensis improves Amyloid-beta 1-42 induced cognitive deficit by enhancing cerebral cholinergic function and protecting the brain neurons from apoptosis in mice. *J. Ethnopharmacol.* **2014**, *153*, 318–325. [CrossRef] [PubMed]
126. Pathania, S.; Mukund, S.; Randhawa, V.; Bagler, G. SerpentinaDB: A database of plant-derived molecules of Rauvolfia serpentina. *BMC Complement. Altern. Med.* **2015**, *15*, 262. [CrossRef] [PubMed]
127. Moga, M.A.; Dimienescu, O.G.; Bălan, A.; Dima, L.; Toma, S.I.; Bîgiu, N.F.; Blidaru, A. Pharmacological and Therapeutic Properties of Punica granatum Phytochemicals: Possible Roles in Breast Cancer. *Molecules* **2021**, *26*, 1054. [CrossRef]
128. Kumar, N.; Kumar, S. Functional Properties of Pomegranate (*Punica granatum* L.). *Pharma Innov.* **2018**, *7*, 71–81.

129. Khodaei, J.; Samimi-Akhijahani, H. Some Physical Properties of Rasa Grape (*Vitis vinifera* L.). *World Appl. Sci. J.* **2012**, *18*, 9–17. [CrossRef]
130. Huamán-Castilla, N.L.; Campos, D.; García-Ríos, D.; Parada, J.; Martínez-Cifuentes, M.; Mariotti-Celis, M.S.; Pérez-Correa, J.R. Chemical Properties of Vitis Vinifera Carménère Pomace Extracts Obtained by Hot Pressurized Liquid Extraction, and Their Inhibitory Effect on Type 2 Diabetes Mellitus Related Enzymes. *Antioxidants* **2021**, *10*, 472. [CrossRef]
131. Krishi, V.; Kendra, I.; Kumar, R.; Kumar, V.; Verma, R.; Kumari, P.; Maurya, R.; Verma, R.; Singh, R. Medicinal properties of turmeric (*Curcuma longa* L.): A review. *Int. J. Chem. Stud.* **2018**, *6*, 1354–1357.
132. Jordan, E.; Wagner, H. Structure and properties of polysaccharides from *Viscum album* (L.). *Oncology* **1986**, *43*, 8–15. [CrossRef]
133. Misharina, T.A.; Terenina, M.B.; Krikunova, N.I.; Kalinchenko, M.A. Influence of the composition of lemon essential oils on their antioxidant properties and component stability. *Chem. Plant Mater.* **2010**, *1*, 87–92. [CrossRef]
134. Siyanova, N.S.; Neustrueva, S.N. Optimization of conditions for growing tissue culture of Rauwolfia serpentine. Scientific notes of Kazan University. *Ser. Nat. Sci.* **2008**, *150*, 201–224.
135. Goryainov, S.V.; Khomik, A.S.; Kalabin, G.A.; Vandyshev, V.V.; Abramovich, R.A. Fatty acid composition of punica granatum L. seeds from pomegranate juice waste. *Bull. Peoples' Friendsh. Univ. Russia Ser. Ecol. Life Saf.* **2012**, *1*, 10–15.
136. Karomatov, I.J.; Murodova, M.M. Kabul myrobalans. *Biol. Integr. Med.* **2017**, *11*, 126–146.
137. Ajala, O.S.; Jukov, A.; Ma, C.M. Hepatitis C virus inhibitory hydrolysable tannins from the fruits of *Terminalia chebula*. *Fitoterapia* **2014**, *99*, 117–123. [CrossRef]
138. Chhabra, S.; Mishra, T.; Kumar, Y.; Thacker, G.; Kanojiya, S.; Chattopadhyay, N.; Narender, T.; Trivedi, A.K. Chebulinic Acid Isolated From the Fruits of *Terminalia chebula* Specifically Induces Apoptosis in Acute Myeloid Leukemia Cells. *Phytother. Res.* **2017**, *18*, 13–16. [CrossRef]
139. Bag, A.; Bhattacharyya, S.K.; Chattopadhyay, R.R. Isolation and identification of a gallotannin 1,2,6-tri-O-galloyl-β-D-glucopyranose from hydroalcoholic extract of Terminalia chebula fruits effective against multidrug-resistant uropathogens. *J. Appl. Microbiol.* **2013**, *115*, 390–397. [CrossRef]
140. Zhang, C.; Jiang, K.; Qu, S.J.; Zhai, Y.M.; Tan, J.J.; Tan, C.H. Triterpenoids from the barks of Terminalia chebula. *J. Asian Nat. Prod. Res.* **2015**, *17*, 996–1001. [CrossRef]
141. Waheed, S.; Fatima, I. Instrumental neutron activation analysis of Emblica officinalis, Terminalia belerica and Terminalia chebula for trace element efficacy and safety. *Appl. Radiat. Isot.* **2013**, *77*, 139–144. [CrossRef]
142. Eshwarappa, R.S.; Ramachandra, Y.L.; Subaramaihha, S.R.; Subbaiah, S.G.; Austin, R.S.; Dhananjaya, B.L. Antioxidant activities of leaf galls extracts of *Terminalia chebula* (Gaertn.) Retz. (Combretaceae). *Acta Sci. Pol. Technol. Aliment.* **2015**, *14*, 33–42. [CrossRef]
143. Wang, H.; Shi, S.; Wang, S. Can highly cited herbs in ancient Traditional Chinese medicine formulas and modern publications predict therapeutic targets for diabetes mellitus? *J. Ethnopharmacol.* **2017**, *213*, 101–110. [CrossRef]
144. Shen, Y.C.; Juan, C.W.; Lin, C.S.; Chen, C.C.; Chang, C.L. Neuroprotective effect of terminalia chebula extracts and ellagic acid in PC12 cells. *Afr. J. Tradit. Complement. Altern. Med.* **2017**, *14*, 22–30. [CrossRef] [PubMed]
145. Velmurugan, A.; Madhubala, M.M.; Bhavani, S.; Satheesh Kumar, K.S.; Sathyanarayana, S.S.; Gurucharan, N. An in-vivo comparative evaluation of two herbal extracts *Emblica officinalis* and *Terminalia Chebula* with chlorhexidine as an anticaries agent: A preliminary study. *J. Conserv. Dent.* **2013**, *16*, 546–549. [CrossRef] [PubMed]
146. Sheng, Z.; Yan, X.; Zhang, R.; Ni, H.; Cui, Y.; Ge, J.; Shan, A. Assessment of the antidiarrhoeal properties of the aqueous extract and its soluble fractions of Chebulae Fructus (*Terminalia chebula* fruits). *Pharm. Biol.* **2016**, *54*, 1847–1856. [CrossRef] [PubMed]
147. Pitkevich, E.S.; Lyzikov, A.N.; Tsaprilova, S.V. Milk thistle—*Silybum marianum* (L.). *Probl. Health Ecol.* **2008**, *4*, 119–126.
148. Tamakhina, A.Y.; Lokyaeva, Z.R. Features of the accumulation of heavy metals by British elecampane (*Inula britannica* L.) in areas with varying degrees of technogenic pollution. *Bull. Krasn. State Agrar. Univ.* **2016**, *4*, 3–9.
149. Tamakhina, A.Y.; Gadieva, A.A. Morphology of excretory tissue of leaves and secondary metabolites of some members of the genus Inula. *South Russ. Ecol. Dev.* **2017**, *3*, 53–63.
150. Suau, R.; Cabezudo, B.; Rico, R.; Nájera, F.; López-Romero, J.M. Direct determination of alkaloid contents in Fumaria species by GC-MS. *Phytochem. Anal.* **2002**, *13*, 363–367. [CrossRef]
151. Chlebek, J.; Novák, Z.; Kassemová, D.; Šafratová, M.; Kostelník, J.; Malý, L.;Ločárek, M.; Opletal, L.; Hošt'álková, A.; Hrabinová, M.; et al. Isoquinoline Alkaloids from *Fumaria officinalis* L. and Their Biological Activities Related to Alzheimer's Disease. *Chem. Biodivers.* **2016**, *13*, 91–99. [CrossRef]
152. Hentschel, C.; Dressler, S.; Hahn, E.G. Fumaria officinalis (fumitory)-clinical applications. *Fortschr. Med.* **1995**, *113*, 291–292.
153. Dul, V.N.; Pupykina, K.A.; Dargaeva, T.D.; Kopytko, Y.F.; Sokolskaya, T.A. Study of the component composition of the lipophilic fraction obtained from grape leaves (*Vitis vinifera* L.). *Bashkir Chem. J.* **2010**, *17*, 121–124.
154. Iskandarova, S.F.; Abdukhalilova, N.S. Characteristics of cumerican long (*Curcuma longa* L.) As a source of biologically active substances. *Sci. Time* **2018**, *2*, 40–43.
155. Guriev, A.M.; Yusubov, M.S.; Kalinkina, G.I.; Tsybukova, T.N. Elemental composition of calamus (*Acorus calamus* L.). *Chem. Plant Mater.* **2003**, *2*, 45–48.
156. Krasnov, E.A.; Avdeeva, E.Y. Chemical composition of plants of the genus *Filipendula* (review). *Chem. Plant Mater.* **2012**, *4*, 5–12.
157. Leusova, N.Y.; Katola, V.M.; Krylov, A.V. Phytochemistry of mistletoe plants (*Viscum* L.) and their medicinal properties. *Bull. Physiol. Pathol. Respir.* **2008**, *28*, 69–73.

158. Dos Reis Nunes, C.; Barreto Arantes, M.; Menezes de Faria Pereira, S.; Leandro da Cruz, L.; de Souza Passos, M.; Pereira de Moraes, L.; José Curcino Vieira, I.; Barros de Oliveira, D. Plants as Sources of Anti-Inflammatory Agents. *Molecules* **2020**, *25*, 3726. [CrossRef]
159. Chen, L.; Deng, H.; Cui, H.; Fang, J.; Zuo, Z.; Deng, J.; Li, Y.; Wang, X.; Zhao, L. Inflammatory responses and inflammation-associated diseases in organs. *Oncotarget* **2017**, *9*, 7204–7218. [CrossRef]
160. Salmerón-Manzano, E.; Garrido-Cardenas, J.A.; Manzano-Agugliaro, F. Worldwide Research Trends on Medicinal Plants. *Int. J. Environ. Res. Public Health* **2020**, *17*, 3376. [CrossRef]
161. Lawrence, T.; Gilroy, D.W. Chronic inflammation: A failure of resolution? *Int. J. Exp. Pathol.* **2007**, *88*, 85–94. [CrossRef]
162. Pharm, M.; Sci, P.; Sami, A.; Usama, M.; Saeed, M.; Akram, M. Medicinal plants with non-steroidal anti-inflammatory-like activity. *J. Pham. Sci.* **2021**, *1*, 1–8.
163. Li, R.; Zhou, Y.; Zhang, S.; Li, J.; Zheng, Y.; Fan, X. The natural (poly)phenols as modulators of microglia polarization via TLR4/NF-κB pathway exert anti-inflammatory activity in ischemic stroke. *Eur. J. Pharmacol* **2022**, *914*, 174660. [CrossRef]
164. Azab, A.; Nassar, A.; Azab, A.N. Anti-Inflammatory Activity of Natural Products. *Molecules* **2016**, *21*, 1321. [CrossRef] [PubMed]
165. Beg, S.; Swain, S.; Hasan, H.; Barkat, M.A.; Hussain, M.S. Systematic review of herbals as potential anti-inflammatory agents: Recent advances, current clinical status and future perspectives. *Pharmacogn. Rev.* **2011**, *5*, 120–137. [CrossRef] [PubMed]
166. Daneshmand, P.; Saliminejad, K.; Dehghan Shasaltaneh, M.; Kamali, K.; Riazi, G.H.; Nazari, R.; Azimzadeh, P.; Khorram Khorshid, H.R. Neuroprotective Effects of Herbal Extract (*Rosa canina, Tanacetum vulgare* and *Urtica dioica*) on Rat Model of Sporadic Alzheimer's Disease Avicenna. *J. Med. Biotechnol.* **2016**, *8*, 120–125.
167. Mehdizadeh, M.; Hashem Dabaghian, F.; Shojaee, A.; Molavi, N.; Taslimi, Z.; Shabani, R.; Soleimani, A.S. Protective Effects of Cyperus Rotundus Extract on Amyloid β-Peptide (1-40)-Induced Memory Impairment in Male Rats: A Behavioral Study. *Basic. Clin. Neurosci.* **2017**, *8*, 249–254. [CrossRef]
168. Sadowska-Bartosz, I.; Bartosz, G. Prevention of protein glycation by natural compounds. *Molecules* **2015**, *20*, 3309–3334. [CrossRef]
169. Locatelli, C.; Nardi, G.M.; Anuário, A.d.F.; Freire, C.G.; Megiolaro, F.; Schneider, K.; Perazzoli, M.R.A.; Nascimento, S.R.D.; Gon, A.C.; Mariano, L.N.B.; et al. Anti-inflammatory activity of berry fruits in mice model of inflammation is based on oxidative stress modulation. *Pharmacogn. Res.* **2016**, *8*, S42–S49. [CrossRef]
170. Fan, W. Epidemiology in diabetes mellitus and cardiovascular disease. *Cardiovasc. Endocrinol.* **2017**, *6*, 8–16. [CrossRef]
171. Kawahito, S.; Kitahata, H.; Oshita, S. Problems associated with glucose toxicity: Role of hyperglycemia-induced oxidative stress. *World J. Gastroenterol.* **2009**, *15*, 4137–4142. [CrossRef]
172. Belinskaia, D.A.; Voronina, P.A.; Shmurak, V.I.; Vovk, M.A.; Batalova, A.A.; Jenkins, R.O.; Goncharov, N.V. The Universal Soldier: Enzymatic and Non-Enzymatic Antioxidant Functions of Serum Albumin. *Antioxidants* **2020**, *9*, 966. [CrossRef]
173. Mishra, V.; Heath, R.J. Structural and Biochemical Features of Human Serum Albumin Essential for Eukaryotic Cell Culture. *Int. J. Mol. Sci.* **2021**, *22*, 8411. [CrossRef]
174. Merlot, A.M.; Kalinowski, D.S.; Richardson, D.R. Unraveling the mysteries of serum albumin—more than just a serum protein. *Front. Physiol.* **2014**, *5*, 10–14. [CrossRef] [PubMed]
175. Safari, M.R.; Azizi, O.; Heidary, S.S.; Kheiripour, N.; Ravan, A.P. Antiglycation and antioxidant activity of four Iranian medical plant extracts. *J. Pharmacopunct.* **2018**, *21*, 82–89. [CrossRef] [PubMed]
176. Choudhury, H.; Pandey, M.; Hua, C.K.; Mun, C.S.; Jing, J.K.; Kong, L.; Ern, L.Y.; Ashraf, N.A.; Kit, S.W.; Yee, T.S.; et al. An update on natural compounds in the remedy of diabetes mellitus: A systematic review. *J. Tradit. Complement. Med.* **2017**, *8*, 361–376. [CrossRef] [PubMed]
177. Fursenco, C.; Calalb, T.; Uncu, L.; Dinu, M.; Ancuceanu, R. Solidago virgaurea L.: A Review of Its Ethnomedicinal Uses, Phytochemistry, and Pharmacological Activities. *Biomolecules* **2020**, *10*, 1619. [CrossRef]
178. Toiu, A.; Vlase, L.; Vodnar, D.C.; Gheldiu, A.M.; Oniga, I. *Solidago graminifolia* L. Salisb. (*Asteraceae*) as a Valuable Source of Bioactive Polyphenols: HPLC Profile, In Vitro Antioxidant and Antimicrobial Potential. *Molecules* **2019**, *24*, 2666. [CrossRef]
179. Tungmunnithum, D.; Thongboonyou, A.; Pholboon, A.; Yangsabai, A. Flavonoids and Other Phenolic Compounds from Medicinal Plants for Pharmaceutical and Medical Aspects: An Overview. *Medicines* **2018**, *5*, 93. [CrossRef]
180. Zaynab, M.; Fatima, M.; Abbas, S.; Sharif, Y.; Umair, M.; Zafar, M.H.; Bahadar, K. Role of secondary metabolites in plant defense against pathogens. *Microb. Pathog.* **2018**, *124*, 198–202. [CrossRef]
181. Sofowora, A.; Ogunbodede, E.; Onayade, A. The role and place of medicinal plants in the strategies for disease prevention. *Afr. J. Tradit. Complement. Altern. Med.* **2013**, *10*, 210–229. [CrossRef]
182. Rashrash, M.; Schommer, J.C.; Brown, L.M. Prevalence and Predictors of Herbal Medicine Use Among Adults in the United States. *J. Patient Exp.* **2017**, *4*, 108–113. [CrossRef]
183. Ekor, M. The growing use of herbal medicines: Issues relating to adverse reactions and challenges in monitoring safety. *Front. Pharmacol.* **2014**, *4*, 177. [CrossRef]
184. Atanasov, A.G.; Waltenberger, B.; Pferschy-Wenzig, E.-M.; Linder, T.; Wawrosch, C.; Uhrin, P.; Temml, V.; Wang, L.; Schwaiger, S.; Heiss, E.H.; et al. Discovery and resupply of pharmacologically active plant-derived natural products: A review. *Biotechnol. Adv.* **2015**, *33*, 1582–1614. [CrossRef] [PubMed]
185. Caesar, L.K.; Cech, N.B. Synergy and antagonism in natural product extracts: When 1 + 1 does not equal 2. *Nat. Prod. Rep.* **2019**, *36*, 869–888. [CrossRef] [PubMed]
186. Mathur, S.; Hoskins, C. Drug development: Lessons from nature. *Biomed. Rep.* **2017**, *6*, 612–614. [CrossRef] [PubMed]

187. Soodabeh, S.; Manayi, A.; Abdollahi, M. From in vitro Experiments to in vivo and Clinical Studies; Pros and Cons. *Curr. Drug Discov. Technol.* **2015**, *12*, 218–224. [CrossRef]
188. Li, Y.; Kong, D.; Fu, Y.; Sussman, M.R.; Wu, H. The efect of developmental and environmental factors on secondary metabolites in medicinal plants. *Plant. Physiol. Biochem.* **2020**, *148*, 80–89. [CrossRef]
189. Owona, B.A.; Abia, W.A.; Moundipa, P.F. Natural compounds flavonoids as modulators of inflammasomes in chronic diseases. *Int. Immunopharmacol.* **2020**, *84*, 106498. [CrossRef]
190. Anand, P.K. Lipids, inflammasomes, metabolism, and disease. *Immunol. Rev.* **2020**, *297*, 108–122. [CrossRef]
191. Mondal, A.; Gandhi, A.; Fimognari, C.; Atanasov, A.G.; Bishayee, A. Alkaloids for cancer prevention and therapy: Current progress and future perspectives. *Eur. J. Pharmacol.* **2019**, *858*, 172472. [CrossRef]
192. Santos, T.N.; Costa, G.; Ferreira, J.P.; Liberal, J.; Francisco, V.; Paranhos, A.; Cruz, M.T.; Castelo-Branco, M.; Figueiredo, I.V.; Batista, M.T. Antioxidant, Anti-Inflammatory, and Analgesic Activities of Agrimonia eupatoria L. Infusion. *Evid. Based Complement. Altern. Med.* **2017**, *2017*, 8309894. [CrossRef]
193. Wenzel, P.; Kossmann, S.; Münzel, T.; Daiber, A. Redox regulation of cardiovascular inflammation—Immunomodulatory function of mitochondrial and Nox-derived reactive oxygen and nitrogen species. *Free Radic. Boil. Med.* **2017**, *109*, 48–60. [CrossRef]
194. Karam, T.K.; Dalposso, L.M.; Casa, D.M.; De Freitas, G.B.L. Broom (*Baccharis trimera*): Therapeutic use and biosynthesis. *Rev. Bras. Plantas Med.* **2013**, *15*, 280–286. [CrossRef]
195. Li, J.J.; Corey, E.J. *Total Synthesis of Natural Products*; Springer Science & Business Media: Berlin/Heidelberg, Germany, 2013; p. 295.
196. Pemovska, T.; Bigenzahn, J.W.; Superti-Furga, G. Recent advances in combinatorial drug screening and synergy scoring. *Curr. Opin. Pharmacol.* **2018**, *42*, 102–110. [CrossRef] [PubMed]
197. Pemovska, T.; Bigenzahn, J.W.; Srndic, I.; Lercher, A.; Bergthaler, A.; César-Razquin, A.; Kartnig, F.; Kornauth, C.; Valent, P.; Staber, P.B.; et al. Metabolic drug survey highlights cancer cell dependencies and vulnerabilities. *Nat. Commun* **2021**, *12*, 7190. [CrossRef]
198. Pavlova, N.N.; Thompson, C.B. The emerging hallmarks of cancer metabolism. *Cell Metab.* **2016**, *23*, 27–47. [CrossRef] [PubMed]
199. Kato, Y.; Maeda, T.; Suzuki, A.; Baba, Y. Cancer metabolism: New insights into classic characteristics. *Jpn. Dent. Sci. Rev.* **2018**, *54*, 8–21. [CrossRef]
200. Martinez-Outschoorn, U.E.; Peiris-Pages, M.; Pestell, R.G.; Sotgia, F.; Lisanti, M.P. Cancer metabolism: A therapeutic perspective. *Nat. Rev. Clin. Oncol.* **2017**, *14*, 11–31. [CrossRef] [PubMed]
201. Rowe, J.M. Will new agents impact survival in AML? *Best. Pract. Res. Clin. Haematol.* **2019**, *32*, 101094. [CrossRef]
202. Vande Voorde, J.; Ackermann, T.; Pfetzer, N.; Sumpton, D.; Mackay, G.; Kalna, G.; Nixon, C.; Blyth, K.; Gottlieb, E.; Tardito, S. Improving the metabolic fidelity of cancer models with a physiological cell culture medium. *Sci. Adv.* **2019**, *5*, eaau7314. [CrossRef]
203. Bisson, J.; McAlpine, J.B.; Friesen, J.B.; Chen, S.-N.; Graham, J.; Pauli, G.F. Can Invalid Bioactives Undermine Natural Product-Based Drug Discovery? *J. Med. Chem.* **2016**, *59*, 1671–1690. [CrossRef]
204. Feng, B.Y.; Shoichet, B.K. The Detection, Prevalence and Properties of Aggregate-Based Small Molecule Inhibition. *J. Med. Chem.* **2006**, *49*, 2151–2154. [CrossRef]
205. Senger, M.R.; Fraga, C.A.; Dantas, R.F.; Silva, F.P., Jr. Filtering promiscuous compounds in early drug discovery: Is it a good idea? *Drug Discov. Today* **2016**, *21*, 868–872. [CrossRef] [PubMed]
206. Khan, A.; Tauseef, I.; Aalia, B.; Khan, M.A.; Akbar, S.; Sultana, N.; Haleem, K.S. Age-related variations in the in vitro bactericidal activity of human sera against Pseudomonas aeruginosa. *Cent. Eur. J. Immunol.* **2018**, *43*, 18–25. [CrossRef] [PubMed]
207. Tam, V.H.; Schilling, A.N.; Nikolaou, M. Modelling time-kill studies to discern the pharmacodynamics of meropenem. *J. Antimicrob. Chemother.* **2005**, *55*, 699–706. [CrossRef] [PubMed]
208. Efferth, T.; Zacchino, S.; Georgiev, M.I.; Liu, L.; Wagner, H.; Panossian, A. Nobel Prize for artemisinin brings phytotherapy into the spotlight. *Phytomedicine* **2015**, *22*, 1–4. [CrossRef]
209. Gong, X.; Sucher, N.J. Stroke therapy in traditional Chinese medicine (TCM): Prospects for drug discovery and development. *Trends Pharmacol. Sci.* **1999**, *20*, 191–196. [CrossRef]
210. Brooks, B.D.; Brooks, A.E. Therapeutic strategies to combat antibiotic resistance. *Adv. Drug Deliv. Rev.* **2014**, *78*, 14–27. [CrossRef]
211. Carmona, F.; Pereira, A.M.S. Herbal medicines: Old and new concepts, truths and misunderstandings. *Rev. Bras. Farmacogn.* **2013**, *23*, 379–385. [CrossRef]
212. Koehn, F.E.; Carter, G. T The evolving role of natural products in drug discovery. *Nat. Rev. Drug Discov.* **2005**, *4*, 206–220. [CrossRef]
213. Montes, P.; Ruiz-Sanchez, E.; Rojas, C.; Rojas, P. Ginkgo biloba Extract 761: A Review of Basic Studies and Potential Clinical Use in Psychiatric Disorders. *CNS Neurol. Disord. Drug Targets* **2015**, *14*, 132–149. [CrossRef]

MDPI
St. Alban-Anlage 66
4052 Basel
Switzerland
Tel. +41 61 683 77 34
Fax +41 61 302 89 18
www.mdpi.com

Molecules Editorial Office
E-mail: molecules@mdpi.com
www.mdpi.com/journal/molecules

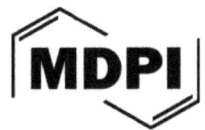